P9-DTF-653

MAN, MIND,
and
HEREDITY

MAN, MIND,
and
HEREDITY

Selected Papers of Eliot Slater
on
Psychiatry and Genetics

Edited by

James Shields
and
Irving I. Gottesman

The Johns Hopkins Press   Baltimore and London

The Johns Hopkins Press, Baltimore, Maryland 21218
The Johns Hopkins Press Ltd., London

Library of Congress Catalog Card Number 75-126802

International Standard Book Number 0-8018-1118-X

CONTENTS

LIST OF TABLES

LIST OF FIGURES

EDITORS' PREFACE

I t was over two years ago, when Eliot Slater's retirement as Director of the Psychiatric Genetics Unit at the Maudsley Hospital was imminent and we were considering ways of commemorating the occasion, that we conceived the idea of putting between hard covers a selection of his best papers on genetics and psychiatry with the intention that they should be published in the United States. In this way we hoped to do better than honour a distinguished friend and senior colleague at this stage of his career by a *Festschrift* of essays by contemporaries and pupils. A short account of work done in his Unit had already been written (Shields, 1968) in a volume surveying the work of the Department of Psychiatry, Institute of Psychiatry, under the chairmanship of Sir Aubrey Lewis. What we hoped to do was to cull from Slater's writings an anthology which would do justice to the wide range of his interests and at the same time be of particular relevance for contemporary workers in the behavioral sciences who are turning in increasing numbers to an examination of the genetic and biological aspects of man's aberrant behavior.

For many years to come, Slater's name will continue to crop up in any informed discussion of genetic influences in the neuroses and psychoses. He has provided more than his share of both data and ideas. Although a few of the papers included here were written over thirty years ago, they are still of interest today. Ideas change — Slater's own as much as those of others — but certain basic problems recur. What are the distinguishing characteristics of the relatives of schizophrenics? How far do psychiatric illnesses in families "breed true"? What types of personality are most vulnerable to stress? Since we do not know the answers to such questions, it is instructive to see how others have tried to deal with them. Although Slater's earlier work on a "diathesis-stress" theory of the neuroses, to borrow Rosenthal's phrase, dates from the years of World War II, the field is still relatively untrodden.

Our selection of scientific papers is framed by two pieces which we invited Slater to write specially for *Man, Mind, and Heredity* — the Autobiographical Sketch and the Retrospect. The former takes him to the age of thirty-five and the outbreak of war in 1939, by which time he was established in his career as a psychiatrist with special qualifications in genetics. This delightfully written account of how he eventually came to combine these two disciplines is insightful, insight-giving, human to a fault, and above all entertaining. The Retrospect is again a brilliantly written personal reflection which will have a wide appeal. It is a powerful, moving statement of his philosophy and values.

After Slater's portrait there appears, in the brief, conventional form of a *Who's Who* entry, the outline of Slater's later career. It includes the Directorship of a Medical Research Council Unit, the authorship of a leading text-book, and the editorship of a leading journal. It is rare for the name of a psychiatrist to appear in the Queen's honours list. We are fortunate in having Sir Denis Hill to write a foreword which adds a warm human note to this bare account of his achievements. An electroencephalographic expert of international repute and the Professor of Psychiatry at the Maudsley Hospital since Sir Aubrey Lewis retired in 1967, Hill has known Slater well since before the war. In his Foreword he takes up the story, from about the time the autobiography leaves off, and tells us something about the man behind the career. It is not a eulogy, but an honest account of a close friend from the writer's own particular angle. As one can see from his Adolf Meyer Lecture of 1968 Hill's approach to psychiatry differs from Slater's in laying much greater importance on interpersonal relationships, including the doctor-patient relationship (Hill, 1968). Sir Denis paints the picture of a dedicated research worker of unconventional opinions, held in high personal regard and affection, and he tells of Slater's influence on British psychiatry today.

We are equally grateful to David Rosenthal, Chief of the Laboratory of Psychology at the N.I.M.H., Bethesda, for the second Foreword. Rosenthal and Slater became acquainted in 1959 through correspondence before Rosenthal published the first of his critiques of twin studies in schizophrenia. Rosenthal was led into genetics when faced with the task of integrating the information on the Genain Quadruplets (Rosenthal, 1963). His later work using the strategy of adoption studies and reported in *The Transmission of Schizophrenia* (Rosenthal and Kety, 1968) has been influential in focusing attention in the U.S.A. on the substance of genetic-environmental interaction for schizophrenia. His Foreword speaks generously of Slater, the man and the scientist, and adds a perspective from the American side of the Atlantic Ocean.

In the U.S.A. increasing attention is paid nowadays to European psychiatry. Three distinguished British psychiatrists, trained at the Maudsley during the years before World War II, have had memoirs or selected papers published recently: Sargant's autobiography (1967) and Lewis's two volumes of papers (1967 *a* and *b*), and now Slater's *Man, Mind, and Heredity*. To some, all three may appear to have something in common in their apparent neglect or scepticism of psycho-dynamic factors and concentration on what their critics would call descriptive, but they themselves would call phenomenological, clinical, or "bedside" psychiatry. Yet it would be difficult to find three more contrasted approaches to their subject. Where Lewis is sceptical, philosophical and critical, Sargant is enthusiastic and therapeutically optimistic. While Slater has been influenced one way or another by both his senior and his junior colleague, he too has made a very individual contribution to the psychiatry of his time, both nationally and internationally.[1] With a greater flair for

---

[1] His textbook, *Clinical Psychiatry*, with Mayer-Gross and Roth, has been (or will be) translated into Chinese, Greek, Italian, Portuguese, Russian and Spanish. His book on *Physical Methods of Treatment* with Sargant has been translated into French, German, Spanish and Swedish.

the science of numbers than either Lewis or Sargant would claim to possess, his speciality has of course been the genetic aspects of psychiatry.

In his Foreword, Professor Hill has told of Slater's willingness to put his methodological expertise at the service of colleagues of different points of view. Another characteristic to which we should like to pay tribute is one that may seem surprising in someone who has himself always been outspoken in expressing his views: this is the latitude which he has always given to colleagues in his team to follow their particular bent. Influential though he has been, he has never forced colleagues to toe the line. For better or worse, there is not a "Slaterian school" of psychiatric genetics.

The thirty-three papers are divided into six parts. Part I contains three papers on Orientation which reflect an attitude to psychiatry that has been described as urbane and wise. They show how reasonable it is to consider both biological and psychological factors in efforts to explain, understand, and treat abnormal behaviour. The next three parts cover the major divisions of psychiatric illness and include reports of original data, theoretical papers, and shorter reviews or discussions. Slater is probably best known in the States for his much cited and criticized but little read monograph of 1953 on psychotic and neurotic illnesses in twins. This is reproduced here in abbreviated form but with special regard to schizophrenia. Two papers present Slater's provocative views on hysteria. The long paper on schizophrenia and epilepsy is given virtually in its entirety. Two papers appear in English for the first time, including his now classical paper on the parents and children of manic-depressives.

The clinical parts are followed by a section on methodological topics which Slater has ingeniously tackled himself. The final part, which we have called Society and the Individual, deals with such diverse subjects as eugenics, the relations between law and psychiatry, and assortative marriage; and it includes a pathography of Robert Schumann. These excursions have meant much to him. A glance through the long list of Slater's publications from 1935 to 1970, to be found at the end of this volume, will give the reader some idea of the variety of papers we have regretfully *not* been able to include. Some of them are referred to in the editorial introductions to each part.

Among the themes which recur in these papers, the following may be noted: the foundations of psychiatry have to be laid on the ground of the biological sciences; the need for careful observation, the value of making a diagnosis, the desirability of coming down on one side of the fence or the other, and the value of numerical analysis in reaching a rational judgment. All-embracing explanations and concepts are of dubious value for Slater, as for Karl Popper, since they do not permit testing and refutation.

Eleven of the papers were written jointly — the names of his co-authors are given below and are also acknowledged on the first page of the papers concerned. Footnotes here give the full source of each paper and indicate any editorial changes made after consultation with Slater. The great majority are reprinted in their original form. References for each paper and for editorial comments have been consolidated into one master list, except those relating to Slater's own works. They are indicated by numbers in brackets which refer to the itemised "Publications of Eliot Slater".

Acknowledgements

The editing of this book was made immensely easier for us through the aid provided by Marjorie Johnson, Joyce Maxwell, Sue Nicol and Elizabeth Shields. We specially wish to thank Magnhild Goodman, who had the task of retyping most of the papers, Vivian Phillips, who helped to prepare the manuscript for the printers, Vera G. Seal for much assistance, especially with the bibliography and index, and Linda Vlasak for judicious copyediting.

For the frontispiece we are indebted to Messrs. Barr, Photographers, of Camberwell, London, S.E. 5.

The following co-authors have kindly given us permission to include the papers indicated below which they wrote jointly with Eliot Slater:

Dr. A. W. Beard (12), Dr. W. H. Craike (6), Mr. Eric Glithero (12, 20), Professor Alfred Meyer (33), Dr. J. A. Fraser Roberts, C.B.E., F.R.S., (26), Dr. William Sargant (2, 15), Dr. Patrick Slater (17), Mrs. Moya Woodside (30), and Dr. K. J. Zilkha (11). (One of the editors, J.S., collaborated on Paper 21.)

We are grateful to the following journals and publishers for permission to reproduce material originally published by them:

The Editor of the *Acta Psychiatrica Scandinavica* (23); the Anglo-Jewish Association (29); Baillière, Tindall and Cassell Ltd. (30); the Editor of *Brain* (6); the Editor of the *British Journal of Psychiatry* (3, 12, 13, 19); the British Medical Journal Publishing Department and the Editors of the *British Medical Journal* (31) and the *Journal of Medical Genetics* (24); Messrs. Butterworths (8); the Eugenics Society (25, 26, 27, 28); the Controller of Her Majesty's Stationery Office and the Medical Research Council (9); Hoeber Medical Division, Harper & Row, Inc. (1); the Editor of the *International Journal of Psychiatry* (14); the Editor of the *Journal of Neurology, Neurosurgery and Psychiatry* (16, 17, 18); S. Karger, Basel/New York, and the Editors of *Acta Genetica et Statistica Medica* (10), *Confinia Psychiatrica* (33) and *Monatsschrift für Psychiatrie und Neurologie* (7); the Editor of *The Lancet* (22); the Editor of *L'Évolution Psychiatrique* (21); E. & S. Livingstone, Ltd. (2); the Secretary of *Modern Law Review* (32); Pergamon Press and the Editor of the *Journal of Psychosomatic Research* (20); the Royal Society of Medicine (4, 11, 15); Springer Verlag, Heidelberg (5).

JAMES SHIELDS
London

IRVING I. GOTTESMAN
Minneapolis

FOREWORD

by
Sir Denis Hill,
Professor of Psychiatry,
Institute of Psychiatry,
University of London

When Eliot Slater went to Germany in 1934 on a Rockefeller Travelling Fellowship to study psychiatric genetics at Rüdin's clinic in Munich, he left behind him at the Maudsley a staff largely influenced by the teaching of Adolf Meyer. This orientation could not have been much to his liking, for the psychological study of personality based on the relationship which the psychiatrist could develop with his patient was not one which his temperament and his particular scientific cast of mind could readily adapt to. It was, however, already being displaced, for Eric Guttmann, Willi Mayer-Gross, Alfred Meyer, and other distinguished refugees from Hitler's Germany had arrived and, by the time of Slater's return a year later, an orientation based on German constitutional psychiatry was already established. By this time neuropathology and genetics seemed the most exciting areas for psychiatric research, with biochemistry and neurophysiology appearing as potential candidates. On his return Slater felt the need to study in greater depth the then comparatively new subject of statistical methods applied to clinical problems, and to this end went to the School of Hygiene where he obtained what he needed under the tutelage of Bradford Hill. Within a very short time he began to collect and study psychiatric twins in the London mental hospitals — the occupation which was to exercise his mind so fully in the years ahead.

When I first met him at the Maudsley in 1938, he seemed a rather aloof man, but kind and hospitable to us juniors, who took pleasure in contentious argument which excited him, and was given to sudden, mercurial bursts of extremely loud laughter. He was already imbued with the aura of the clinical scientist — having knowledge and techniques in a field which was unfamiliar to most of us. His work on the inheritance of manic-depressive disorder was already well known. In a sense, he was a prototype of what was to become the necessary requirement of the academic psychiatrist in Britain in the postwar years — a man of intellectual distinction, a man of scholarly habit, a sound and experienced clinician, but above all a man who had made himself expert in some branch of applied science which he could use in

xiii

psychiatric research. To be a good clinician, a pleasant colleague, even a good teacher was not enough. The psychiatrist as clinical scientist was nevertheless a new phenomenon in the academic scene, and there can be no doubt that Eliot Slater was one of the first of the new breed. Within a few years he had established the reputation of being the leading clinician in psychiatric genetics in Britain.

When war came and when the Maudsley Hospital was evacuated, the staff were divided into two groups, half going to Sutton, half to Mill Hill. It seemed natural that Slater should lead the team who went to Sutton in South London. The emergency hospital established there was to meet the enormous numbers of expected air-raid casualties which of course did not occur, and it soon became for practical purposes a military one. During the war years twenty thousand psychiatric casualties, mainly from the army, were admitted to it. While the administration was the responsibility of Louis Minski, Slater was appointed Clinical Director. He had a team of men (among whom were William Sargant, Alexander Kennedy, Geoffrey Tooth, Joe Shorvon, Gilbert Debenham, and myself) of varying orientations, decided opinions, and different interests. It was a very busy, noisy war; the hospital was evacuated twice — once after it had been bombed, another time to meet the emergency of the Normandy invasion in 1944; throughout, the Clinical Director managed to pursue his genetical research with a ruthless determination while doing his full share of the clinical work — and to persuade and help others to do theirs. Slater's direction was unobtrusive, but his scientific enthusiasm and his great willingness to help, particularly on methodological and statistical problems which were beyond the ken of many of his staff, are remembered by many who still owe him a debt of gratitude. It was during this time that Slater's own stable temperament and courage as well as his scientific distinction became apparent. There are of course many stories told about him. There are those who recall the Clinical Director playing chess against himself on his pocket-set during the worst of the bombing while those of different genetical constitution got under the heavy table at which he sat. There are probably more soldiers than one who, having arrived in the night at Sutton for admission after a long journey across England, can remember being met by a tall donnish figure who asked him only one question, "Are you a twin?"; and, on replying that he was not, being told to go to bed and that he would be interviewed in the morning.

While I believe all his colleagues in the war years regarded Slater with personal affection and esteem and deferred to him for help with their clinical and research problems, there were many who could not share his orientation to the subject. At least one of the first papers (not reproduced in this book) on the subject of war neurosis was the product of an uneasy compromise by authors of different orientation who could not share Slater's essentially biological approach to psychiatry — his preoccupation with the interaction of genetical constitution and environmental stress, the latter viewed by him in what they regarded as over-simplified terms. There seemed to be no place for a psychology of personality; all the important and identifiable differences between men must, it seemed, be due to endogenous or genetical differences. It was the nature of the vulnerability to "stress" and his belief in its genetical basis which occupied Slater's mind. The mass phenomenon of "war neurosis" provided him with problems which he believed could be tackled by the techniques of psychiatric genetics; the issues were essentially biological ones. The accumulated research of those years led to the two important papers, on the neurotic constitution and on the heuristic theory of neurosis, published during the war.

These papers excited little interest at the time, but the second paper, written with his brother Patrick, remains an intellectual achievement of high order. It presents a logical analysis of the available data relevant to biological thinking and examines the evidence for each theory, its practicality and probability. It concludes that a poly-genic theory fits best the facts—each of many genetic components has a small effect and each reduces resistance to some form of environmental stress; these effects are additive and "so facilitate the appearance of neurosis." The evidence that the various components were genetic in origin still seemed an act of faith, although the normal distribution of some of them in the population was known. Slater's conclusion that the neurotically predisposed has a more than average susceptibility to environmental stresses put the neurotic at one end of normal curves of human variation. Neurosis was therefore not a disease, but a product of multifactorial deviance. In this respect it was therefore quite unlike manic-depression and schizophrenia. Because of Slater's insistence that the degree of vulnerability must be due to genetical variation little attention was aroused by his work at the time. It also seemed barely relevant to the psychiatrists who had espoused a psycho-dynamic theory of neurosis, and being a general biological theory based on massed statistical data, it had no relevance to the treatment of clinical cases with which all the energies of psychiatrists were engaged at the time.

Nevertheless, this theory should be seen in its historical context. As a general theory of neurosis it bridged the gap between the earlier period when many believed neurosis to be due to the operation of specific psychological traumata in childhood and the neo-Freudian concept of ego-psychology with its emphasis upon the strengths and weaknesses of ego-structure which determine adaptive capability, and the later realisation that neurotic phenomena are ubiquitous and general. It also can be seen as the theoretical precursor to the modern psychological and psycho-physiological techniques of studying individual differences to stress.

In 1946, after the conclusion of hostilities, Slater was appointed Physician in Psychological Medicine to the National Hospital for Nervous Diseases, Queen Square. This famous neurological hospital had for years had a psychiatrist on its staff. Bernard Hart had been a predecessor. Now, however, a department was to be established with its own ward accommodation and outpatient clinic. Slater entered his new appointment with enthusiasm, for he believed that the psychiatry of organic diseases of the C.N.S. was very important. He assembled around him a group of young research workers of talent, including Alick Elithorn, Malcolm Piercy, George Ettlinger, John McFie, and persuaded Oliver Zangwill from Cambridge to set up within the department a section of clinical psychology to promote research. From the first it had been anticipated that when the opportunity arose the subject at Queen Square would be represented by a professorial unit. But the hospital was slow in accepting academic units even in neurology and neurosurgery, and when a voluntary foundation finally offered to provide the financial support for a chair of psychiatry, which Slater was so eminently suitable to hold, the hospital rejected the offer under the terms in which it was made — to the great dismay of many, but particularly of Slater himself, who in consequence resigned prematurely in 1964.

The post at Queen Square had always been one of great potential, but was not without its hardships. To meet the needs of his colleagues Slater was persuaded to engage in some private practice, which he disliked greatly, feeling he was not very good at it and that his temperament was unsuitable for its objectives. While Slater's main interest always lay in his genetical work — and this he was able to pursue throughout the whole period by his appointment at the Maudsley and at the Institute of Psychiatry — the Queen Square period, largely as the result of his clinical experience, elicited the study on hysteria (given as the Maudsley Lecture in 1960), the work on leucotomy for intractable physical pain, and, most important of all, the comprehensive description and analysis of the schizophrenia-like psychoses of epilepsy. As usual these studies provoked controversy. In claiming that hysteria was "not a syndrome," he based his belief on the demonstration that he could not find concordance for the condition in either identical or non-identical twins. It could not therefore be a genetically-given form of behaviour, and therefore hysteria seemed to be nothing very much at all. This to Slater's critics was a form of psychiatry without a psychology with a vengeance. The fact that, after years of follow-up, patients who had presented with hysterical symptoms were later found to have other conditions, including organic disease of the C.N.S., schizophrenia, and other functional psychoses was no surprise to him.

There can be no doubt that through his general writings Eliot Slater has influenced British psychiatry very profoundly. The publication with William Sargant of the small text on *Physical Methods of Treatment* soon after the war, came as a boon to a generation of young psychiatrists who based their thinking on the medical model of psychiatric illness, and provided a concise, practical and very readable guide to therapeutic practice in this developing field. More important and more influential was the appearance, with Willi Mayer-Gross and Martin Roth as co-authors, of the large text on *Clinical Psychiatry* in 1954. This was the most up-to-date, erudite, and brilliantly written account of the subject as it had developed from the work of the German and Scandinavian schools of psychiatry which were based upon the Kraepelinian system. It became essential reading, and a valuable source of reference to every psychiatrist in training in the country. The neglect of the psycho-dynamic and social determinants of personality, the study of personality itself, and — as some saw it — the savage and ill-informed attack on psychoanalysis could all be forgiven. The book contained the most comprehensive, brilliant account of the clinical phenomena of schizophrenia and other psychotic conditions which had yet been written in the English language. It was the epitome of a psychiatry based on the natural sciences. In 1961 the Royal Medico-Psychological Association appointed Slater Editor-in-Chief of the (then) *Journal of Mental Science*. The journal had fallen into decrepitude, the published papers were of a very varied quality, its reputation was low. In Slater's hands this Journal, now the *British Journal of Psychiatry*, has been transformed into one of high scientific quality — I would claim one of the world's leading psychiatric journals. Slater has of course given it the impress of his own orientation — his own high standard of what constitutes scientific evidence, his demand for new knowledge based on measurement and verification rather than description and supposition, his deep antipathy to what he conceived as the "crazy structure" of psychoanalysis and the "panpsychic" explanation of psychodynamic formulations of aetiology. Few papers by psychoanalytical authors have appeared in the Journal. Perhaps few have been submitted; yet I know from having served with Slater as co-editor for a period, no paper with this orientation has been rejected by him upon his own responsibility alone.

It is of course for his original and far-reaching investigations into the genetics of schizophrenia that Slater has won an international reputation. Despite the evidence from successive studies by other authors that show a lesser concordance of the condition in identical twins, Slater holds to his original monogenic theory of aetiology. Without the pathogenic gene, schizophrenia cannot occur, and this claim would seem vital to sustain the strongly held view that the search for the biochemical anomaly or abnormality in schizophrenia must be pursued — research which has hitherto been so disappointing. In 1959, the Medical Research Council, recognising Slater's pre-eminence in his subject, invited him to form a Psychiatric Genetics Research Unit, and to head it as Director. This was given a home at the Institute of Psychiatry, and he collected around him a small group of workers, which included James Shields and Valerie Cowie. Upon his retirement from the Directorship it was decided to publish the present volume of his selected works.

This is not the place or time to attempt any assessment of Slater's place in the scientific history of our subject. He is still actively pursuing his research; he is still a great influence in psychiatry both nationally and internationally. He has always been a controversial figure — a clinical scientist dedicated to the pursuit of biological knowledge, but also a man concerned about the social and political ideas of the times, always seeing them as a biologist equipped with his own skills and insights and his own frame of reference. But there are ambiguities and contradictory aspects of his personality. The personal problems of individual patients cannot rate high in the work of the clinical scientist, yet Slater has nevertheless always felt a deep sympathy for them. Surprisingly, in 1967 he reviewed Konrad Lorenz's book *On Aggression* with great enthusiasm. In accepting with Lorenz that human aggression is a biological drive which must be "discharged," that present day civilized man suffers from an insufficient discharge of his aggressive drive, Slater finds himself in a new position, not so different from that which Freud first adopted in his first account of instinctual activity in man. Slater has never lacked critics, even among those who most value his friendship; and even when the differences go deep, the integrity and quality of the man ensure that disputation does not affect personal relationships — indeed it is of the essence of his intellectual life.

This book will be valued by the many who know of his work, but have never had the opportunity of seeing it in the round. To many more it should prove a source of stimulation and knowledge — the account of an intellectual journey in pursuit of biological understanding in psychiatry, a record of achievement over thirty-five years in which the author has always applied to his data and to his own hypotheses the same scientific rigour and criticism which he has expected from others.

DENIS HILL
London

FOREWORD

by
David Rosenthal,
Chief, Laboratory of Psychology,
National Institute of Mental Health

My association with Eliot Slater has been neither very long nor very close, but it has been professional in the best sense of that term. When one day I found myself responsible for carrying out studies of the MZ schizophrenic Genain Quadruplets, I quaked a little inside because I hadn't the foggiest notion about genetics, or, more pointedly, about the genetics of schizophrenia. It took only a cursory reading of the literature to recognize that among the most able of the investigators in this field, Eliot Slater ranked high indeed. I pored over his monograph on twins and found it a treasure of information. Among other things, it stimulated me to test the hypothesis that there might be two kinds of schizophrenic disorder, one where the genetic loading was high, the other where the genetic contribution was minimal, and to carry out the test on his own case material! This was certainly a presumption for a rank novice, and it carried the implication that the investigator hadn't analyzed his data thoroughly. But I took courage and sent a preliminary manuscript to Dr. Slater. In it I described the hypothesis and the data analyses designed to test it. I expected a stinging reply, but instead I received from him a kindly letter of encouragement, generously sprinkled with helpful comments and suggestions. As a matter of fact, he was delighted that someone had tried to use his data productively, whether he agreed with the conclusions or not. Imagine my gratitude. After that, we kept up a correspondence in which the flow of benefit was almost entirely from London to Bethesda.

In subsequent years, I developed my own views about the etiology of schizophrenia, and Dr. Slater and I did not always see eye to eye. In his Retrospect, which he wrote for this book, he advocates abolition of the adversary system in trials of criminal offenders, and proposes instead to substitute an investigatory process to determine fact and cause. I believe that what he is saying here is simply a carryover from his views regarding science and research. These views are based on a genuine interest in the search for truth and understanding. Let no one think that he has any distaste or ineptitude for the role of adversary! For a week-long "confrontation conference" organized by S. S. Kety and myself, we invited leading investigators, who had opposed views regarding the roles of heredity and environment in schizo-

XX   DAVID ROSENTHAL

phrenia, to present and defend their positions. From the outset, no one was more embroiled in the fray than Eliot Slater. With characteristic eloquence, he led the exposition of the genetic view repeatedly and incisively, in regard to clinical phenomena or group research findings, citing case material or statistics, which he knew intimately. When others posed alternate views, he was quick and ready to point up weaknesses and errors in supportive data or argument. He was a formidable opponent indeed, and on a number of occasions I was myself on the receiving end of his trenchant criticism. But his debate was always joined to the issues and never involved personal rancor. When the meetings were over and we had a few moments alone together, he said simply in his own patrician way, "We will have our battles, won't we?"

Apart from my deep respect for Dr. Slater's thorough command of his area of interest, what I admire most about him is that he is uncompromising in his principles. On one occasion, a minor — almost trivial — matter arose which might have had a seriously deleterious impact on an enterprise which involved not only Dr. Slater and myself, but other persons and a publishing house as well. Dr. Slater not only insisted that the matter be resolved in the way he thought correct, but he was unyielding as well in affirming that he would not tolerate any well-wisher subverting the proper manner of resolving the matter, even if it was trivial. It would have been easy and politic to avoid the fuss, but that was not his way. How badly the world of today needs such men who think clearly, generate principles based on such thought, and hold to and speak out in behalf of such principles, unafraid of the consequences.

From the professional side, I think that his most important contribution has been his monumental twin study and his theorizing about the etiology of schizophrenia. Although he was not the first to propose a major dominant single gene as the principal etiologic agent in schizophrenia, his exposition of the theory was the most elegant and the best-documented. During the sixties, polygenic theory caught on and Dr. Slater's closest colleagues, Shields and Gottesman, took the lead in expounding this theory. My understanding is that they had a real impact on his thinking, and he was willing to admit that they might be right, but he has never really conceded that his monogenic theory was incorrect. I, too, have leaned toward a polygenic theory, but a cursory look at some of my recent data suggests that Dr. Slater may well be right after all. In a way, I hope he is. He deserves to be.

DAVID ROSENTHAL
Bethesda, Maryland

MAN, MIND,
and
HEREDITY

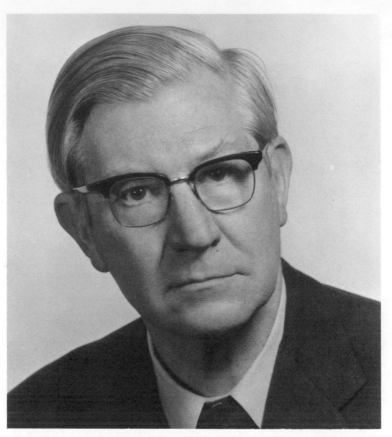

Eliot Trevor Oakeshott Slater

C.B.E., M.A., M.D. (Cambridge), F.R.C.P. (London), D.P.M.

Editor-in-Chief, *British Journal of Psychiatry*
Director, 1959–69, Medical Research Council (MRC) Psychiatric Genetics Unit,
Maudsley Hospital, London, England

Born, August 28, 1904; son of Gilbert Slater, M.A., D.Sc.; educated at Leighton Park, Cambridge University, and Saint George's Hospital, London.

Medical officer, Maudsley Hospital, 1931–39; Rockefeller Foundation Fellowship for study in Munich and Berlin, 1934–35; Medical Research Council research grant, 1935–37; Gaskell Gold Medallist in Psychiatry, 1938; Clinical Director, Sutton Emergency Hospital, 1939–45; Physician in Psychological Medicine, National Hospital, Queen Square, London, 1946–64; Member of the Royal Commission on Capital Punishment, 1949; Senior Lecturer, Institute of Psychiatry, University of London, 1950–59; President, Psychiatric Section, Royal Society of Medicine, 1958–59; Director, Medical Research Council Psychiatric Genetics Unit, Maudsley Hospital, 1959–69; Litchfield Lecture, Oxford University, 1959; Galton Lecture, 1960; Maudsley Lecture, 1960; Editor-in-Chief, *British Journal of Psychiatry*, since 1961; C.B.E. (Commander of the British Empire), 1966.

Genetical Society; Eugenics Society (Fellow; Vice-President 1963–66); American Psychiatric Association (Honorary Fellow).

Books: *Introduction to Physical Methods of Treatment in Psychiatry* (with W. Sargant), 1944; *Patterns of Marriage* (with M. Woodside), 1951; *Psychotic and Neurotic Illnesses in Twins*, 1953; *Clinical Psychiatry* (with W. Mayer-Gross and M. Roth), 1954; *Delinquency in Girls* (with J. Cowie and V. Cowie), 1968; *The Genetics of Mental Disorders* (with V. Cowie), 1971.

AUTOBIOGRAPHICAL SKETCH

THE ROAD TO PSYCHIATRY

It must have been about 1919, when I was fifteen, that my father came to see me at my boarding school while on leave from India. At that time he was Professor of Indian Economics in the University of Madras, a post that kept him out of England over a critical period of my career. As I remember it, we went for a walk about the school grounds, and he asked me what I wanted to do with myself in life. I told him I wanted to be a doctor, and I think he must have sighed. My parents were never well off, and it must have been a grievous task to put three sons through fee-charging "public" schools and a university afterwards. To be asked to undertake the additional cost of supporting a son during the years he was a medical student must have been hard. Yet he did not attempt to persuade me out of it.

I do not know what had made me pick on medicine at that age, and I cannot believe I had any solid reasons. Such decisions, one would think, should really be taken by adults on the basis of a fully informed appreciation of the boy's intelligence, aptitudes, and interests. However, the decision in favour of medicine could claim the support of some good sense. A medical career offers such a variety of occupations, and presents such a variety of niches for personalities of any imaginable kind, that once started on it a young man should be able to find his way to the right spot for him in the end. It was also a good choice from the point of view of what the school had to offer. Leighton Park was a small public school with only about a hundred and twenty boys at the time I was there. It had been chosen by my mother, who had been given the decision by my father away in India, mainly because she was a Quaker and this was a Quaker school, and because she was a pacifist and this school had no military training for cadets. The teaching was somewhat uneven, and was extremely weak on the classical side. The best teaching was in biology, and Mr. Unwin our biology master also ran a Sunday evening discussion group for sixth form

Specially written for *Man, Mind, and Heredity*.

boys, the S.I. or Synthetic Iconoclasts, in which we read and discussed such books as *Thus Spake Zarathustra*. Biology was very attractive, and if one went into biology medicine became the natural final goal — then at least, if it would not now.

I do not think my mother's choice was a wise one; but since I have no regrets for the form that my career finally took, I cannot regret the separate steps that took me there. Half the boys at the school came from Quaker families, that is to say predominantly from very prosperous middle-class backgrounds. There were many representatives of the big Quaker chocolate manufacturing firms, Cadburys, Rowntrees, and Frys. These boys had no need for scholarship, and after school most of them would go into a secure place in the family business. Very few of them went to a university, and the school had no facilities for educating boys up to university scholarship level. On the mathematical side they had a Wrangler (a first-class-honours man from Oxford), but the time allotted to maths was small and I was never taken any further than the first few exercises in calculus. My lack of mathematical training has been a source of regret to me all my life.

To cope with its clientele, the School regarded it as its main task to train not for scholarship but for character. The ultimate aim was that the boy should become a good citizen, a God-fearing Christian, and a solid asset to the community. Prowess in learning met with no rewards. Annual examination lists were posted on the school notice board, but were the occasion neither for praise nor punishment. Solid financial rewards were reserved in the form of prizes for the results of leisure-time hobbies. The annual hobby exhibition included such things as items of carpentry, maps, collections of butterflies, etc.; and prizes were given for these and for stories, poems, recitations, public speaking, and so forth. I think we got a very peculiar view of what really matters in life — but who is to say? Maybe the School was right.

Despite my negligible training in scholastic competitiveness, I succeeded when the time came in winning a minor exhibition (a sizarship) to St. John's College, Cambridge. This was worth only £30 a year, and would not do much better than take the edge off the sharpness of the financial difficulty for my father. I always felt rather uncomfortable about being a sizar, since in the middle ages sizars had been a lowly order of creature who earned their remission of fees by doing domestic duties for their College in spare time. There was, however, the opportunity of converting my sizarship into a full scholarship, worth say £100 per annum, if I succeeded in getting first-class honours in the examinations at the end of the first academic year.

This was not to be. I went to the prescribed lectures and lab courses and dissections not finding great interest in them and spending practically none of my spare time in working on the textbooks. My tutor might have kept my nose to the grindstone if he had been worth his salt, but he wasn't. In fact most of my friends were fairly carefully looked after, and not only had a weekly tutorial, but also had a supervisor who looked after their reading and set questions. When the Mays examinations came along at the end of the first year, I only got second-class honours, and did not get any promotion.

Later on I resented this experience, perhaps more on my father's behalf than my own, and sometimes would say to myself that if I met that man I would give him a piece of my mind. The opportunity came, not once but twice. This tutor and I both went into psychiatry after Cambridge years, and in the fullness of time ran into one another at a tea-party of the RMPA (Royal Medico-Psychological Association). He recognised me, and we had some conversation in the course of which he asked me what kind of a guide and teacher I had found him while I had been under his tutelage. I asked him whether he really wanted to know, and when he said he did, I told him. He was greatly surprised, but did not seem to lose his affability. As he was practising as a psychotherapist, the *sang froid* may have been professional. Anyway, as fate would have it, we met again only a few months later, this time finding ourselves sitting next to one another at an RMPA lunch. Once more he turned to me and said, "Ah, Slater, I thought I recognised you. Tell me, weren't we at Cambridge together? I fancy I was your tutor." It was quite clear that he had totally forgotten the previous occasion and that the wasp-sting I had endeavoured to stick through his thick skin had taken no effect. This was quite a lesson to me; on future occasions when I found something rankling I would try to shrug it off, and abandon the absurd dream of one day giving a tit for tat.

The low classes I got in the Mays examinations did not spur me to do better in succeeding years. Instead of cramming, or engaging in athletic pursuits as so many, I spent nearly all my spare time in the excellent library of the Cambridge Union Society, reading works of English literature and some of the easier French classics. English drama particularly attracted me, and I read everything I could lay hands on. That, and poetry. I also tried my hand at writing stories of both a romantic and fantastic kind to take me into another world, and poetry as an attempted abreaction of my miseries in this one. During the whole of my Cambridge career I felt lonely and out of place. I had a few good friends among the boys who had come up to Cambridge with me from my school; but I made few new ones. Above all, I lacked a girl friend. Much of my reading was with a view to finding out what kind of creature the female of the species is, and what was meant by a love relationship. I am inclined to think now that in this way my time was better spent than it would have been if I had worked at my anatomy, physiology, and chemistry with the good will I ought to have had.

Scholastically, the most mediocre successes continued to attend me. This did not stop my being ambitious. Many medical students were contented with passing their strictly medical examinations and otherwise collecting only a pass degree for the diploma of B.A. I had to try higher. At the end of my second year I took the Natural Sciences Tripos Part I in anatomy, physiology, and chemistry. During the chemistry practical I had one of the attacks of complete gormlessness which afflict me at times. I found myself presented with a bottle of colourless, limpid, aromatic-smelling fluid and asked to identify it. Such a task had never yet been given to me, and I was flummoxed. How on earth could one analyse the chemical constitution of an organic compound? With the aid of my sense of smell I identified it as ethyl ether, and found that it was to inspection not distinguishable from the fluid in the bench bottle of ether. This had to be the substance of my report. It never occurred to me to measure any of its physical characteristics, such as the boiling point; and I think it quite probable that I didn't even discover whether it was inflammable. I still do not quite understand how I achieved second-class honours in that exam.

Despite these indifferent results, it was still a matter for decision whether I should go on with science or turn entirely to medicine. I still felt that chemistry was a fascinating field and that biochemistry was a promised land. My father visited me at Cambridge and together we went to see the Professor of Biochemistry, Frederick Gowland Hopkins, famous for his discovery of vitamins. By his advice I opted to do Part II of the Natural Sciences Tripos in biochemistry, which only that year became a possibility. Those few medical students who went as far as a Second Part of the Tripos practically always did the course in physiology, which was very well regarded;

and this was, for instance, the part chosen by the star pupil of my year, John StClair Elkington who won all the prizes and got a double first.

Elkington became a neurologist and went on to the honorary staff of St. Thomas's Hospital at an earlier age than anyone before him. I later became a colleague of his at Queen Square. He was one of the small number of neurologists I have known who have had any respect for psychiatry; and it was to a considerable extent his support which enabled my friend Will Sargant to establish such a flourishing department of psychiatry at St. Thomas's. Though he was most benign to his students and juniors, Elkington resembled many other neurologists in being very cool and remote with patients. It was said of him that in his own consulting room he put his patient in a chair that was screwed to the floor, as he so much disliked the way some patients have of edging their chair closer and closer to the doctor's.

There were only four of us who took Biochemistry in the Second Part of the Tripos; and at the end of it, two got firsts and two thirds. Needless to say I was one of the thirds. Hopkins was much too much tied up in his own researches to pay much attention to the course, and it was mainly organised and run by J. B. S. Haldane. He didn't take to me particularly ("What, Slater, studying astral physics?"). Haldane was a man of genius, but he was no organiser. There wasn't any syllabus for the course, no set books, and no one knew what would be asked about in the finals. My colleagues who got firsts no doubt did so by working hard and systematically reading everything that came their way; this was more than I could or would do, left to myself. I am afraid that I would never have made a good lab worker. On one occasion we were given the material and instructions to carry out a colorimetric estimation of one of the constituents of a specimen of human urine (J.B.S.'s, diluted ten times). We all had to use the same colorimeter, and I noticed that after I had had my turn one of my first-class colleagues who followed me carefully washed out the glass container with distilled water. I asked him why he did this, since distilled water was colorimetrically less like his test material than my test material was. My recollection is that he didn't have a good answer to this question (though the answer is obvious enough); but he did know intuitively, as I did not, that to leave a trace of other test material in the chamber could not possibly be good practice.

I had now reached the end of my third year at Cambridge, and it was clear that I should never make a scientist. I put my name down in the books of the University Appointments Board, but when I told them that nothing would persuade me to take up teaching, they seemed to think that, if that were so, for a third class man there was little left. Some months later I got my first and only notification of a vacancy, for the post of biochemist in one of the dependencies in Africa, salary £500 per annum. But by that time I had at last made some progress with my medical studies.

Up till the end of my last term at Cambridge I had been dogged by lack of success in examinations on anatomy. I was a messy dissector, and had such a poverty of visual imagery that I had the greatest difficulty in grasping the relation of one structure to its neighbours. I passed in physiology and came down in anatomy in the 2nd M.B. examination at the end of my fourth term and again at the end of the sixth term. It was now the end of the ninth term, and somehow or other I had to pass. If I could not learn things by sight I might learn them by sound. My technique was to attempt to learn more or less by heart the condensed statements in "Aids to Anatomy". On the morning before the written examination in anatomy at 9 A.M., I rose at six (I had meant to get up earlier), and turned over the pages of *Gray's*

Anatomy looking over as many as I could of the more important pictures, trying to imprint something on my mind firmly enough to last there for the few hours necessary. The gamble came off; one whole question and a large part of another could be answered with confidence on the basis of what I had seen that morning. I had some hope that I might yet pass, but there was still the oral to come. Here luck continued to smile on me. I found myself facing the external examiner, for whom I was only a number. The first question he gave me was not too bad, and the second was about the shoulder joint. This too I was able to parry, and then I thought I might chance my arm. I asked him whether I might put a question to him about something I had never been able to understand. When he gave permission, I asked him about the way the biceps tendon ran through the shoulder joint quite freely, covered only by the joint endothelium, or whether it had a kind of "mesentery" or membrane connecting it to the joint capsule. I have no idea what his answer was (and I still do not know the answer to my question), but for the next seven or eight minutes or so dizzily and happily I listened to him discoursing about the minutiae of the shoulder joint, which must have been some kind of a pet subject for him.

I did get my pass, and my father could look forward to the pleasing prospect of supporting me in my studies for an additional two and half years. My last term at Cambridge, the tenth, was for eight weeks in the long vacation in the summer of 1925. There were only a few students up, mostly medicals, doing "bugs and drugs" (bacteriology, pathology, pharmacology). We all lived in college, and indeed had to be within college walls by 10 P.M.. This was a painful restriction, as there were half a dozen of us who liked to play bridge in the evenings and would not enjoy having to break off much before midnight. By good luck I was given a set of rooms with one window from which I could step onto a broad ledge over the window below, from there onto the top of a wall, and from there onto a pile of builder's rubble beyond which there was level ground and only one easily scaled gate separating me from the freedom of the Backs, the college gardens alongside the river. My last term at Cambridge, with studies which now came easily to me, with the companionship of friends, and with a reprieve from anxieties, was the only really happy one. Certainly the little town in its summer sleep, shut down at night, with few and dim street lamps to compete with the moon, showed all its magic in those late hours. In the narrow lanes between the black silhouettes of ancient buildings there would be hardly a footfall; and out on the Backs no other soul with whom to share the wide lawns and the great trees and the black and silvery river. Momentarily one was submerged in a cloistered mediaeval town, perhaps a fellow student with Christopher Marlowe.

At the end of the summer I came up to London, having won a minor scholarship to St. George's Hospital. Once again I was the victim of quite unsuitable ambitions. The really prestigious branch of medicine was surgery, and if I were to be a surgeon I should do well to take the primary examination of the F.R.C.S. diploma. Instead of getting on with the job of learning to be a doctor, I took three months off working at the Primary course at St. Mary's Hospital. The medical school there was full of young men who had been given scholarships for athletic prowess (Will Sargant was later to be one such), all very beefy and boisterous. The general atmosphere of the most aggressive type of heartiness didn't suit me a bit. Of course I failed my Primary examination, being totally unfitted for work along this line; and it was with great relief that I discovered what a soothing place a medical school could be when I went to St. George's.

5

Here the atmosphere was quiet, well-bred, almost genteel. There was a cult, proceeding by contagion from the more to the less senior students, of wearing fancy waistcoats, cravats and tiepins, and spats even with, say, a light grey suit. If one wore the short black jacket with pinstripe trousers, then one's sombre tie was relieved with a white slip just showing from inside the waistcoat. I never aimed so (expensively) high, though in due course I acquired an umbrella, a gold-headed ebony cane, and a monocle; more importantly I became aware of the necessity of wearing in immaculate state the dresser's clean white jacket and of having clean hands and spotless finger-nails. This was a lesson that I learned, but I cannot claim a faultless standard of practice.

The teaching at St. George's was excellent, at a rather humdrum level. Such a standard would not be acceptable nowadays. In fact, we were all apprentices, and were there to learn the art and practice of medicine from teachers to whom we were individually assigned. Medicine as a field of enquiry only existed in a few holes and corners, mainly perhaps behind some partition in one of the labs. St. George's men for the most part got through their exams without difficulty and went into suitable private practices. They had the reputation of becoming very successful general practitioners in the West End of London, recommending themselves to their aristocratic or influential or wealthy patients by their polish and address no less than their competence, kindness, and good sense. The ultimate product of this scheme of apprenticeship and training was not always to be in every way admirable. At a later time I met at the bedside of a wealthy widow one of my contemporaries who was known to be very successful in this little world. The way in which he handled the lady, her parlourmaid, the other consultant, and myself, easy and self-effacing as it was, seemed to me indistinguishable from that of the upper servant or an old family retainer.

When I came up to London for hospital work, my father suggested that it would be much better than living in lodgings to become a resident at Toynbee Hall, a very famous institution just about at the border between the City and the East End of London. Communal life at Toynbee had many resemblances to life at a college; even the architecture and the small individual bed-sitting rooms conveyed that impression. In the evenings the residents would sit down to dinner at a long table in a dining hall, at one end of which there were a few comfortable chairs and a cheerful coal fire. It was in one of these chairs that I would sit after dinner reading the latest work of fiction I had borrowed from the "Times" Lending Library. This wasn't really quite the done thing. I should have been up and about the Lord's work. University graduates were there to take their share in the social work of the neighbourhood, and to do their best to bring one kind of a light or another into the lives of the vast arrays of the underprivileged which swarmed around us to north, east, and south.

It was brought home to me that I must do my bit; and the first suggestion made to me was that I should help to run one of the several boys' clubs associated with Toynbee. This would only mean spending one or two evenings a week in the company of rather rough boys at a club a mile or so from the Hall in, admittedly, a squalid neighbourhood. This was at a time when such clubs ran quite easily, and encountered no disagreeable attentions from hooligans as has been the case in recent years. Nevertheless I was terrified. I would not have the least idea how to communicate with such persons. I imagine I had a suspicion that, as soon as they would become aware of me as a foreign body, a gang of them would set on me and beat me up. But what held me back was not so much a physical fear as a mental one; the torturing shyness I suffered from at this time effectively cut me off from practically everyone but my old friends and fellow medical students.

Running a boys' club would have been a very soft option in comparison with what I chose. This was to give a course of lectures to prisoners in Pentonville Gaol; my subject, English literature. This meant a long tram-drive at night, through a dreary neighbourhood, entering through the frowning gates of the prison, being conducted by a warder to a room in which some thirty prisoners were awaiting me. Once into the room, I heard the door clang to behind me and the lock slammed, leaving me alone with my pupils. What followed was frightful. I would endeavour to make my voice heard above the hum of conversation on all sides, and make pathetic attempts to keep order. What the men were there for was to have the chance of a gossip, and I was pretty well ignored except, I remember, by one sycophantic clerkly fellow who seemed to listen and want to draw me out. I knew that I was making a fool of myself, and that if this was what social work was then it was not for me. I put in an application to the Warden and Residents' Committee to be permitted to regard my work at the bedsides of the poor and sick and dying as a sufficiency of social work, and this specious plea was actually allowed though I think with a poor grace. I was not well regarded after that; and when the residents at their dining table heard my fits of laughter (over Gerhardi's *Polyglots*, I remember) and saw me at ease in front of the fire, my image suffered further damage. Some years later an ex-resident wrote a history of Toynbee Hall, in which as an appendix there was a complete nominal roll of all the residents up to that date — complete, that is to say, but for my name, which had been omitted like that of a criminal.

About this time I developed a craze for gambling. There were about four or five of us who indulged this taste at Toynbee, and we would meet in the most spacious of our bed-sitting rooms at least once or twice a week. Bridge was soon thought too slow, poker followed, and then the nakedly gambling games like crown and anchor and roulette. It was at this game that I learned a lesson which stayed with me ever after. Typically of my nature, I was trying to get the better of the odds; instead of taking the slim chance of a big win, I wanted the maximum chance, certainty indeed if attainable, of some win, however small. In pursuit of this, starting with a small stake on an even chance, say red or black, I doubled it every time I lost until at the end I should have recovered the initial stake plus its equivalent. Unfortunately with this cautious technique, a long run of ill luck can be murderous. Sweating, I was finding I had bet all the money I had and was now venturing my next month's allowance; what would happen if that went I did not even envisage. Fortunately, the last bet won and I only found myself out of pocket by that small amount occasioned by rounding off when passing by doubles from pennies into shillings and shillings into pounds.

I was not entirely cured of the itch to gamble, but after this confined myself to games with an element of skill (particularly poker, when I was a resident at St. George's). In post-graduate years in London I also played a good deal of bridge; and in general I fancied myself at games of skill. Here too I have been taught lessons of humility. I gave up poker after a game in the emergency hospital I was seconded to in the war years; at this there was one good player, who took the money of all the rest of us and gave me the clearest demonstration of my incapacities. I have had exactly the same experience at bridge, and indeed from the same man, a well-known ear surgeon; but here I was more put off the game by playing with a married couple who bickered through the evening and were so passionate in their addiction to play that there could be no interval for conversation or even for refreshments which had to be consumed at table. Most instructive of all was when I met someone very much my master at chess, in a postal game in which one had all the time one needed for reflection and calculation. This was a bewildering experience. After the opening development, in which my opponent chose almost from the start a little-played and unorthodox line, I found myself becoming more and more unclear about what his intentions were. Time and again, the reply I expected was not made, perhaps indeed one different from all the possibilities I had considered plausible. On the other hand, each of the possibilities I considered for my own play disclosed itself as having objections and weaknesses. Eventually I had entangled myself into a cramped position in which instead of developing my own game I was restricted to holding off the enemy attack. It came, indeed, from an unexpected quarter; the gap in the armour was exposed and the knife came through.

Somewhere in his recollections Bertrand Russell has spoken of what it was like to meet on the intellectual level someone considerably more able than oneself, in his case Maynard Keynes. In my chess game I felt as if I was living in a thick darkness out of which cobwebs were descending on me, always thickening the dark and hampering my movements. My opponent, I knew, was in the light. The impression one gets at a scientific meeting is not quite like that. More than once I have heard J. B. S. Haldane enter the discussion of a paper presented by myself (and others too, of course) and shine like some kind of firework. Squibs are let off in all directions, exploding among one's cherished ideas, and one thinks again and again "how dull of me not to have thought of that." But I fear we can learn only from our intellectual equals or near equals; and those to whom we are as mental defectives can neither instil us with any of their brilliance nor even give us perhaps the line that we in our inferiority should choose in which to go on with our work. I certainly learned no chess lesson from my victor and I fear that in the course of my connection with genetics I never learned much from Haldane.

In my day it was possible to qualify after only 21 months of hospital practice, with the "Conjoint" examination; the university diploma of M.B. required one more year. I succeeded in getting my qualification in minimum time, but once again it was not without a smile from fortune. One such came to me in the written examination in medicine.[1] There before me stood the question, demanding that I should tell the examiners what I knew about "dementia praecox." I looked at it aghast. I had never heard of this disease. After some hesitation I went up to the invigilating examiner and asked "Please, sir, is this another name for G.P.I.?," to which he replied "You can't very well expect me to answer that question, can you?" I retired to my desk for another think. Clearly this could not be another name for G.P.I., since if it had been a rarely used synonym, he would surely have told me. It was then something different, apparently a dementia and coming on in young people. I sat down and wrote. I threw in everything I had ever heard of. The disease was commonly insidious and progressive but could be interrupted with acute attacks, mania, melan-

---

[1] The reader may be surprised at so much preoccupation with examinations. In fact, for a great part of my life, say from 13 until my M.D. at 36, they constituted most of the major challenges. Of those that have been or could have been critical I can remember 25: 4 public examinations in general education, 12 medical, 7 for scholarships, and 2 for prizes. Despite some facility in this kind of test, I do not much respect it: those who markedly lack the special ability which is needed to cope are at a great and unfair disadvantage in the pursuit of a professional career.

cholia, delusions, hallucinations, confusion, homicidal and suicidal outbursts, remissions that did not last, a tendency to relentless deterioration of mind and character. The pathology, I wrote, was unknown (it had to be, since I had never heard of it); some thought that it belonged to the group of progressive disorders for which Gowers had advanced his hypothesis of abiotrophy. I feel sure that on this question I scored at least a pass. I dare say that the examiners themselves, necessarily none of them psychiatrists, knew no more than I had invented. Clear proof of widespread ignorance was given me a few years later when I tried to look up the subject in a well known textbook of medicine. I was a neurological house physician at the time, and I was trying to find what might be the matter with a very odd patient, who showed nothing abnormal neurologically, who seemed sometimes to be bright and at other times answered so oddly that you might take him to be mentally deficient. After a thorough study of the chapter on psychological medicine, I came to the conclusion that my patient might be suffering either from schizophrenia or from dementia praecox. The two disorders seemed to have much in common, but they were distinct since each had its own section, with a number of pages separating them (1930).

After qualifying I had a brief experience of general practice. A G.P., ex-St. George's, who must have had an extraordinarily confiding disposition, let the School secretary know that he wanted a holiday locum for about ten days. I went out to see him, in a nice house in a pleasant leafy residential part of Bucks, about twenty-five miles from the centre of London in the Oxford direction. The experience should have been idyllic. I was living in the doctor's house, waited on by his domestic staff, driven around by his gardener-chauffeur. It was hell. I was called to patients who had something the matter with them, pains in the tummy, unexplained fevers, a sprained (or was it fractured?) ankle, which I was usually unable to diagnose, and if able to diagnose did not know how to treat. The only patient of all those I visited whom I could recognise as suffering from a familiar syndrome, was an emaciated young man in a poor cottage with lumps all over his belly to be felt through the thin abdominal wall. That I had seen in the wards at St. George's, and knew it for tuberculous peritonitis.

The doctor had warned me that there was one baby case coming up, in a young primipara and no complications to be expected; if there were, I could call in his partner who lived a couple of miles away. I regarded this prospect with sinking sensations, since despite all the regulations I had only delivered one baby, and that in the wards and under supervision. My hopes that the baby would be delayed were disappointed, and in due course I was sent for. There at the cottage was the district midwife, who should have been able to manage the whole affair without my help. I asked her whether she had examined the patient and what was the lie of the baby's head. She said yes, and it was one of the two normal positions with the baby's occiput to the front, either right or left. In the course of my examination I thought it was an occipito-posterior presentation, but thought that I must be wrong as I was so inexperienced. To cut a horrid story short, it was an occipito-posterior and it never corrected itself. All that day the patient continued in labour, without advancing. I came and saw her, and went away, and came again, and walked about in the doctor's garden in the delicious early summer weather, sweating and groaning and wishing I were anywhere but there. It would be too impossibly bad luck to have my first delivery an abnormal one! In the end I was injecting pituitrin in a kind of panic, and did not have the courage or the cold common sense to call in the partner until the early hours of the following morning. He was most kind, and accepted this abysmal conduct as just a manifestation of the natural irrationality of mankind. He found the baby's head stuck, applied forceps, and dragged it out face to pubes, dead.

General practice would not be for me, and I should have to work for some time with the shadow of the hospital's authority behind me. I was lucky in getting my year of hospital appointments at my teaching hospital, and for four months in turn was casualty officer, house surgeon, and house physician. My period as house surgeon was spent with Mr. (later Sir) Claude Frankau, who rapidly became allergic to me. I do not know quite what it was about this long, gangling (189 cm, 70 kilo), ham-handed youth that put him off; I always imagined that it was because he sensed some lack of respect when, in the course of those long bed-side discussions on the Surgeon's round, I edged my behind onto the corner of a locker, instead of standing dutifully fully erect, to save some of my blood from sinking into my belly. Every house surgeon regarded it as one of his rights to be allowed to perform one operation on an inguinal hernia and one operation on a quiescent appendix under the supervision of his chief. In the last week of my tenancy of the appointment, Mr. Frankau placed the knife in my hand and indicated where I was to make the skin incision. However, no sooner had I taken hold of it than he exclaimed: "That isn't the way to hold a scalpel! Here, let me show you!" With that he took the knife back again, and completed the operation himself.

My period as a House Physician with Hugh Gainsborough was much more rewarding. I was still capable of failing miserably to carry out an air-replacement of a pleural effusion (to the confusion of the Registrar's class of students in the afternoon who all mistook the "hyperresonant" chest for a "dull" one); but I enjoyed the sustained excitement of working through the night to save the life of a patient in diabetic coma, and of demonstrating by my own preparation the pneumococci in a sample of cerebrospinal fluid I had taken. I don't know quite how good or bad I was. Gainsborough advised me not to try to take the Membership of the Royal College of Physicians, which would be the portal of entry for a career as a specialist.

My year came to an end. I was enjoying life so much in the "Cottage" (the residents' quarters) that I could not bear to leave. I applied for and got six months as resident anaesthetist. I should think I must have been the worst ever. My predecessor was an extremely able man, and he had been practically the first at St. George's to use gas-oxygen machines and introduced the technique of intubation (passing a catheter into the trachea). I tried to follow in his footsteps, but would have been better advised to do just what all the Hospital's senior anaesthetists did — just pour the mixture of chloroform and ether onto an open mask.

After that they threw me out, and what was I to do now? Hospital it had to be. I thought first of paediatrics and then of neurology. I was turned down for the paediatric job I applied for but got the neurological one, and so became junior house physician at the West End Hospital for Nervous Diseases, and resident in the small in-patient department in a converted mansion in its own grounds in the very substance of Regent's Park — probably the most delightful quarters of any hospital in London. I had been attracted to neurology by the clinical demonstrations of James Collier, with all the elegance that neurologists, the prima donnas of the medical profession, aspire to and so frequently attain. Now, in practice, I found that neurology suited me well, although my lack of feeling for anatomy would have been a serious handicap if I had proceeded with it.

During my year at the West End I succeeded, despite Hugh Gainsborough's opinion, in passing the examination for the Membership of the Royal College of

Physicians. This was then a ferocious ordeal in which at three successive stages one had to report to receive an envelope in which there would either be a notice of dismissal or a request to present oneself for further examination. I failed at the first hurdle on the first attempt, and on the second went through all stages up to the final terrifying oral in which one faced not only the four Censors but the President of the College himself, in his robes of office. The strangest stories circulated among candidates about the out of the way, or ironic, or utterly bizarre questions that had been asked and might be asked. My toughest nut was a question about psittacosis, an infection then current which had been passed to mankind from parrots. All I knew about it was that it somewhat resembled typhoid fever. In the vaguest terms I dared I described, as the symptoms of psittacosis, the leading symptoms of typhoid. My questioner grumbled "Sounds rather like typhoid to me," but fortunately did not cross-examine me further.

After this, my ambitions revived somewhat and I determined to try to get to Queen Square. At that time there were three neurological hospitals in London, of which the National Hospital at Queen Square was sublime, the one at Maida Vale respectable, and the West End despised. The reason for the contempt in which it was held lay in the fact that, very sensibly, it had psychiatrists on its staff to help with the large numbers of psychiatric patients which, then as now, are attracted to neurological clinics; and a neurologist, who allows himself to associate with such borderline citizens, must be badly in need of a hospital appointment. In due course a vacancy for a house physician at Queen Square was advertised. I made my application, and went the rounds of the doors in Harley Street, Wimpole Street, and Queen Anne Street calling on the demigods who had my fate in their hands. My reception was every bit as forbidding as I could have feared. Both Kinnier Wilson and Gordon Holmes (names that were glittering with fame, in that little world) implied that it was really rather impudence on my part to be applying for such a wonderful job, and Gordon Holmes told me it was a senior appointment for which I was quite insufficiently prepared. However, I heard later that I had been a second choice when it came to the decision, the man who got the job having worked at Queen Square in a voluntary capacity for some months. I meant, then, to have another shot, and considered how I might prepare myself better for it.

Now, for the first time, it seemed to me that I ought to know something about psychiatry. Everyone knew that the neurologists drew most of their income from consulting on psychiatric patients, and it would be well then to have some understanding of them. I wrote to Edward Mapother and asked him whether he would be able to take me on at the Maudsley. This time the response was encouraging. He asked me to come over to see him, and at the end of the interview told me he would like to take me on but that there was no vacancy now or for some time to come. Looking through the advertisements in the *Lancet*, I next saw a vacancy for an Assistant Medical Officer at Derby County Mental Hospital, residence and £350 per annum. I applied for it, was summoned north (a hundred and thirty miles) for an interview with the assembled committee of the local authority and the medical superintendent, and was appointed. I had been the only applicant.

There now began an extraordinary interlude in my career. The hospital was shut off from the world in its own extensive grounds by a high stone wall, through which the main egress was by a great pair of iron gates, fronted by a weighbridge, at the side of a lodge. Foot-passengers went through the lodge; cars, vans and lorries through the gates which were specially opened for them. Now the great stone wall has disappeared, and the patients are made at home in villas instead of those long halls, lined by shuttered side-rooms, that housed them in my day.

Most of the patients who were allowed some liberty were restricted to ground parole, but there were a few who were allowed at times to go down to the village, and execute small commissions for fellow patients. The little world inside was governed by the medical superintendent, and the medical assistance, at the time I was there, consisted of the deputy medical superintendent whose wife practised as a general practitioner in the neighbourhood, an elderly bachelor "locum," and myself. It was difficult to find someone to make contact with, but I did get some human companionship from the dispenser.

The day's routine consisted of rising at 9.30, in time to put in an appearance at the superintendent's "office" at 9.45. Here we three doctors stood lounging in front of the desk, at which sat the superintendent, his clerk at his side, while the morning's mail was opened. Answers, mainly about patients to questions from their relatives, were dictated to the clerk, on information provided by the doctors. The affair was over by 10, when I went upstairs again to eat the breakfast still lying rather coldly on the table and read the paper. At 10.30 I would start on the morning round, which was confined to male chronic wards. The acute reception centre was looked after by the super himself, the female wards (notoriously more difficult than male wards as well as having a heavier case load) by the deputy and the locum. My round consisted in walking briskly from one ward to another, initialling a diet sheet put before me by the charge nurse, asking him whether there was anything else, and moving on. Sometimes an annual clinical note was required, and sometimes a statutory recertification. The annual note would be written by me, the charge nurse standing at my elbow telling me what to say: "He is very melancholic and depressed, sir, and believes his insides are being eaten up by lice. He is extremely dependent and devoid of initiative, and still in need of hospital care". The recertification was too responsible a job for a beginner, and the patient would be sent to the office for one of the two seniors to do it. There were also periodical physical examinations, and the visit of the ward for the sick and bedridden. The whole thing, though it involved perhaps three quarters of a mile of walking, would be over by 11.30 to 11.45, when would come my visit to the hospital dispensary, a cup of coffee, and a gossip with the dispenser. On four afternoons a week I would be off duty, and so able to take a bus into Derby, where my principal errand was to go to the Boots lending library and change my book. The two half-days on which I was on duty, most of the time would be spent, when the season advanced, in playing tennis. Two week-ends out of three I was off, and would have been able to go away on a visit, if Derby had not been, as it seemed to me, lost in the unknown northern parts of the country, and an unmanageable sum in travel money from the genial south.

It could not be said that the clinical work demanded of a junior psychiatrist in the chronic wards was of a stimulating or educative kind. There was nothing that one could do for the chronic patients; and when from time to time, in the course of writing the required six-monthly notes, I settled down to a talk with the patient, and found that he was much saner, happier and healthier than one might gather from his records, my efforts to get him considered for discharge were not well received. My seniors relied in the main on a security argument; the man might seem to have recovered, but underneath he would show some residuum of his old illness, let us say a lingering belief in the reality of delusional experiences of the past, or a degree of emotional lability and a liability to get down-hearted. Such men were not safe.

Practically always, of course, the relatives of these patients had long reconstituted their family lives without him and would not be over-enthusiastic about his return. In quite a few cases, the patient himself had become happily adapted to hospital life. I remember particularly the groundsman who loved the cricket pitch as if it had been his own lawn, and though long since recovered from a single attack of an affective psychosis, was reluctant to face the insecurities of the outside world.

In due course, another vacancy for a house physician at the National Hospital was advertised, and I applied. I might have spared my effort. It was for nothing that I invested in a short black jacket and waistcoat and pinstripe trousers, came up to London, and went from door to door in the Harley Street area. I had touched pitch and had now become defiled. I imagine that I was quite written off, and did not receive even that degree of consideration which had met my first application.

My position now was extremely discouraging. I could not bear the life I was leading, and I even thought of applying for a post as a ship's doctor, in order to see some of the world before I settled down to whatever fate I should have to meet in the end. However, even in my state then, I could not voluntarily enter such a blind alley as that. I had heard nothing from Mapother, but clearly could lose nothing by writing to him again. I did so, and poured out my heart. Work in the mental hospital, I wrote, was completely stultifying. One was not even a doctor who could try to help his patients, but only a custodian. Any clinical discussion of the strange and ununderstandable case material was out of the question, since my colleagues were not interested. As for the possibility of research — !

This last point may have been made more because I knew that research work was highly regarded at the Maudsley than because I myself felt any strong spontaneous urge. In fact, I did not have the least idea what research was. None of my clinical teachers had been research workers and few, very few, had made any original contribution to medical knowledge. This instinctive appeal, however, did touch Mapother on a soft spot. He replied, almost by return, that there would be a vacancy for a locum to do holiday duty, if I liked to come south and try it, without any guarantee for the future. I remember still the last journey by train from Derby, on a Sunday evening in the beginning of October 1931, giving myself the treat of a dinner in the restaurant car, and hugging myself all the way with joy.

THE ROAD TO GENETICS

Life at the Maudsley was all and more than all that I could possibly have hoped. We were quite a small body of doctors, in order of seniority Thomas Tennent, the Deputy Medical Superintendent; Aubrey Lewis; Edward Anderson; Louis Minski; Mildred Creak; Desmond Curran; William Hubert; and another young man who died quite soon after of bacterial endocarditis. Those who were not married and wishing to go home for lunch, sat down to a long table with the principal lab workers. This was one of the places where the art of conversation flourished, and not always about shop. Nevertheless, a good deal of shop was talked, also at dinner if one stayed in for an evening on duty, and also over a rather prolonged coffee break in the mornings. The day's routine ran: 10 A.M. into the wards, 11.15 knock off for coffee, 12.00 back to the wards, 1 P.M. knock off for lunch, 2 to 4.15 back to the wards, 4.15 to 5 tea, 5 to 6.30 or even later once more in the wards; and it was not unknown for the enthusiastic to stay on for dinner and after it return once again to the ward if he was wanting to study in depth a more than usually interesting patient. Many as the breaks were in the day's routine, the time they took was not wasted. I certainly learnt from my fellow students, only a year or two more advanced along the road than I was myself, during those interminable, fascinatedly interesting discussions, as much as from text books and papers.

If most of us were keenly vocal, there can still be no disputing that Aubrey Lewis was the leading spirit. He had more than a touch of deviltry at this early stage in his career, and delighted in pulling the legs of anyone he could make a victim of. His supreme achievement in this line was to persuade a junior colleague that (despite his small and very slender physique) at one stage in his life, when practically down and out, he had earned his living as an all-in wrestler. Hardly less noteworthy was his successful persuasion of a whole lunch table that, when he had been working as an anthropologist in the Australian outback, he had lived in a settlement fortified with a zareba against the raids of the black pygmies who surrounded them. In the same spirit he would from time to time flabbergast us with his learning. I remember one lunchtime when the conversation drifted haphazardly from one theme to another till it ended up with Queen Elizabeth, Mary Queen of Scots, and the complicated intrigues of their conflict. Lewis came out with fascinating items of history, and dazzled us with a breadth of knowledge and a grasp of recondite items of detail that might have done credit to an earnest student of the period. That, in fact, was what for a few short days he had actually been. At the very time of that conversation there was lying on the table of one of the residents' sitting rooms a library copy of a contemporary work on the subject. Edward Anderson, Lewis's fellow resident, who himself had been reading the same book, sat all the way through that lunch hour, never by a blink giving his colleague away. The same whimsical spirit led to a test of olfactory powers to which he subjected the rest of us. In half a dozen small phials he had a few drops of faintly discoloured water, one of them carrying a very faint smell of, say, lavender. We were asked to identify them, and it was left open to us to suggest to ourselves any odour we might care to think of. The test was, in fact, one of suggestibility. While some of us, in another environment, might have resented such an intrusion into our human failings, at the Maudsley we became trained to accept the role of S as well as E, and bear as well as we might the penetrating regard of those brown and beady eyes.

Lewis was an adept in the art of disputation, and there were very few who could stand up to him. Bill Hubert was one of these few — a man of consummate fantasy, cheated of his normal career at the Maudsley by his failure to pass a higher examination, this itself being caused by landing himself with a never terminated training analysis at the hands of a lay analyst who later became psychotic. He was a genuine eccentric, who tried to do all too much with his life, psychiatry, and psychoanalysis, and marriage and children, and a very active bohemian social life on the fringe between artistic Chelsea and the "bright young things" of the social world of the glossies. His final end as a drug addict was one of dreadful tragedy. At the time at which I knew him he was finding it difficult to make ends meet (and, for instance, wore spats to cover up the fact that he had no socks), but was full of an abundant life and humour. He could keep Lewis in play by producing some bizarre quirk of fantasy at the critical moment of a keen debate, after which Lewis would dash with the enthusiasm of a hound at the doubling of a hare. My own fortune with Lewis was somewhat different. Though he was at times most stimulating, he exasperated me by his keenness to exact a precise definition of terms used as counters, by his deliberate mistaking my meaning to show the falsity of what I had actually said (rather than listening to what I had tried to say); this unprogressive toing and froing over the same bit of territory had the aim of defeating you in formal terms rather than advancing to a higher level of understanding. In debate with him I would become more and more excited. Automatically, my hand would reach into my pocket where I kept the medical officer's massive keys, in my case tied to a length of stout cord. These I would play with and swing as a pendulum to and fro. Eventually at the top of my excitement, when the keys were whirling round my head or whizzing through the air in a vertical circle at my side and threatening to fly off at high speed in an unpredictable direction, Lewis would begin to blench, to lose the current of his thought, to hesitate in utterance, and perhaps abandon the topic.

Though an immensely hard-working man, Lewis was not very productive. His creativity was in due course to be shown in the organisational field, and the present Institute of Psychiatry at the Maudsley Hospital is largely his creation. At that time (1932), his contribution to our thinking about psychiatry was essentially in giving us much needed criticism. He gave me to read his own thesis for a doctorate in the University of Adelaide, on the subject of melancholia, in two parts, one historical and one clinical. This has since become a classic and has been influential, I think, in a retrograde way. Needless to say when I read it as a newcomer to psychiatry I was immensely impressed and, in fact, devoured it. At the end I could not but feel a sense of disappointment; it seemed to me indeed that it did not end. He asked me what I thought. I told him how persuasive, how convincing I had found his arguments, and could quite see all the faults, the inconsistencies and insufficiencies of all the aetiological theories advanced by earlier psychiatrists. But I had found myself at a loss to see what his own theory was. He told me rather shortly that with such an abundance of theories in the field it was not necessary to find a new one or adopt one of the old. In course of time I came to consider this unwillingness to take a positive line, whether it arose from a reluctance to meet those critical weapons which he himself wielded with such skill, or merely from a lack of personal need to identify himself with a point of view, as a fault of character which was his greatest weakness as a scientific worker. The sceptical approach to psychiatry is not enough.

However, in those days it was a wonderful aid to teaching. Lewis organised fortnightly evening meetings in his sitting-room, where one of us would produce an essay based on some personal work. Quite early on it was my turn, and I had not the slightest idea what to tackle as a theme. Lewis offered me a subject – hypnagogic hallucinations. I should read up what I could about the subject, and should think how I could investigate it clinically. I did so. For some weeks, as my turn to talk approached, I talked to the Maudsley outpatients, asking them whether they ever had such experiences, and what their attitude to them was. Many did, and the numbers had to be correlated with age and sex and educational background, intelligence and capacities for visual imagery, diagnosis, time relations to illness, etc. I am sure my report was not a good one, but it provided a good deal of new matter to the group, and it was essential discipline for me. This was Lewis's greatest contribution: teaching us to define our operational terms, to define problems so that they would be subject to empirical attack, to consider the tools necessary for such an attack, to proceed in an orderly and purposeful way. In clinical psychiatry we were taught to examine our patients, to look and listen and record accurately and without presuppositions, to resist interpretations that were not based on observational data. Although Lewis had received training at the hands of Adolf Meyer, much of what he passed on to us came from his earlier apprentice experiences in Heidelberg.

In this benign environment I developed fast. Lewis suggested that I might like to attempt a parallel investigation of the incidence of mental disorders in Britain to complement and to contrast with the several studies which had already emerged from the Munich school. As a way of sampling the general population, arrangements were made for me to be able to visit the surgical wards of King's College Hospital, and ask the patients there about nervous and mental disorder in their first degree relatives. I soon discovered the disadvantages of this approach. To begin with, the sample was not an unbiased one. It was quite clear that a proportion of the patients had been admitted in part for psychiatric reasons; for example, patients there for the removal of a "chronic appendix" were rarely suffering the effects of any local pathology. The sample was unsatisfactory in age distribution, the propositi peaked in middle age and their children were not yet into the ages of greatest psychiatric risk. The information obtained was not only incomplete from ignorance or reluctance on the part of the informants, but was probably also both unreliable and biased by unwillingness to admit psychiatric morbidity. The informants were not a captive group, and I had no lever to use to extract information. I did not take very long to reach the conclusion that some other way of approach was necessary.

I enquired whether the national statistics kept by the Board of Control might be made available. Mapother and Lewis received this request with understanding, and the necessary official contacts and consents were obtained. Now figures were made available to me which lacked nothing in objectivity and precision; the one big trouble was the antiquated diagnostic classification in which they were arranged. Another problem was the way in which risks from year to year and from age group to age group could be cumulated to give a life-time risk. At this, I had the temerity to write to R. A. Fisher to ask for his help. He gave it at once, and in a completely satisfying way; and it was in his journal that my paper was eventually published. Fisher helped me on many occasions, in investigations I carried out in later years, and never grudged time or trouble. I came to have for him the greatest admiration and a strong affection.

Looking back, it is interesting that after giving me a method of approach, Fisher did not trouble to see that I carried it out as exactly as I should have; and he accepted for publication two papers with logical errors. One of them was this paper about incidence. The risk of admission to a mental hospital was, as I worked it out, about 5 per cent by the end of a life time. This probability of 0.05 was the result of accumulating much smaller risks over a total of, say, fifty years. These year to year probabilities should have been turned into probabilities of survival from year to year without admission to hospital, and these survival probabilities multiplied together to give a total chance of escaping admission. What I did was to arithmetically sum each of these small probabilities; this was quite incorrect but probably made no difference of any magnitude, and Fisher let me get away with it.

Life was now something close to heaven. I liked psychiatry, I loved playing with numbers, and I revelled in the give and take, even the cut and thrust, of intellectual interchange. I was determined to stay at the Maudsley, and was prepared to go through some long and extremely impecunious months that winter when my holiday locum job ran out and I had to hang around as an unpaid voluntary worker, waiting for the vacancy for an additional medical officer caused by the opening of the "Villa," a small block in the Hospital garden for the nursing of disturbed and noisy patients.[2] I had taken a half share in a flat with an old school friend, and had begun

---

[2] Methods of treatment in those days were extremely limited. Apart from such standby drugs as paraldehyde, the main nursing treatment was by keeping the patient continuously in a luke-warm bath. The din and the antics and the cascades of water that one might meet on the morning

to enjoy the social life available in London to a young man, provided he had enough to live on. This I had, once my position at the Maudsley was stabilised. Above all things the Maudsley was a "happy ship" and the team spirit was tremendous.

Nothing was wanting to make for strong loyalties. Regarded by medical colleagues in the better established specialties and general medicine with a good deal of derision, we had to face on the other side a variety of unorthodox practitioners that shaded off into quackery. Our institutional enemy (how absurd it seems now!) was the Tavistock Clinic whose workers, as we saw it, had abandoned the scientific approach entirely for a system of therapy derived from dogma and applied intuitively. With these therapists, led by J. R. Rees and Ronnie Hargreaves, interpretations of the patient's behaviour would be made without basis in close clinical observation, and theories would be applied which had never been tested in open-ended enquiry. Our champion was Edward Mapother, and he it was who led us against the heathen. If the enemy had captured the Medical Section of the British Psychological Society, we had a firm grip on the Psychiatric Section of the Royal Society of Medicine. Neither group paid any attention to the effete and recumbent Royal Medico-Psychological Association, which was regarded as just a club for medical superintendents!

I do not think there was one of us who came under his influence who did not develop a passionate loyalty to Mapother. He was a man of great vision but at times incredibly wrong-headed. Life under him was not easy. Not more than one of us was allowed to go away on holiday at the same time, so that juniors found themselves taking their holidays at very odd times in the year. Doctors off duty at public holiday weekends had to return for half an hour in the afternoon to meet any relatives of their patients who might want to see them. Men who came to the Maudsley accustomed to handle even dangerous emergencies in previous house appointments found themselves deprived of the discretion to take the simplest measures without the approval of a senior. An intensely anxious man, Mapother could never have enough security. One of his whims was that the two hospital residents must be the two most senior, and not the two most junior, of the unmarried medical staff. When in the course of time I attained the seniority to be dragged from my delightful flat in the West End to a hospital bedroom and sitting room in the purlieus of Camberwell in south-east London, I resented it very keenly. This was a fate that would presumably continue as long as I was unmarried, and I could find my way from one prison only by entering another.

During those years there was one cloud that overshadowed all lives, mine as well as everyone else's. For the first time, and very much against the grain, we were being forced to think about politics. In the continent of Europe, unspeakable men had seized the levers of power in nation after nation, and the reaction of our own statesmen was to pay lip service to the collective security which, enthusiastically and realistically sought, would have given us the peace and security which they sought to buy by accommodations with the devil.

The Germans in their mass hysteria began to expel the Jews. With characteristic liberality and vision, Mapother secured from the Rockefeller Foundation grants to support three of the most distinguished fugitives from oppression, Eric Guttmann,

round added some light relief to the predominantly depressing task of trying to treat illnesses that obstinately responded only to their own occult intrinsic laws. The preoccupation with exact observation and description was also, of course, in part a method of preserving one's own equipoise when surrounded by such hopelessness.

Willi Mayer-Gross, and Alfred Meyer. Guttmann and Mayer-Gross were the clinicians, and the new insights into the reach of clinical observation and the application
to concept building, diagnosis, and systematics which they brought with them were
to some of us, to me at least, like a view into a new world.

The Rockefeller Foundation had for long been generous to the Maudsley in
other ways. Every year one travelling fellowship was made available to us, and
Mapother's nomination (made always, I think, on Lewis's advice) was all that was
required. Just as my turn had come for slavery as a resident, so now came my
opportunity. I remember a discussion with Lewis about what my plan should be.
Very sensibly he was against sending yet another man to study everyday psychiatry
at the feet of Adolf Meyer. As he saw it, the clinician of the future who would hope
to make a personal contribution to the advance of knowledge should have a training
in another specialised field of enquiry which might serve psychiatry. There were, he
thought, two fields that came in question, neuropathology and genetics. To which
did I feel the greater attraction? There was no hesitation in my answer.

I think they were rather disappointed, when I arrived that autumn of 1934 in
Professor Rüdin's genealogical department of the *Forschungsanstalt für Psychiatrie*
in Munich, to find that my command of spoken German was so poor when my
letters from England had been not only faultless but even stylish. Of course it was
my German friends, mainly Eric Guttmann,[3] who had aided and corrected my
German, and they were not here now to help me. However, everyone was pleasant
enough, and I was assigned to the care of Bruno Schulz, who would see that the
facilities were made available for my proposed study into the genetics of manic-
depressive disorder and would supervise my work. Bruno Schulz was not impressive
to meet, but a delight to have the privilege of knowing. He was a tubby little man,
his cheek bearing the scars of German-style fencing, with a great fondness for
Munich lager, the wines of the Rhine and Pfalz, and evenings out with the colleagues
from the department. From my point of view he was perfect, warm, friendly,
endlessly helpful, acutely intelligent, hard-working, with a fine sense of research
discipline. These were the days before anyone thought of double-blind diagnoses,
and the only way to scientific integrity was to set the standards of evidence for a
firm diagnosis, and for a "probable" diagnosis, and try to abide by them consistently, even when one saw the evidence going against the working hypothesis.
Schulz's political integrity was the equal of his scientific honesty. He could not
stand the Nazi ideology and never compromised with it. This meant that there could
be no future for him other than static continuance in the job he held, where no one
would be likely to call on him for declarations of loyalty to the regime he detested.
It was not until after the war, when he had only a few years to live, that the
University gave him the titular rank of Professor. In fact, in that one job in Munich
he stayed till the end of his days.

Life in Munich was very strange. Schulz told me when I first appeared that he
would not recommend me to arrive at the Institute before a quarter to eight in the
morning, as up till that time the cleaners might still be about in the rooms. I was
aghast, since in the Maudsley I was not accustomed to starting work before ten
o'clock. I compromised with arriving at work by about a quarter past nine, and my
recollection tells me, perhaps untruly, that I succeeded in keeping to about that time

[3] Eric's kindness and patience were endless. He it was who touched up all the German papers I
wrote about this stage in my career.

fairly consistently. Nevertheless, in the first few weeks it seemed very early, and breakfast, consisting of a couple of rolls, butter, honey and a cup of very weak coffee as provided in my "pension" or boarding house, had also to be taken in the chill of the early morning. On my first morning I was feeling hungry by ten, famished by eleven, and in increasing danger of fainting with inanition as the hours of twelve, one and two succeeded one another. I had been told that I would be collected for lunch, and I wondered what on earth could have happened. However, at last, about half past two, Schulz did appear to conduct me upstairs to the "casino," a spacious room with great windows looking over the fields, where lunch was taken. This was cooked on the spot in the adjoining little kitchen by a Fräulein who served us schnitzels sizzling straight from the pan, *Kartoffelsalat* and, in fact, top quality home cooking. On the walls were pictures by Leonid Pasternak (father of the poet Boris), which had been lent by his daughter, Lydia, who was at that time working in the Institute as a research chemist. This was the lady I eventually married. Other research workers also drifted in as they finished the main part of the day's work, among them the Scheid brothers and Karl Stern. Karl eventually went to Canada to a chair in psychiatry, and in his book, *The Pillar of Fire*, he has given an account of life in the Institute at that time. Franz Kallmann was at the Institute for about a fortnight while I was there, getting help from Schulz in the statistical analysis of his great Berlin material which went into *The Genetics of Schizophrenia*. When I arrived, the Institute was full of talk of the engaging personality of the Swedish research fellow who had preceded me and had only just left, Erik Essen-Möller, a man with whom I was eventually to develop the warmest friendship.

We did not see very much of Professor Rüdin, our departmental head. In fact, apart from my original reception, I can remember meeting him in any kind of social interchange only on a single occasion — the day, once a year, when the members of the department were invited to dinner in his home. We all arrived by arrangement together, one of our number carrying a large bouquet of flowers to be presented with a "Küss' die Hand, gnädige Frau" to the Frau Professor when she graciously received us. The dinner and the evening's conversation which followed were fitting to the somewhat ceremonial nature of the occasion.

If I had known that one day I should be working with twins, I should have paid more attention to Conrad. He was a man of exceptional ability, and his twin investigation into the genetics of epilepsy was methodologically by far the most advanced piece of twin work of its age. In many ways it has still not been equalled, and it is now most unworthily neglected. Conrad was an Austrian, and like a number of Austrians who were working about the *Forschungsanstalt*, an enthusiastic Nazi. For these expatriates Hitler represented a great hope for the future, when all Germanic peoples would be united. This it was that made it difficult for me to get to know him. His after-history was a sad one. In the end he became disgusted with what demagogy had made of genetics, and he abandoned the subject for good. In the chair of psychiatry in Homburg, Saar, he turned his mind to the application of Gestalt theory to phenomenological and clinical analysis. Those who have studied his work have found it highly original and interesting; but it was in a field into which I could never penetrate. Here, too, he has not received the appreciation he has deserved.

To the Scheid brothers I was especially indebted for a thorough-going discussion of all my basic psychiatric concepts. What I brought to Germany from the Maudsley was a very loosely conceptualised and articulated psychiatric framework, mainly derived from Adolf Meyer's teaching which had been taken over by all the British teachers including David Henderson, R. D. Gillespie, Edward Mapother, Aubrey Lewis, and Desmond Curran. It did not prove strong enough to stand up to dissection at the hands of K. F. Scheid, and bit by bit it was replaced by something much closer to the teaching of Kurt Schneider, who was the Institute's Professor of (clinical) Psychiatry. This proved a very much firmer basis on which to build an approach to the genetical aspects of psychiatry, but of course it has had its disadvantages. It always predisposed me to think that the distinctions we draw in our theories correspond to equally certain distinguishable "phenomenal appearances." It should be perfectly possible, for instance, to distinguish clinically between an "endogenous" and a "symptomatic" schizophrenia, something which I have been later led to doubt; and it strengthened a tendency to ascribe insufficient importance to psychological and social causes of variation in the life histories of individuals. Nevertheless, every scientific worker has to work out his own scheme of things entire by which to guide himself, and all such schemes must have faults. One does well to choose a scheme which offers adequate ways of trying to understand the phenomena with which one is concerned, and to remember always that it may be wrong in ways not yet to be recognised which may be fatal.

By Christmas time I was desperately homesick for England; but after a fortnight's leave returned to Germany and was not affected in that way again. This was despite the fact that the shadow of the Nazi Goliath was beginning to dim the light in the research institute. As the year wore on, guest workers in uniform began to appear, and imperceptibly "Grüss' Gott" came to be less heard than "Heil Hitler." By the time I had come back from a few months of travel towards the end of my fellowship, the old way of life had gone, the casino was invaded by brown-shirted "scientists," and the Jewish pictures had been taken down from the walls. My last day there Theo Lang (known for his studies of the sex ratio in the sibs of male homosexuals) took me into the lift for a talk, and kept it moving from the top of the building to the bottom so as to be sure of speaking without being overheard.

I wanted to see something more of Europe during my year, and applied to the Rockefeller Foundation for permission to visit Zurich and Vienna. This resulted in a lunch with the Rockefeller Foundation European representative, on his next visit, to check whether such expenditure could be allowed. Dr. O'Brien seemed rather doubtful of this, and thought that some further opinions were called for. I was accordingly instructed to take leave and given my expenses to visit experts in Scandinavia for their advice. No doubt the journeys involved seemed trifling to an American, but they were vast, romantic, and exciting to me. I went to see Jens Christian Smith (author of valuable genetical studies in mental subnormality and atypical psychoses) in Roskilde near Copenhagen; Professor Tage Kemp who was then building up from its foundations the *Domus Biologiae Hereditariae Humanae Universitatis Hafniensis*, which housed the national registration centre for hereditary defects in Copenhagen; and in Sweden Torsten Sjögren and other psychiatric workers at Gothenberg, Dahlberg at Uppsala and Essen-Möller at Lund. I did not meet Erik Strömgren at this time, although I did on many occasions after the war. Although temperamentally I think we are very different, in our intellectual approach we share much in common; in one bit of statistical methodology we both hit on the same idea independently.

This was a wonderful trip. Apart from the delights of the journey and the wonders of strange lands, to cross the Nazi frontiers felt like coming out of an unventilated dark-room into the air. Above all, in meeting these immensely able and distinguished men, I had the feeling of being welcomed as a neophyte into a body of dedicated people searching for the truth along paths I felt myself capable of follow-ing.

The Scandinavian referees vindicated my desire to visit Zurich and Vienna,[4] and permission was given. Ironically enough, I got very little out of those visits. At Burghölzli, H. W. Maier was a capable but as far as I was concerned not an inspiring teacher. At Vienna, the greatest chance of getting some new ideas was given me when I attended the Professorial visit to the neurological-psychiatric clinic. Here all the bums and roughs and prostitutes and alcoholics who had been picked up by the police and thought in need of a psychiatric opinion were lined up on a bench, and very briefly interviewed for a decision on treatment and disposal. From that time, and also from my experience in an English "observation ward", it has always seemed that the case material that life itself throws up as a detritus on the psychiatric beach has much more instructive value for the young student than the carefully selected sample of "prognostically favourable cases" that came our way in the wards of the Maudsley Hospital.

At that time Sakel was working at the Vienna clinic and had been given facilities to treat a limited number of schizophrenics with his insulin coma therapy. I am sorry to record the fact that I regarded this pioneer effort, in due time to be the thin end of a wedge which broke a way through an impassable barrier, as so much absurdity. I thought to myself, the Viennese have done it once, with the senseless but successful malarial treatment of G.P.I., and they think they can pull off just such another wild shot.

If my own ideas for improving myself did not bear much fruit, I continued to benefit from the wiser advice of others. My Scandinavian friends had warmly recom-mended that I should have some training, even if time was available only for the slightest, in general genetics. As a result, when most of my work was done in Munich, I went to Berlin-Buch to the *Institut für Hirnforschung*, with the aid of a three-month extension to my year, to study genetics under Timoféeff-Ressovsky. Here I was trained in breeding Drosophila, in practical work at the bench, and in genetical theory by reading very widely under instruction, and in many conversa-tions with Timoféeff. Timoféeff was a typical Slav, genial in both the English and the German sense, and became in turn a greatly admired teacher, a loved friend, and eventually godfather to one of my sons. He was one of the earliest workers to explore gene interactions and to show that the manifest effects of a gene could be greatly modified by other non-specific genes, the "genotypic milieu." This was an idea that I carried away with me, and used it to show that with its help the intractable non-Mendelian proportions of affected and unaffected in psychiatric sibships could be reduced to some kind of order — all too easily, as the critics of monogenic theories would say.

---

[4] I also visited Frankfurt am Main and spent a couple of weeks in Kleist's clinic there, seeing also von Verschuer's research institute which was occupied with a large twin sample from the general population. A short visit to Prague was also fitted in, with tragic memories later: I did not see or hear again from the Dr. Sekla I met then until the Rome Genetics Congress of 1961. While in Berlin I visited Curtius, who was more of a neurological than a psychiatric geneticist. I also visited Kallmann in his large Berlin mental hospital, an occasion heavily overcast with tragedy. Shortly he would have to emigrate to no such settled and welcoming home as was offered to our Maudsley refugees, and of all his savings allowed to take with him only ten marks for himself, ten for his wife.

The end of that story was tragic. Timoféeff received an offer from the U.S.A. to go there to work, an offer attractive in every way except that it would mean uprooting his family and settling down in a new world, the language of which he only poorly understood. He was not a Jew, and so in no danger from the Nazis, but he was a man of liberal principles and should have heeded the warning they might have given — that from that detestable ideology evil must come. He preferred to stay in Berlin and, as I have heard, was in the fullness of time overrun by the Russian occupation. To the Russians he was suspect as an emigré, and later no doubt doubly so, after the disgrace of Vavilov, as an adherent of the condemned Darwinism-Mendelism. However, he and his family did survive, though he never reappeared as one of the leaders of thought in genetics.

At the end of 1935 I returned to England, bringing with me Lydia Pasternak who was now my fiancée; she stayed in my parents' house until we were married at Christmas time. It was not so long afterwards that her elderly parents gave up their home in Berlin and followed; and again not so very much later that her cousin Frederick Pasternak, who had married her sister Josephine, brought his family to England to make a new home there. It was a source of peculiar satisfaction to me to be showing what I thought of Nazi *Rassenhygiene* by marrying a Jewess, a member of an inferior race by their standards, a lady of the highest genetical aristocracy by mine.

It was always foreseen that, after the generous training I had been given, I should continue with research; and in due course I was given a personal research grant by the Medical Research Council to carry out an investigation based on psychiatric patients, born one of a pair of twins, and with the twin surviving into an age of psychiatric risk. For this research I was given leave from my appointment as an assistant medical officer of the Maudsley Hospital, and for two years spent my days at one or another of the London County Council's mental hospitals. This proved to be a valuable experience at the clinical level. Once again, as previously in Derbyshire, I was brought into contact with patients showing the effects of years of mental illness, but this time with a background of knowledge and experience, as well as with a number of fundamental questions in my mind, which gave me the attitude and some of the understanding which the experience needed. I also got to know a considerable number of psychiatric colleagues working in the slow moving and often melancholy world of the outlying mental hospital, and to appreciate their ambitions and frustrations. When I eventually got back to the Maudsley I often thought, in conversation with the luckier colleagues there, that work in chronic wards was a piece of training that every psychiatrist should have, and that without it a real picture of the long-term development of the psychoses could not be obtained.

At that stage in the investigation I had only a clerk to help me, who sat in the hospital office and sent off cards to relatives to ask whether the patient had been born a twin or no. I had to do all the field work myself; and going round and calling at people's homes was something new and difficult, which I never learned to like. In Munich I had indeed done a little of it; but there, the well trained population could be expected to present themselves at the research institute for interview if called on to do so by an official letter — an attitude different indeed from the one I met in the relatives of British schizophrenics.

During those years the shadow of the German armed colossus spread and deepened across Europe, which seemed to be sliding into a pit at its feet. For me the bottom of the pit was reached with the Munich agreement of 1938, when I felt my country was eternally disgraced. I was always glad and grateful that my father died before that compact with the devil was made, a death that also put an end to a long and debilitating illness. In fact, the deaths of both my parents have shown me death in the form of a friend and a deliverer, and since then I have ceased to feel, as I did in my youth, an uneasy sympathy with the poet's "Timor mortis conturbat me."

My personal grant from the M.R.C. ran out, and I returned to clinical duties at the Maudsley, trying to keep the investigation going in my spare hours. It was not so easy. As acting deputy medical superintendent I was asked to carry out functions for which I had no natural gift; and when it became necessary to make far-reaching plans for the welfare of hospital patients in the event of air-raids and for the emergency evacuation of the hospital, I felt this was something someone else would do much better. At my suggestion Mapother gave these duties into the capable hands of Aldwyn Stokes. The evacuation of my own family to Oxford took place in good time before the war, and the evacuation of the Maudsley Hospital was carried out the day before the declaration. The official view was that immediately after the outbreak of war there would be intensive air-raids on London, and that psychiatric casualties would be running up to tens of thousands a day; the civilian population, in fact, was expected to go half-mad. All our patients were sent home, or into outlying hospitals, and our medical and nursing staff divided into two teams, going severally into emergency hospitals at Sutton in Surrey and Mill Hill at the northern fringe of London. Lewis was to be "Clinical Director" at Mill Hill, and I at Sutton, these being clinical and research appointments rather than administrative ones. For the actual running of these hospitals, Mapother brought in Louis Minski and Walter Maclay, both of them ex-Maudsley men no longer on the staff. However, Lewis and I picked the two teams, turn by turn, like two captains on a children's playground, each of us using his own criteria of desirability. This resulted in two groups of doctors widely different from each other in team personality and team spirit. With our group at Sutton, under Minski we had an exceedingly happy ship, since he let us ward workers run our own affairs, but saw that we got what we needed administratively, and protected us against too much interference from the hierarchy of officials that towered above us, tier upon tier, to its apex at the War Cabinet.

The last morning of peace, a lovely Saturday morning in early autumn, saw the charabancs gathering in the drive in front of the Hospital and, watching them fill and drive off, Mapother in his wheel-chair, a man broken in health who had now himself pulled down the great structure he had built. The next morning I was one of a party sent from Sutton to pick up equipment left behind which could be rescued. And as we fetched and carried, through the sparkling blue air came the sound of the air-raid warning. War had been declared.

That was thirty years ago.

London, 1969.

I

ORIENTATION

EDITORS' COMMENTS: This section consists of three papers, spanning a period of 27 years. The main theme is the relationship between the biological, psycho-dynamic, and social approaches in psychiatry. In the first paper, the value of diagnosis and clinical observation is stressed. One of the features of Konrad Lorenz's work (Paper 3) that appealed to Slater was the careful observation of animal behavior; Slater believes that ethology has a considerable contribution to make to psychology. One thing we may learn from the ethologists is the means of controlling and channelling phylogenetically adapted instinctive behavior such as aggression. The longest paper in this section consists of the final chapter of Sargant and Slater's pioneering *Introduction to Physical Methods of Treatment in Psychiatry* which stresses the complementary nature of psychological and somatic methods. There is not the slightest need for those who are interested in genetics to take a nihilistic view of treatment. Dr. Sargant, in giving us permission to include this chapter, wrote to Slater: "It should include a note to the effect that this last chapter was written while the buzz bombs were flying overhead, and the roof was falling in on you. It is like one of Beethoven's symphonies, written as Napoleon was entering Vienna."(!)

1

AREAS OF INTERDOCTRINAL ACCEPTANCE:
A BIOLOGIST'S VIEW

The problem we are called on to consider is the major contemporary problem of psychiatry. There are dangers that psychiatrists may split into mutually irreconcilable schools, unable to understand each other's languages. We must build a synthesis; and although in our several parties we are working on separate parts of the building, we should be aware of the ground plan, in which space is allotted to the other fellow, whose work will eventually join up with ours. From this point of view, the detail of the other fellow's work will be of no great interest or importance to us, but the skeleton on which his superstructure is raised will be vitally important, as it will have to interlock with our own.

Looking at psychiatry from the organic point of view, which I take to include also the genetic viewpoint, I think that the modern organicist is fully aware of the limitations of his field and the insufficiency of his methods. He knows that his work must be complemented from other sides. He has discovered, for instance, that a particular genic mutation provides the predisposition for the disease we call Huntington's chorea, after the American discoverer who found it in certain families living on Long Island a century or so ago. But the geneticist is quite unable to say what it is that makes the condition appear early in life in some cases, while in others the onset is retarded to the presenium, why some people who are gene carriers never develop the condition at all, why in some cases the disorder leads to gross abnormalities of behaviour, sexual misdemeanors, and the like, while in others there is only a flat dementia. The organicist knows that there are some forms of depression which have a specific genetical basis; that in other cases what matters most is a structural lesion of the brain; and in yet others it is the psychodynamic causes which predominate. In any particular case his methods will probably be sufficient to elucidate only part of the story. The coordinated use of other technics will be needed to understand the

Originally published as "Areas of Interdoctrinal Acceptance: an Organicist Speaks," in *Integrating the Approaches to Mental Disease*, ed. H. D. Kruse (New York: Hoeber-Harper, 1957), pp. 41-43.

case in all its complexity. When we are called on to deal with the individual patient, we must try to decide how far causative factors of all these and many other kinds are involved. This brings me to the importance of diagnosis.

It is sometimes maintained (Lidz, 1952) that if organic disease of the brain is present, there is always a degree of intellectual defect. I do not believe this is true. Certainly many lobotomised patients show no degree of intellectual defect which can be detected clinically or measured psychometrically. Their predominant defects may be shown in the temperamental field, along lines which we are accustomed to classify as neurotic or psychopathic. There is no single psychological symptom, of which I am aware, which cannot be caused by an organic or by a psychodynamic factor. The deviation of personality in the direction of irritability and aggressiveness will be associated here with a train of frustrating circumstances, there with an old brain contusion, and in a third case with a temporal lobe epilepsy. But for purposes of prognosis and treatment it will be of paramount importance to decide whether or not there is an epilepsy, whether or not a history of a knock on the head meant that the patient has had a cerebral contusion, whether or not the frustrating circumstances, which can no doubt be found in his life, are to be regarded as the predominant cause. Our means of reaching such a decision will be provided by clinical tools, psychometric, physiological, psychosocial, and not least by the tools of descriptive psychiatry and the phenomenological approach which are today so much out of fashion.

Once we have allocated a patient to a particular diagnostic group, we do not pretend to ourselves that we know all we need to know about him. But we have simplified our problems. We have reached the point where certain lines of inquiry and certain practical procedures are in the center of our field of attention, and others have passed into the periphery, or have been left behind. If we discover that a mentally ill man, however adequate the psychodynamic factors which could explain his illness may be, has many cells in his cerebrospinal fluid, a positive Wassermann, and a paretic gold curve, then the first thing we shall do is to give him penicillin. Whether or not he is to have psychotherapy has become a secondary issue.

When we come to the problems of classification in psychiatry, the same concepts will continue to provide a useful guide. Causes of a particular kind are of greater frequency and importance in some conditions than in others. In the genetic field, this is particularly obvious. In my own investigations on twins (63), the genetic factor was found to be much more important in the schizophrenic psychoses than in the field of neurotic disturbances and behaviour disorders. In close agreement with the findings of Kallmann (1953), three out of every four pairs of uniovular twins were adjudged as concordant in respect to schizophrenia. But only one out of four were concordant in respect to neurosis. Among the schizophrenics, binovular twins were no more alike than one might expect ordinary sibs to be; in the neurotic group there were pairs of binovular twins who took very similar delinquent or aberrant paths despite large differences in intellectual and temperamental make-up, owing to the fact that they shared a bad environment and disturbed home life. This does not mean that in the schizophrenics the genetic factor was the only one that mattered; after all, one in four of those who had the necessary genetic equipment never fell ill and must have been protected from the environmental side. There were also often large differences in age of onset. In one uniovular pair, for instance, one twin started on a slow progressive hebephrenic deterioration at the age of sixteen, while the other fell ill with a more stormy paranoid psychosis at forty-nine, having, as far as we could tell, been quite normal until then. If we could discover what exactly were the environmental differences between two such individuals, we would be a long step toward finding reliable methods of treatment.

In the neurotic group it is easier to tell what are the decisive psychodynamic factors than in the psychotic group. Let me instance one pair, a uniovular pair of boys. They were of good intelligence, and in addition had some artistic abilities in painting, modeling, music, and writing. One of the two was of a slightly more passive but steadier personality, made nothing of his little talent, and settled down contentedly to the humdrum life of a commercial traveler. The other twin, the leader of the pair, was ill content with life as a city clerk, changed from job to job, but wrote stories and succeeded in selling some of them so as to make a worth-while addition to his income. He fell in with a Bohemian set and eventually married a girl who was even less emotionally stable than he was. There were frequent quarrels and threats of violence and of suicide; and eventually, on the part of our twin, a hysterical fugue which landed him in a psychiatric clinic. In such cases as this we see a chain reaction between constitution and environment which leads to a decisive departure from the normal. The causative factors are laid out, as if on a dissecting dish; genetic constitution, results of early environment and the psychological inter-twin relationship, and even sheer fortuitous accident in the form of the marriage lottery.

I hope I have said enough to show that, from the organic point of view, there are wide areas where we are ready for interdoctrinal acceptance. I do not anticipate that there is cause for any very hot disputes between the organic and the psychometric schools. What I am hoping for is that those who approach psychiatry from the psychodynamic and the psychosocial angles will concede that we on the organic side have some glimmer of the light that illumines their paths, that we too can contribute something useful to the structure of psychiatric theory. A recent paper by Sandor Rado (1953), which I have had the privilege of reading in manuscript, gives me hope that that may be so.

2

THE RELATION OF PSYCHOLOGICAL
TO SOMATIC TREATMENT

In this book we have tried as far as possible to avoid theory and to deal in terms of empirically established facts, even if they were founded on clinical experience and not on the basis of planned experiment. If the reader has found the approach a mechanistic one, this will be because, in our view, both psychological and physical methods of treatment converge, and by different channels impinge upon the same processes, mechanisms and functions. The crude emotional shock of a revivalist meeting can be as disruptive of established functional patterns as that caused by the electric shock machine. Either psychological or physical methods or a combination of both may be used to produce these heightened emotional states in which suggestibility is increased, and old habits which have broken down may be re-established or new ones implanted. Under these circumstances it is often a matter of mere convenience which method one employs. An open-minded attitude on the part of the therapist will contribute towards that synthesis of view-points and practice for which we must hope.

It is not easy to delimit the roles to be played by the psychological and the somatic approach to treatment. The attitude taken by any psychiatrist to this problem will be determined by his views of the aetiology of nervous and mental illness. As we conceive it, it is not helpful to think of psychological events of any kind occurring without some physical or physicochemical change. On the other hand, any such change produces effects in the psychological field, which may be large enough to be observed. Individual differences which make one man particularly liable to the development of a conversion hysteria, another to an involutional depression, are primarily to be sought in differences of physiological, and therefore also psychological make-up. Such a view directs attention to the physical aspects of psychologi-

By William Sargant and Eliot Slater. Originally published as Chapter 12 in *An Introduction to Physical Methods of Treatment in Psychiatry* (Edinburgh: Livingstone; and Baltimore: Williams and Wilkins, 1st ed. 1944). Text given here is from 3rd ed., 1954, pp. 306-15.

cal changes as the point where a possible cause may be found, or, even if this is not so, where treatment may at times be most usefully applied. It is fair to point out that this view is not shared by all psychiatrists and that in what follows some will consider that the field of psychotherapy has been unduly restricted.

In the last twenty years [1934–54] we have seen a great change in the methods of psychiatric treatment. Before that time the malarial treatment of general paralysis was the only form of physical therapy that was more than symptomatic and expectant. Psychotherapy represented for the bulk of nervous and mental disorders the only approach that offered the possibility of a radical interference, and the hope of attacking actual causes. We have, however, now passed beyond the stage when the treatment of the mentally ill can be solely along psychological — or somatic — lines. On the one hand the last war [W.W. II] re-emphasised the incapacity of highly individual and time-consuming methods to deal with a large-scale problem. On the other hand, it brought out the importance of morale. Since then we have seen, therefore, the application of physical methods of treatment to the neuroses, and also the development of group methods of psychotherapy, by which considerable numbers of men may be handled together. In the graver psychiatric states, schizophrenia, depression, and the more recalcitrant and incapacitating forms of anxiety and obsessional neuroses, the development of somatic methods has been at the expense of psychotherapy. The former have shown their advantage in three essential qualities, speed, convenience, and certainty.

These are merely practical considerations. Of more fundamental importance has been a shifting of emphasis in our conception of the pathogenesis of mental disorder. Symptoms which were once thought to be psychogenic have now been found to rest on a deeper physical deviation. Dynamic interpretations of the development of a mental illness can be misleading even when they are plausible. What appears to be the psychologically precipitating cause is not infrequently the first indication that an attack has started. A careful examination of the earliest difficulties experienced by our patients before the gross onset of mental disorder will often show that they have only arisen because powers of adaptation were already in decline. The organic causation of apparently psychogenic symptoms is very easy to miss clinically. Only in recent years have physicians acquired sufficient knowledge to become suspicious of the neurotic symptoms of pre-clinical pellagra. Today we are probably still struggling along psychological lines with other organic illnesses, whose nature is unrecognized and whose appropriate treatment is unguessed.

Psychogenic interpretations do not lose their validity with the discovery of a physical aetiology; they merely lose in importance. Psychotherapists, however, have too often devoted the whole of their interest to the psychogenesis, and have too wholeheartedly linked with it their conception of the modifiability of the symptom. The discovery of a real or apparent psychogenesis may be an inadequate guide. The mechanisms by which symptoms develop are an attribute of the human make-up, and to show that they are at work is not to explain their appearance. It is not helpful for any medical purpose to find and demonstrate identical mechanisms in depressives, schizophrenics, and neurotics. The preoccupation with what is common to every one has obscured the significance of individual and class differences, and has sometimes led the psychotherapist into an undue faith in his powers to make of any man what he will.

It is not every one who is liable to neurotic symptoms under stress, even after physical deterioration has taken place. But if the patient is now showing a liability to psychogenic symptoms which was previously foreign to him, if there is evidence of a change of constitution, the suspicion arises that the alteration is based on a physical factor. Certain types of organic disorder seem to be particularly effective in producing neurotic symptoms, others much less so. Hysterical symptoms are common in disseminated sclerosis, rare in syringomyelia; they are common with lesions of the frontal and rare with lesions of the occipital cortex. Broadly speaking, interference with bodily well-being makes a man more, not less, liable to be disturbed by psychogenic stimuli. In the war neuroses, the psychological causes of anxiety and hysteria, till then relatively inoperative, began to have a greater effect when the man had lost severely in weight. The change in physique had altered his disposition and his ability to adapt. Head injuries illustrate the same phenomenon. Psychiatrists and neurologists are very apt to discover in the headaches of the post-concussive the operation of psychological factors, and to conclude therefore that the proper treatment is psychotherapeutic. The change that has escaped notice is that the psychogenic stimuli which now produce symptoms would not have been effective before the injury. The real disability is not a hysterical headache, but an increased susceptibility to hysteria; not the faints, attacks of giddiness, or ill temper, which are so clearly due to the circumstances of the moment, but the raised autonomic lability.

Similar changes of disposition are also common in early senility and cerebral arteriosclerosis. Syndromes of this kind are seen more frequently than their causes can be elucidated. In persons showing acute anxiety states, it is sometimes found that the symptoms are in part due to a recent increase in a fluctuating susceptibility to anxiety. But their aetiology remains obscure, and so far it has only been possible to link the menopausal anxiety state with an oestrin deficiency, and the premenstrual tension state with water retention by the body and glandular disturbance.

Genuine psychogenic symptoms are, of course, quite likely to occur in the course of organic or endogenous psychoses. As a rule they are transitory, and can frequently be neglected once their nature is recognized. They represent mere superficial manifestations and have little relation to the main current of change. Remedial treatment of the underlying process takes precedence, as the ordinary methods of dealing directly with such symptoms leaves the patient open to their recurrence. Nevertheless it may be difficult, and accordingly important, to reach an explanation for them. They may be the only visible sign, at least upon superficial enquiry, of a basically physical disorder, e.g. the neurasthenic symptoms of myxoedema or nicotinic acid deficiency. If they are misconstrued, valuable time may be lost.

When we are dealing, not with a change of disposition which has been produced by some specific cause or causes, but with a developmental anomaly, there are likely to be serious difficulties in the way of treatment by either psychological or physical means. But this is no reason for despair. One of the outstanding qualities of the chronic neurotic is a lack of general drive; some psychopathic people have an excess of energy which may lead, after the building up of tension, to an explosive outburst. These seem to be primitive biological qualities that may have comparatively simple physical correlates. No very great degree of advance, for instance in endocrinology, may perhaps present us with the means of directly influencing them. Methods of increasing or diminishing the instincts of hunger and sex will overcome many neurotic symptoms. Modified insulin treatment, by creating intense hunger in the hysteric, may make him eat in a few days, while months of analysis may be needed to achieve the same end by eliciting the psychological causes of a refusal to eat. The operation of prefrontal leucotomy does effectively alter the bodily and mental constitution; its disadvantages lie in the fact that it may do both more and less than we want. But the problems of psychotherapy of, for instance, an obsessional before and after leucotomy are quite different. A complicated psychological problem may sometimes be by-passed by a simpler and more direct physical approach. Psychotherapy would have a part to play in adapting the hypertensive patient to a necessary alteration in his mode of life. But if the hypertension is due to destruction by disease of one of his kidneys, while the other is still healthy, a surgical operation may render any re-adaptation superfluous. Unfortunately this is only rarely possible. If there were a means of raising the intelligence of the defective, special schools would no longer be needed. Until we can do so, this form of psychotherapy remains a necessity.

Although the possibilities of advance along these lines are important, they are still speculative. Physical treatment has established itself in the psychoses, and is becoming nearly as important in the neuroses. But the scope for psychotherapy remains enormous and will probably still expand. It will be long before constitutional peculiarities can be regulated or predetermined, and before the organic aspects of hysteria, anxiety and other psychopathic behaviour problems are cleared up. There will never be a time when there are not people at odds with themselves or their circumstances, and in need of the help of the trained psychotherapist. In the meanwhile patients must be helped to the best of our ability along whatever lines lie open, regardless of personal predilections. Where we cannot alter the constitution we must try to vary the environment, or the manner in which the environment is dealt with by the individual. The patient can never show the clarity of insight and impartiality of judgment that the physician can, and is often unaware that his symptoms are being caused by factors that lie within his power to alter. In other cases the effective causes of the illness may be clear for all to see, but the co-operation of the physician may be needed for effective action to be taken.

A psychogenic aetiology is not a *sine qua non* for successful psychotherapy. Even where the symptoms are springing from causes beyond our interference, and are themselves unalterable, much may be done to reduce their disabling effect. Psychotherapy does not consist merely of suggestion and re-education, but may involve a re-orientation of fundamental drives, and, when successful, bring about a far-reaching alteration of the patient's attitude to himself and to his environment. There are few patients who have found the best way of exploiting their positive advantages and of protecting themselves against their defects. Where some organic change has occurred, help in re-adaptation may be imperative. The patient who has undergone leucotomy is often much in need of psychotherapy, even though it be other than of an intensive or analytic kind.

To be effective psychotherapy, like other methods of treatment, must be realistic. It must set its goal within the compass of what is possible to the individual. Environmental circumstances are often very rigidly set and refractory to modification. What is possible for the intelligent may be out of the question for the dull. The mode of expression of temperamental tendencies may be alterable, while the tendencies themselves are beyond our reach. There is no evidence that psychotherapy will provide a personality with qualities it lacks, however frequently these qualities are shown by other persons. The best guide to a fair judgment of a man's capabilities is gained from his own past history, not from a comparison of his present state with that of the "normal" individual.

Furthermore, particular symptoms will be capable of treatment in certain settings, in others not. In certain settings they may demand treatment, in others not be worth bothering about. We have seen great pains taken to deal with the functional impotence of a middle-aged man, when it was merely the expression of a not very obvious depression. With attention to the underlying mood change the impotence could have been safely ignored. But in a young man whose marriage is being wrecked by a conditioned ejaculatio praecox, the emphasis might have to be the other way round, and treatment of the impotence regarded as the main method of attack on the associated depression as well. In such cases the very successful mechanotherapy devised by Loewenstein (1947) offers an almost perfect example of a physical method of psychotherapy. Providing the patient with a penile splint, so that, whatever the state of the tissues, coitus will be possible, gives him artificially a sense of security in which natural self-confidence can grow.

All methods of treatment involve interfering at some point in the vicious circle that keeps a conditioned response or behaviour pattern alive. Deep psychotherapy may be no more effective than simpler methods, somatic or psychological. Even where the intervention is at a superficial level, it may succeed in abrogating symptoms that follow primitive physiological paths. A girl student, the patient of one of our colleagues, suffered from hyperhidrosis of the hands whenever she sat in the lecture room with men students. It was so excessive that she could not write or touch a book. This symptom was dealt with by a few hypnotic sessions, and deeper conflicts were left for the time being. She was an intelligent girl, and solved most of her problems for herself without help. But the more ingrained a behavioural pattern becomes, the more likely it is that a physical method of treatment will be required to unseat it. Leucotomy may be necessary after years of illness in the chronic anxiety neurotic, who could have been cured by psychotherapy in the earliest stages.

The type of psychotherapy chosen must be balanced against the patient's constitutional disposition. The hysteric often dislikes going over his past failures and seeing himself exposed as the sport of his own make-up; or, on the contrary, he may delight in confessions of his weakness but with ironclad complacency defeat all attempts to alter his ways. Psychotherapeutic measures directed primarily towards increasing insight are likely to run up against the blank wall of obstinate self-deception. On the other hand, the hysteric is suggestible, and his suggestibility may be turned to account in procedures of another kind. The obsessional, intellectually over-scrupulous, will not accept the same crude suggestion and persuasion that are willingly absorbed by the hysteric; and though a more analytic approach will not make any difference to the given fact of his obsessional temperament, it will allow him to come to terms with himself, to adjust his life to his limitations, and to exploit his positive qualities, for instance, in types of work that appeal to his liking for detail and accuracy.

The main aim of a psychotherapeutic approach is to alter the attitude of the patient to himself and to his environment. But the aim of psychiatric therapy in the widest sense is to procure the optimal adjustment of the patient and his environment to one another. In the coordinated totality of treatment, therefore, psychotherapy has a defined but almost inevitable part. It should indeed precede, accompany, and terminate physical therapy, not only in psychiatric but all medical and surgical disorders. Psychological and somatic methods are not mutually exclusive, but should be made complementary to one another. The "bedside manner" and, for instance, the general medical handling of a case of gastric ulcer, involve the same psychological principles as the treatment of the neurotic individual. An interest in the personalities and lives of patients as human beings should be fostered in medical schools. To attend to the neurotic aspects of bodily disorders, which constantly face the physician and the surgeon, we do not need more psychiatrists. We need rather a wider diffusion of the psychiatric attitude and of psychiatric knowledge among the general medical public. Psychosomatic medicine will do itself no good if it takes yet more patients from a general medical attack. The failure to find a physical pathology for effort syndrome has turned the minds of workers to the psychological side; but this has in turn proved almost as barren of the possibility of therapeutic advance. An attack along physiological and constitutional lines has scarcely begun.

Religious teaching and inspiration have made many neurotics and psychopaths from burdens on their families into benefactors of mankind. The drive that is provided by a faith or an idea may be contrasted with that given by nature to the hyperthymic pyknic. The one is well-directed, but is liable to fail outside its own field; the other is capable of direction to almost any end, but is in danger of dissipation. A somatic approach is only capable of improving the instrument that is in our hands; psychotherapy may have something to say of the aim towards which it is directed. Both an efficient instrument and a worth-while aim are needed for a satisfactory life.

The main claim of the physical approach, that is the assumption that mental disorders are dependent on physiological changes, is that it is a useful working hypothesis. It has made great advances and looks like making more. It is in line with the main front of biological advance. It is here where psychiatry belongs. There is a tendency today to expand its field unduly, and for the psychiatrist to regard himself as a universal expert. Psychiatry is a young science, and in many fields where it is now being introduced it has more to learn than to teach. We should be more sure of the ground on which we daily tread before we venture too far afield. We are not the sole arbiters on the designing of a brave new world. It is our function as doctors to provide the health with which it may be fought for and enjoyed when won.

3

ON KONRAD LORENZ'S "ON AGGRESSION"

This is a very remarkable book. The author is famous as an expert on the behaviour of animals; he is also an extraordinarily gifted observer, and in prose which it is a pleasure to read (for which our gratitude goes also to his translator) he conveys a vivid picture of what he has seen in an underwater world and in the life of reptiles, mammals, and birds. In this book he expounds the insights he has derived from these observations, as penetrating as any which psychiatrists have based on the study of humankind. Distance and objectivity are combined with warmth and empathy. One finds to one's astonishment and delight how relevant an understanding of animal behaviour is to an understanding of man, and how many and how important are the lessons which one may derive from it. This particularly relates to the universal primary drive of aggression, perhaps the motivational field which in our own kind we understand least of all, with potentially the most dreadful consequences.

Lorenz contrasts intraspecific aggression with the aggression shown between members of different species; in animal economy the latter plays much the lesser role. By and large, members of different species can live contentedly together. Even when one species lives by preying on another, the relationship, though it is one of occasional hunting and killing, does not mobilize in the predator an aggressive mood; expression and behaviour are much nearer to those of aggression in the prey that turns at bay to defend itself. In general, members of different species do not compete in a struggle for survival; predator and prey live in equilibrium. What threatens a species is not its "enemies" but its competitors: the mammalian dingo has ousted the marsupial wolf from Australia.

On the other hand intraspecific aggression, the instinctive hostility that springs up, though perhaps only in narrowly definable circumstances, between two members

Originally published as a review of *On Aggression* by Konrad Lorenz, translated by Marjorie Latzke, with a foreword by Sir Julian Huxley (London: Methuen, 1966), in the *British Journal of Psychiatry* 113: 803-6 (1967).

of the same species, has an enormous role in nature's economy. Thus a stretch of coral reef, which harbours perhaps thousands of species living in amity, may be able to support one only of any given species of coral fish. Endowed with brilliant colours to warn the stranger off, the little fish attacks and tries to ram at its first appearance only a similarly coloured member of its own kind. One wonders how these creatures are able to mate. Some of them live permanently in pairs, and then the pair of mates is likely to be even more aggressive than single fish are. In other species at spawning time the fish lose their brilliant colours and become dull, permitting mutual approach. Colouring, aggressiveness, and sedentary territorial habits all go together. In such species intraspecific aggression plays a useful survival role; the territorial animal that drives off his rivals helps to spread them around the countryside and so helps towards a wider and a balanced distribution.

Lorenz demonstrates most convincingly that aggression is instinctive and wells up spontaneously; it is not primarily reactive, and for its appearance it does not depend finally on appropriate stimuli. Lorenz illustrates this principle by describing a common error of aquarium keepers who find, after putting a number of young fish into a large aquarium to give them a chance of pairing naturally, that when one couple have paired they become set on driving out all the others.

> Since these unfortunates cannot escape, they swim round nervously in the corners near the surface, their fins tattered, or, having been frightened out of their hiding places, they race wildly round the aquarium. The humane aquarium keeper, pitying not only the hunted fish but also the couple which, having perhaps spawned in the meanwhile, is anxious about its brood, removes the fugitives and leaves the couple in sole possession of the tank. Thinking he has done his duty, he ceases to worry about the aquarium and its contents for the time being, but after a few days he sees, to his horror, that the female is floating dead on the surface, torn to ribbons, while there is nothing more to be seen of the eggs and the young.

This error may be avoided by providing a tank big enough for two pairs and dividing it in half by a glass partition, putting a pair on each side.

> Then each fish can discharge its healthy anger on the neighbour of the same sex — it is nearly always male against male and female against female — and neither of them thinks of attacking its own mate. It may sound funny, but we were often made aware of a blurring of the partition, because of a growth of weed, by the fact that a cichlid male was starting to be rude to his wife. As soon as the partition separating the "apartments" was cleaned, there was at once a furious but inevitably harmless clash with the neighbours and the atmosphere was cleared inside each of the two compartments.

A general principle can be formulated, that the damming up of aggression will be the more dangerous the better the members of the group know, understand and like each other. The validity of this is appreciated by men living in isolation, e.g. in Arctic exploration.

Lorenz notes, somewhat sardonically, that this principle has been forgotten by educationists. "It was supposed that children would grow up less neurotic, better adapted to their social environment and less aggressive if they were spared all disappointments and indulged in every way. An American method of education, based on these surmises, only showed that the aggressive drive, like many other instincts, springs spontaneously from the inner human being, and the results of this method of upbringing were countless unbearably rude children who were anything but non-aggressive."

Social animals, who have to live together, have to find some way of surmounting the dangerous effects of intraspecific aggression, which still has its part to play (as in the solitary territorial animal) in securing advantages for survival. The fighting of rivals for a mate advances the selection of the strongest; parental aggression serves for the defence of the young against a careless or hungry neighbour, or against the predator; and within the society aggression leads to the working out of a ranking order on which peace depends. Lorenz has a warning for the youthful rebel and for those who tend to see only the evil side of the "Establishment," to the effect that without rank order every turn of the social machinery would grate against friction and resistance.

Species after species in the process of phylogenetic development have worked out their own ways of guiding aggression into harmless channels. Within the species the manifestations of aggression are ritualized; mock battles take the place of real ones; submissive gestures, perhaps based on infantile behaviour patterns, or on the soliciting behaviour patterns of the female, have at once an inhibiting effect on the aggressor. The gesture, as in the wolf who turns his unprotected throat towards the aggressor, may in effect put one animal completely at the mercy of the other. The more dangerous the animal is, the more effective and absolute are the prohibitions imposed by the appeasing gesture; and the most bloodthirsty predators have the most reliable killing inhibitions. It is unfortunately in the animals who are but weakly endowed with natural weapons of offence that these inhibitions are weakest. However, mankind, who can only with difficulty kill his fellow with his bare hands, has invented for himself tools to do so, and moreover ones which, by acting at a distance, have a much reduced effect in awaking such inhibition of a murderous attack as nature has given him.

Lorenz discusses the different means which have been taken by different species towards the aim of keeping intraspecific aggression within bounds. In some species of social animals aggression is reduced to a minimum; but then one finds that the flock is a very loose structure with little internal organization. The shoal of fishes has no structure at all. In general, the ethologist does not know of a single species which is capable of friendship and which lacks aggression. On the other hand, aggression may dominate intraspecific relationships too far when the inhibiting stimuli are confined to, say, the immediate group or clan. Rats are biologically an extremely successful species, tough, courageous, adaptable in their ways, and (one of the few species who can do so) able to pass on information from one generation to the next. But intraspecific aggression constitutes a major danger for them.

Rats living together recognize their common allegiance by smell, and the stranger rat who exhibits the wrong smell is attacked and destroyed as soon as he is recognized. When two clans of rats are living in proximity they are constantly at war; and such warfare must exert a huge selection pressure in the direction of ever-increasing ability to fight. A parallel in man is offered in Sydney Margolin's studies of Prairie Indians, particularly the Utes, who suffer from an excess of aggression drive which under the ordered social conditions of today in the North American Indian reservations they are unable to discharge. At one time Prairie Indians led a life almost entirely of war and raids, when selective pressures must have favoured an extreme aggressiveness. Ute Indians are said to suffer from neuroses more than any other human group, the cause of the trouble being undischarged aggression.

A section of the book, of a strangely attractive and indeed moving kind, is given to the phylogenetic processes which have mobilized the aggression drive into being the instinctual basis of the bond which unites animals by ties which, at the highest level, are those of love and friendship. A very detailed account is given of the triumph rite of geese, which forms the bond between members of the same family and also between the pair when a young male goose falls in love with a young female. Mistakes can be made, and then the triumph rite may unite by accident two males; despite the fact that copulatory attempts prove vain, their relationship becomes as close and as intense as the normal lifelong heterosexual one. The prestige of the male pair in the total society of geese is just as high as that of a married pair. Following on this, a female may fall in love with one of the males. With great patience and assiduity she may eventually seduce him into coitus, after which he immediately flies back to his partner to go through the triumph rite with him. Bit by bit the female may become the sexual partner of both males; and then there is happiness for all. No other couple in the flock can stand up to such a united trio; they are always at the top of the ranking order, they are never driven out of their nesting territories, and they are highly successful parents.

It does not seem to this reviewer that Lorenz goes beyond the support available from biological observations when he applies his theories to man. Human behaviour is not rational, but it is understandable as phylogenetically adapted instinctive behaviour. The nature of the laws which control such behaviour can be learned from studying animals. Present-day civilized man suffers from insufficient discharge of his aggressive drive. Lorenz considers that intraspecific selection is still working today in the direction of increasing aggressivity. Aggression is to be controlled by ritualizations and by redirected activity. Hitting the table instead of the other man's jaw, would be a simple example, and another more complex one is what Grzimek has called "bicycling"; the "bicyclist" is the man who bows to his superior and treads on his inferior. Every culture has its own ways of channelling aggression. Cultural rites and social norms are indispensable. It is highly dangerous to mix cultures. To kill a culture it is often sufficient to bring it into contact with another, particularly if the other is higher or has a higher prestige. In aping the "higher" culture, the people of the subdued side may lose an invaluable heritage.

On this basis, at the present time, with races and cultures in the melting-pot, we are facing grave dangers. Lorenz points to the coinciding factors which threaten the continuity of Western culture; diminishing cohesion of the family group, decreasing contact between the generations, the greatly diminished tolerance of the young for the values held in honour by their seniors.

What preventive measures can we take? A number are suggested: the ethological investigation of ways and possibilities of discharging aggression on substitute objects; the psychoanalytic study of sublimation; the encouragement of personal friendships between members of different ideologies or nations; the intelligent channelling of militant enthusiasm. Remedies doomed to failure would be any attempt to breed out aggression, the attempt to suppress it by moral vetoes, or to starve it by depriving it of appropriate stimuli. But a simple principle offers an apposite line of approach. Aggression can find complete satisfaction by the use of substitute objects, in fair fighting, in sport, and in dangerous undertakings. The race for space flight may be indeed an inestimable safety valve.

There are points in this book where one would wish to part company with the author. The reviewer, for instance, would demand more evidence before he would accept the view that in civilized societies aggressiveness, which may admittedly tend towards wordly success, tends also to a higher differential survival rate. Nevertheless, the unspoken claim that ethology has an enormous contribution to make to human psychology must be conceded. This book should be read by every clinical psychiatrist, and it should be a set book for the D.P.M. The student's task in reading it will be a most grateful one. It is full of magic, full of profound concepts and vivid illustrations, full of wisdom.

II

MANIC-DEPRESSIVE ILLNESS

EDITORS' COMMENTS: In 1934-35 Slater spent nine months at the Research Institute for Psychiatry in Munich, studying psychiatric genetics under Bruno Schulz. By means of personal interviews and research based on the records of the Institute, he studied three generations of manic-depressive families — a defined group of 315 probands with recurrent illnesses, their parents and their children.

On his return home, two papers (4, 5) were published in English on the provisional results of this study. The first of these, read at the Royal Society of Medicine, is given here in full as Paper 4. Although not the definitive version, it contains the most complete account of the material and methods and the most general discussion of the problems of the genetics of manic-depressive psychosis at that time. Editorial footnotes indicate in which respects the final report, translated from German and appearing here as Paper 5, differs materially from the provisional account.

4

THE INHERITANCE OF MANIC-DEPRESSIVE INSANITY: PROVISIONAL REPORT

Attempts are frequently made to base theories of the method of inheritance of psychiatric abnormalities on the statistics obtained from family investigations. For these theories to be worth consideration, it is necessary that the preliminary investigations should fulfil certain elementary requirements:

(1) In the gathering of the material there should be no process of selection that is not scientifically justified, and clearly understood and stated by the author. (2) The original material should be, as regards the character investigated, genetically uniform. (3) The numbers of relatives investigated should be sufficiently large to reduce the errors of random sampling within reasonable limits. (4) All persons covered by the terms of reference should be included, and exhaustive, up-to-date, and reliable information should be obtained about each and all of them. (5) The diagnosis of presence or absence of the character examined for should be sufficiently well founded to command general agreement among those qualified to judge. (6) The statistical working out should be free from objection.

Judged by these criteria there is no family investigation in psychiatry known to me that passes the test. Certain grave difficulties lie in the nature of the material itself. It is impossible to assure oneself of the genetic similarity of the material, but it is quite possible to attempt as close as possible a phenotypic similarity. Most authors do not take this nearly far enough. I may mention the many family investigations that have been made in schizophrenia, where practically no attempt has been made to attempt similarity of material. It is in the nature of work on human material, particularly in psychiatry, that exhaustive information about any one individual is really only to be obtained when he has been observed by experts over many years in a hospital. Anything less than this is only an approximation to what would be scientifically desirable. Nevertheless many authors are contented with much less information than would be available with more intensive work, and are

Originally published in the *Proceedings of the Royal Society of Medicine* 29: 981–90 (1936). Subtitle and headings added.

ready to publish figures on such a basis, with the implicit assumption that their material is complete. When one considers that in only a minority of cases is the investigator lucky enough to obtain what knowledge he can in a short interview, and that in the often great majority he is compelled to rely on secondhand information, one is in a position to appreciate how shaky are the "facts" on which the grandiose superstructure of psychiatric genetic theory has been built. These are what one might call the genetic difficulties. To them must be added the difficulties that arise from our lack of knowledge of what is fact and what is theory in psychiatry. Genetic investigations of twenty years ago would have included numbers of cases of "delusional insanity." This term has little meaning for us now. We have little right to assume that "schizophrenia," for instance, will have much more for our psychiatric descendants. Above all, we have little ground for supposing that the clinical entity, which is a matter of conception and convenience, and the supposed underlying genetic entity correspond. To all these difficulties, genetic and psychiatric, must be added the practical difficulties of the investigation itself, the necessity for the investigator to reach a diagnosis on inadequate material, the impossibility of excluding the influence of preconceptions on judgment, the highly inadequate and often frequently slipshod statistical methods so often employed. The criteria I have outlined above would be difficult to satisfy in their entirety, but much of the unsatisfactory character of family investigations in psychiatry hitherto is due to the investigators either having little idea that these requirements should be filled, or in any case making but a poor approach to their fulfilment.

PREVIOUS WORK

The present knowledge of the inheritance of manic-depressive insanity is based on the work of Rüdin (1923), Hoffmann (1921), Banse (1929), and on the work of Luxenburger (1932) summarizing and editing the data of others, including those of Entres and Röll (unpublished). The investigations of Rüdin have never been published, and cannot be criticized. The work of Hoffmann is especially important, because of the very heavy incidence of manic-depressive psychosis he gives for the children of manic-depressives. Judged, however, by the criteria I have suggested above, his work fails to satisfy one of them. There is no sign that Hoffmann made any attempt to secure uniformity of material; his numbers are small and unsatisfactory for statistical working out; not more than one member of the family was seen in any case; the amount of information obtained, at least that which he prints, is very inadequate; above all, his diagnosis of manic-depressive insanity among the children he investigated is such as to command general disagreement. Apparently led by a Kretschmerian psychiatry, he includes among manic-depressives all persons in any way subject to swings of mood, however socially well adapted and unremarkable they may be, and he includes among slighter degrees of hypomanic and depressive temperaments such persons as he describes as "quiet humorists." It is possible that such people as quiet humorists are found more frequently among the relatives of manic-depressives than in the general population; this remains to be proved; but it gives no right to rank them with persons showing well-marked cyclic character traits as carriers of manic-depressive hereditary elements. The very heavy incidence of manic-depressive insanity among the children of manic-depressives found by Hoffmann seems to me to be largely explained by his tendency to exaggerate normals into abnormals, and mild character deviations into psychoses. The most cogent criticisms on psychiatric grounds have already been made on Hoffmann's work by

44

Wilmanns (1922) and Mayer-Gross (1925), and I will not go into the matter further. Finally, Hoffmann did not attempt any adequate statistical evaluation of his material, and though Luxenburger has subsequently attempted to treat his figures so as to make them comparable with the figures obtained by others, I do not think that Hoffmann's material can stand the strain.

Banse's work on the cousins of manic-depressives is free from the psychiatric objections to which Hoffmann's work is open, but is of dubious statistical value. Banse admits that among the 1,586 cousins he includes in his material he obtained personal information about less than two-fifths; data about the rest were obtained from the use of records, family trees collected in previous years, odd facts jotted down in the case records, etc. This limits the value of his work very much. Luxenburger collates his work with that of Hoffmann, Rüdin, and other workers in the following table:

TABLE 4.1. INCIDENCE OF MANIC-DEPRESSIVE INSANITY AMONG RELATIVES OF MANIC DEPRESSIVES (AFTER LUXENBURGER, 1932)

Relationship	Number of persons investigated	Percentage of manic-depressive psychosis
Children	165	30.2
Nephews and nieces	452	2.6
Cousins	867	2.7
Brothers and sisters	263	12.6
Parents	170	10.6
Uncles and aunts	559	4.8

PRESENT MATERIAL

The investigation that forms the basis of this paper was carried out at the *Deutsche Forschungsanstalt für Psychiatrie* in Munich, with the kind permission of Professor Rudin, who placed the resources of his institute at my disposal. I should first like to pay a tribute to the magnificent organization of this research institute, without which it would have been unthinkable for a foreigner to attempt such an investigation in a strange land. Summaries of all the cases admitted to Kraepelin's clinic in Munich between the years of 1904 and 1922 are kept on file at the psychiatric research institute. Of these records some 3,000 referred to cases diagnosed as manic-depressive. I read through these records and selected cases which fulfilled certain conditions. It was my hope at that time to investigate that group of manic-depressives who show in the appearance and remission of illness a certain ordered rhythm. There seemed to be a possibility that these persons might show peculiar relations in the matter of heredity. Unfortunately, though there were such cases, they were extremely few in number, and insufficient for statistical work. Accordingly I was reduced to selecting any cases which showed some degree of phasic recurrence, the conditions at last decided on being that they had had at least either one clear manic and one depressive attack, or three separate depressive or manic illnesses. I neglected all cases in which the first illness had appeared in the fiftieth year or subsequently, so as to eliminate the dubious involutional and arteriosclerotic cases. About half-way through the investigation, a few more cases filling my conditions were obtained from Eglfing, the Munich mental hospital. Of such cases I collected, in the end, 315, of whom 114 proved to be childless. The relatives of the remainder were then written to, and I saw as many of the children of the original case in every family as I could. Of the 201 families with children I was able in 41

45

cases to get no direct information from any member of the family. Although in one or two of these cases this was due to every member of the family having died, and in others very complete information was available on file at the institute, I have thought it better to exclude them all from my statistics about the children. In the remaining 161 families I obtained information from 157 personal interviews and 62 written communications (in 172 cases from children and in 47 from other members of the family). In most instances these interviews and letters served to complete the very extensive information already in possession of the institute. For information about parents I have not restricted myself to these personally investigated cases, as the documentary evidence was already complete, and could in any case be but little supplemented by information from grandchildren.

I have, however, subjected my material to other processes of selection. In the original selection of the cases I was satisfied in taking the Kraepelinian diagnosis as it stood, without paying close attention to the symptomatology. It is, however, well known that at one time Kraepelin purposely expanded his diagnosis of manic-depressive insanity to include as many cases as possible, subsequently testing the validity of the diagnosis by follow-up records. When, after a few months, I attempted a provisional estimation of the material, I was surprised to find a number of schizophrenics among the children. It seemed possible that this might be in part due to incorrect diagnosis in the original cases. It is, for instance, only in recent years that the attention of clinicians has been drawn to remitting forms of schizophrenia, and the course of an illness is now no longer considered sufficient as the only criterion for the diagnosis of manic-depressive psychosis. Accordingly I completed the collection of my material, and have subsequently attempted to subclassify it according to the clinical picture presented by the propositus, so as to isolate out cases where error might be introduced through incorrect diagnosis. In this process I have availed myself extensively of the help of colleagues, particularly of Drs. Mayer-Gross and Guttmann, and have in no case ventured myself to decide on the final diagnosis of a case, where I knew of the presence of a schizophrenic child, but, to avoid any possible partiality, have in every such case relied on the judgment of others.

The incidence of any abnormality appearing late in life is to a great extent dependent on the age-distribution of the population in which it occurs. It is essential to employ some statistical device to remove this disturbing factor. The method in use in Germany is, in the case of manic-depressive insanity, to neglect all members of the population in question who have not reached the age of 20, as having had no chance of developing the illness, to count as half all those between the ages of 20 and 50, and to count in full all those above 50. For this to be fully justified, no persons should develop the illness before 20 or after 50, while the chance in the intermediate years should be about the same for any year, and the population in question should show a similar even distribution between these years. Although the fundamental assumptions for this device are difficult to justify, it seems likely that the employment of this method does not give rise to any gross source of error, at any rate not comparable to the many other grosser sources of error which I have pointed out above. As my cases, however, showed in some groups a somewhat uneven distribution between the ages of 20 and 50, I have preferred to divide them up into five-year groups, and take the number in each group as being concentrated at its mean. Thus a group of people between the ages of 20 and 25 would be reckoned as of age 22½, and considered to have lived two and a half of the thirty years in which they might show themselves as manic-depressive, i.e. their number would be divided by 12. Similarly the number of those in the 45 to 50 group would be multiplied by the fraction 11/12.[1]

The exact clinical interpretation of the cases with children necessitated obtaining the full record from the psychiatric clinic, and the clinical records from many other mental hospitals, and an up-to-date catamnesis on every case. As a result of this I was eventually placed in possession of an immense amount of clinical material which I hope to be able to use for other purposes. As a result of this more exact examination of the material, I have eliminated from the 201 families 20 in which the diagnosis of manic-depressive insanity seemed to be altogether incorrect, and I have further separated a special group of 41 cases in which both manic-depressive and schizophrenic symptomatology was shown clearly in the record. It is hoped to subject these last to special study. The remaining 140 cases I divided into two groups: firstly a group of 72 cases (Group I), in which the symptomatology was not only clearly manic-depressive, but purely so, and unaffected by organic or schizophrenic-like disturbing elements; and secondly a group of 68 cases (Group II), in which such disturbing elements did enter, but not in any sufficient amount to throw the diagnosis of manic-depressive insanity in any doubt.[2] Among such foreign symptoms I included greater irritability than usual, a somewhat paranoid attitude to the environment, exaggerated hypochondriasis, any episode of apparently exogenous origin, such as a period of confusion accompanied perhaps by delirious hallucinations. Cases where there were hallucinations in a state of clear consciousness are not included.

FINDINGS

My material falls, then, into three groups of parents — those of the childless manic-depressives who were subject to no special investigation, and the parents of Groups I and II; the children are classified in Groups I and II only. I give the results in Tables 4.2 and 4.3.

TABLE 4.2. INCIDENCE OF PSYCHIATRIC ABNORMALITY AMONG PARENTS OF MANIC-DEPRESSIVES*

	Childless group (225)		Group I (141)		Group II (129)		All groups (495)	
	%	S.D.	%	S.D.	%	S.D.	%	S.D.
Manic-depressives	15.6	2.4	13.5	3.0	17.1	3.3	15.4	1.6
Cycloid psychopaths	9.1	1.1	2.5	1.3	5.1	1.7	3.8	0.7
Schizophrenics	1.3	0.8	0.7	0.7	0.0	0.0	0.8	0.4

TABLE 4.3. INCIDENCE OF PSYCHIATRIC ABNORMALITY AMONG CHILDREN OF MANIC-DEPRESSIVES

	Group I (116)		Group II (93)		Both groups (209)	
	%	S.D.	%	S.D.	%	S.D.
Manic-depressives	15.5	3.4	16.1	3.8	15.8	2.5
Cycloid psychopaths	11.4	2.3	15.6	2.8	13.4	1.8
Schizophrenics	1.4	1.0	4.2	1.8	2.6	1.0

*S.D. = Standard deviation of percentage in preceding column. The figure given in brackets under the name of the group is the statistical size of the group for the purpose of estimating the incidence of manic-depressives in the group.

[1] In the final report (Paper 5 in this volume) a different method was preferred. — *Editors.*

[2] In the final report the cases were reclassified; 138 remaining cases were divided into 84 "A"-probands (typical cases) and 54 "B"-probands (with disturbing elements). — *Editors.*

It is necessary to note that the figure given in brackets under the name of the group, indicating its size for estimating the percentage of manic-depressives, does not represent its real size, or its statistical size for the estimation of the frequency of other abnormalities. For instance, the number of children of Group I was 269. For the purpose of estimating the frequency of "cycloid psychopaths" I have reckoned only those over 20 years of age, 193 in number. For the estimation of the frequency of schizophrenia, those between the ages of 20 and 40 were counted only in part, according to the principle I have already described for the estimation of manic-depressives, but giving in this case a population of 146 persons; while for manic-depressives themselves the figure is further reduced to 116. It is with some hesitation that I have used the term "cycloid psychopath." Under it I have included all persons who have shown well-marked swings of mood lasting considerable periods, varying from over-activity and elation to inertia and depression, or varying from normal in one of these directions only, or persons of a permanently depressed or boisterous overactive temperament, these abnormalities of mood being so marked as to be frankly obvious to friends or relatives, but not being so extreme as to lead to illness or temporary or permanent incapacity. In the latter event I have included such persons among the psychotics, using therefore a purely social criterion as to what shall necessitate a diagnosis of manic-depressive insanity — that of social incapacity of such a degree that it has necessitated medical treatment.

It will be seen that this investigation fails in several particulars to fill the requirements which I gave earlier in the paper. It cannot be claimed that thoroughly adequate information has been obtained about all the persons investigated. Their number is really inadequate to base any certain figures on my findings. It is on this account that I have given the standard deviation of all the percentages. It is generally assumed that the true figure will lie within the limits given by the observed figure, plus or minus twice its standard deviation. Thus the frequency of manic-depressives among the children of Group I was probably between $15.5 \pm 2 \times 3.4\%$, i.e. between 8.7% and 22.3%. Such a large possible margin of error indicates the rather unsatisfactory character of this type of investigation. Further points of possible criticism are that my diagnosis of manic-depressive insanity in parents and children might well be questioned in many cases by competent psychiatrists, usually on the grounds of insufficiency of information. To this the only reply is that to class such persons statistically under such titles as "mental illness, of unknown nature, but with affective features" would hardly make informative reading, and that it is sufficient if one accepts the figures with the proviso that in a high proportion of cases the diagnosis has not been certainly established. Finally, it cannot be claimed for this work that the statistical working out is free from all source of objection.

DISCUSSION

In discussing what conclusions one might draw from this investigation it is necessary to underline these points. The inadequacy of material, its insufficient ascertainment and not irreproachable working out have not prevented previous authors from putting forward complicated theories of the genetic basis of manic-depressive insanity. Hoffmann has built up a theory involving three independent genetic factors, each as it were carrying different weights, and a total weight being necessary to precipitate the individual into a psychosis, a lesser weight being sufficient to make him a cycloid or cyclothymic personality. Rosanoff, Handy, and

Plessett (1935), in their study of manic-depressive twins, propose a theory involving two independent factors, a cyclothymic autosomal factor and an activating factor in the X-chromosome, both factors being dominant. Rüdin proposes a theory involving one autosomal dominant and two autosomal recessives. Luxenburger favours a similar theory with one recessive and one dominant. From our present knowledge it would appear that all these theories are quite premature. Such speculations may certainly be possible, but are improbable, unsupported by any real evidence and serve no useful purpose.

In our knowledge of the genetics of manic-depressive insanity only two things stand out as fairly certainly established, firstly that it is inheritable, and secondly that the inheritance follows a dominant type. The simplest possible theory to account for the facts is that the inheritance depends on a single dominant autosomal gene. Once dominance is assumed, this theory must be shown to be inadequate before any other is even provisionally accepted. There are not sufficient facts at present to reject this theory.

On this theory the expectation of manic-depressives among the parents, brothers and sisters and children of manic-depressives would be 50%. Luxenburger gives the percentage of manic-depressive insanity among the parents and siblings as 10.6 and 12.6%. For the children he uses Hoffmann's figures, which I think must be rejected. I have found corresponding figures to Luxenburger's, though slightly larger, for parents and children. They are all far below the 50% level, a fact which is usually held to be sufficient for the rejection of a theory of simple dominance. There are however many reasons why the figures actually found should be so much below theoretical expectation. No genetic factor works in the void, but in an environment which may help or hinder its expression. Rosanoff and his co-workers found that only 70% of the probably uniovular twins of manic-depressives themselves developed the illness. This gives us a direct measure of the influence of the environment, and at the same time reduces the theoretical expectation of 50% to 35%. A large part of the remaining difference may well be accounted for by the very serious difficulties of ascertainment, and to the probability that many persons who have true depressive psychoses are not sufficiently severely or sufficiently long ill to require even perhaps the advice of a doctor, still less incarceration in a mental hospital or psychiatric clinic. There are however theoretical grounds which make it probable that a part also of the difference between theory and expectation is itself genetically determined. These genetic influences are conveniently included under the term "genotypic milieu."

The gene or genes responsible for the appearance of any character have to work not only in an external environment, which as Rosanoff's work has shown, may have a very large influence, but also in the internal environment of all the other genes which go to make up the hereditary structure of the individual. This genotypic milieu is the same for both individuals in the case of uniovular twins, and so does not find expression in Rosanoff's figures. That it can be very important is shown by recent work on Drosophila. Timoféeff-Ressovsky (1935) has shown that the recessive gene "vena transversa interrupta," which brings about an interruption in the transverse vein, shows itself normally in homozygotic culture in only 1 to 5% of the flies, all of whom should exhibit the change. This percentage is raised to 40 to 100% if a second recessive gene is present also homozygotically, which by itself has no effect on the transverse vein, but shortens one of the longitudinal veins. This is a good example of a "weak" gene, and weak genes are so common, that in spite of difficulties of investigation in their case, they are already held to be more frequent than the "strong" ones. Timoféeff remarks that it is absurd to speak of one gene as being the only one affecting a given change. Every single gene known in Drosophila can be shown to have an influence on several different qualities; and there is no change which is not affected by several different genes. In any single quality one is not dealing with a single gene, but with the totality of genes. Dominance and recessivity are not absolute but quantitative characters. All genes can be ranged on a scale passing from almost complete recessivity to almost complete dominance, and on quite another scale passing from very bad to very good manifestation. The two scales are not, however, related, and weakly manifesting dominant genes are very common.

These considerations are important for human genetics. It seems possible that we are dealing in manic-depressive insanity with just such a weak dominant gene, that manifests itself in only a proportion of its carriers. To say that the degree of manifestation of such a weakly dominant manic-depressive factor is also affected by other genetic factors, is an entirely different thing from saying that manic-depressive insanity is governed by two or three or more separate factors. The latter is a statement that the psychosis does not appear without all the factors being present, when 100% manifestation results. It seems quite possible that only one gene is responsible for the change, but the degree to which it manifests itself will be governed by a variety of circumstances, genetic and environmental.

In manic-depressive insanity besides the genetic and the purely external environment, there is the environment represented by the body itself. It is a remarkable fact that women tend to develop manic-depressive insanity more frequently than men. Some authorities have tried to explain this by the assumption of a factor in the X-chromosome. Unsupported by accessory hypotheses, this theory does not fit the facts. It seems more likely that the female constitution, involving among other things quite a different endocrine balance, forms a more suitable medium of expression for this particular hereditary factor.

There are, however, other criticisms of a theory of simple dominance. How on this basis are we to explain the bewildering variety of clinical syndromes? In the present state of our knowledge this criticism has no weight. Apart from the predominant mood change, we have no idea what are the primary and what the secondary and inessential features of this illness. The great symptomatic variety is likely to be caused in part by the inclusion of what are not really manic-depressive psychoses. Further, it is probable that in such a condition, in which the whole psyche is involved, many of the varying features are due to other qualities of temperament and character, which are conditioned by other and independent genetic factors. There is no convincing clinical reason for rejecting the theory of one single factor, as the main one responsible for this type of psychic breakdown.

There is one curious fact which is in favour of a theory of simple dominance. It is a remarkable fact that parents, siblings, and children all show about the same percentage of manic-depressives, namely in the neighbourhood of 15%. I can imagine no other theory which would give this relation, which is just what one would expect on a theory of simple dominance. Furthermore Banse's figure for cousins, given in his paper as 3½% (corrected by Luxenburger to 2.7%) is just about one-quarter of the empirical expectation for parents, sibs and children, a figure that also fits in well with this theory.

Before leaving this aspect of the subject, there is an important observation to make. Geneticists have shown that in the majority of known heritable abnormalities, of Drosophila for instance, the same change may be brought about by a number of quite different and independent genetic factors. Similarly in man it has been shown that there are a number of different genetic types of syndactyly, polydactyly, etc. It may well be that the same holds for manic-depressive insanity. All that I would assert at present is that in the typical recurrent manic-depressives there is sufficient evidence to believe that this is governed in the majority of cases by a dominant type of inheritance, and that there is insufficient evidence to show that the hypothesis of a single dominant autosomal factor as the main responsible agent is insufficient.

Any theory of the inheritance of manic-depressive insanity must take into account the problem of its relationship to schizophrenia. In the children of Groups I and II together, there was 2.6% of schizophrenics (in the total of all the children there was about 6%). This is a very high figure, as all that one can expect, were manic-depressive insanity to have no relation to schizophrenia, is about 0.85%. In the German literature, the matter is usually represented as just the opposite. Luxenburger gives the liability of sibs of manic-depressives to schizophrenia as 0.9%, less than that of the general population. These figures are based on Rüdin's work, and require confirmation. Similarly Luxenburger gives the probability of children of manic-depressives developing schizophrenia as nil. This is based on Hoffmann's work, who omits to state in his statistical analysis that he found among his 162 children five cases of schizophrenia. On further partial examination and catamnesis on this material two more cases of schizophrenia have been discovered, raising the percentage of schizophrenics among these children to over 4%. In previous years Krauss (1903) found among the children of cyclic parents schizophrenic more frequently than cyclic children. Luther (1914) found among the children of manic-depressives as many other psychoses as manic-depressive ones, and most of these other psychoses were schizophrenic. Smith (1925) found that in cyclic-schizophrenic crossings, schizophrenic children were commoner than in crossings between normals and schizophrenics. All these findings point to a special relation between manic-depressive insanity and schizophrenia, which is supported by my finding of 2.6% of schizophrenics among my children, when all possible incorrect diagnoses had been eliminated. This figure is of no great statistical significance; yet I am inclined to believe that it represents a real tendency.

In attempting to explain this finding one might be led to examine the family trees of these cases to see whether schizophrenia appeared in other members of the patient's family and perhaps of the family into which he married. Of the fifteen families in which manic-depressive subjects had schizophrenic children, in ten cases I could find no other schizophrenic in either the patient's family or in that of the husband or wife. In one case the patient had married into a family with a schizophrenic member, in the other four cases there was schizophrenia already in the patient's own family. I do not think that these findings, even if they had been much more positive, could give any explanation of why manic-depressives should have more schizophrenic children than normal parents do.

It seems established that manic-depressives are scarcer than might be expected among the relatives of schizophrenics, so that the positive correlation, if it exists, is in one direction only. It is this sort of finding that has led some authorities to an acceptance of the now somewhat discredited theory of anticipation. Others would explain the relationship between manic-depressive insanity and schizophrenia by holding that both are due to a general neuropathic tendency. Others again would endorse the theory that both manic-depressives and schizophrenic psychoses are dependent on two or more genes and have one or more of these in common, that there is in fact a common hereditary factor. The facts, however, particularly the one-sidedness of the relationship between the two psychoses, would not appear to support any of these theories.

Manic-depressive insanity, however, does not stand alone in this peculiar relation to schizophrenia. The relatives of general paralytics and epileptics also show an increased incidence of schizophrenia, and it would seem undesirable to assume the presence of common hereditary factors in each and all of these cases. A more plausible explanation would lie in alteration of the capacity of manifestation. It would not seem improbable that the carrier of any hereditary factor which shows itself in disturbance of the psyche will not only be more predisposed to that special kind of disturbance, but also to the more profound and destructive disturbance of schizophrenia, or in other words that the gene or genes responsible for the development of schizophrenia find it easier to manifest themselves in a genotypic milieu, which includes other hereditary factors which predispose to psychic disorder, such as manic-depressive ones, whether those other factors have actually manifested themselves or not.

One is tempted to take this possible explanation further and make the following suggestion. There is in genetics no very hard and fast line between dominance and recessivity. This quality also of the gene frequently depends on environmental factors as well as on the genotypic milieu. It seems quite possible that the presence of a manic-depressive gene might, when present in the same individual, have the effect of lending the schizophrenic gene a semi-dominance, so that this might manifest itself in a heterozygotic individual. It is conceivable that some process like this is responsible for the strange atypical psychoses half way between manic-depressive psychoses and schizophrenia in symptomatology and course, which as a matter of clinical experience are not infrequently seen. I should hesitate very much to advance this sort of speculation, but that there is a way in which it could be tested.[3] If the manic-depressive gene does have any activating influence on the schizophrenic factors, then one would expect the majority of the schizophrenic children of manic-depressives to be themselves masked manic-depressives. An investigation of their children would then show the reappearance of manic-depressive insanity. In my material I have five cases where something is known both of the generation preceding and of that following a case of schizophrenia appearing in a manic-depressive family, and in one of these that is the case. Here the patient, a woman, had a perfectly typical recurrent manic-depressive psychosis, with complete recovery after the attacks. Her mother had, at the age of 34, an acute psychotic illness with many manic features. From this, however, she never recovered. She developed a chronic hallucinosis with many paranoid ideas and passed at last into a chronic schizophrenic state in which she remained until she died at the age of 79. Her mother, the patient's maternal grandmother, was at various times in her life four times in a mental hospital with recurrent melancholia, and her mother, the patient's great-grandmother, also had one or more psychotic illnesses, of which no details can be obtained. One sees here four generations showing the typical dominant type of inheritance, with a schizophrenic suddenly appearing in the middle, but capable herself of continuing the manic-depressive line. Research on this point might well bear fruitful results.

Many explanations have been advanced for the occurrence of atypical endogenous psychoses, having some of the features of schizophrenia, and others more

[3] In Paper 5 Slater considers this speculation to be unjustified. — *Editors.*

manic-depressive in nature. Many authors recognize no hard and fast boundary line between these two principal types, but speak also of remitting schizophrenic psychoses which fail to show any destruction of the personality, and chronic psychoses, manic-depressive in symptomatology, which do. It seems premature to suggest any genetic explanation of these phenomena which will require a fuller clinical study and analysis. It has been suggested that they are due to the concurrent presence in the same individual of both manic-depressive and schizophrenic hereditary factors, drawn in part separately from paternal and maternal sides. My material does not very strongly support this view, and cases of these unusual kinds appear in some of my families where a manic-depressive taint is the only one apparent. Another explanation is that a schizophrenic psychosis appearing in a person constitutionally of the pyknic and cyclothymic type will tend to show manic-depressive features, particularly relatively good preservation of the affect. It would seem likely that in some cases one of these explanations may be the true one, and in others the other; and further likely that some of these atypical psychoses are peculiar in themselves and are due to quite different genetic factors from those of the manic-depressive and schizophrenic psychoses, that they may in fact be found to breed true. Some families published by Leonhard (1934) are especially suggestive of this possibility.

This is a fundamentally opposed attitude to that of Bleuler, who thinks that the qualities of being schizoid and cycloid appear in every normal man in varying proportions, and are, so to speak, functional antagonists. This view-point would be of little help in genetic research, and likely to lead only to such pieces of research as Hoffmann's (1921). What facts we have seem to be against the view that there is an infinite series of gradations between the normal and the psychotic, and if English psychiatrists adopt this view, they should be clear on what grounds they do so.

EDITORS' COMMENTS: Slater's second paper in English on the inheritance of manic-depressive insanity (5) is devoted largely to a trenchant criticism of a paper (Duncan, Penrose, and Turnbull, 1936) which claimed to show a positive relationship between manic-depression and mental defect.

The first of the German papers reporting his research project (9) is on the subject of the periodicity of manic-depressive insanity. Though we do not reproduce it here, its relative inaccessibility to English-speaking readers justifies a brief summary. His Munich material confirmed previous reports of a peak incidence of the disease in early summer and a small secondary peak in early autumn. Individual patients had a significant tendency to fall ill at the same time of year. There was no general tendency for intervals between attacks to become shorter. The most original contribution of the paper was methodological: this was probably the first time an analysis of variance was ever applied in psychiatric research. Slater used this technique to examine whether or not a patient tended to have his individual pattern of illness. Variation within individuals in respect of the interval between attacks was found to be less than variation between individuals. The difference was ten times the standard error, and Slater concluded that the phases of each patient did in fact have their own natural rhythm.

The main paper describing the findings in the manic-depressive study (10) is a long one of 47 pages, including 17 pages of case histories and over 20 tables, several of them stretching over two sides of the page. It has, with the author's permission, been abridged as well as translated for presentation as the fifth paper in this volume. The case histories, including some occurring in the course of the text, have had to be excluded, some tables and figures have been left out or condensed, and three sections have been omitted altogether. These are the first section describing material and methods, which is largely repetition of information given in Paper 4, and the two following sections on causes of death and on social class. To summarise them briefly, Slater found a raised frequency of arteriopathic illnesses as causes of death in the parents (29%) and probands (36%). Compared with the general population risks, cancer and tuberculosis played a relatively small role. A table was provided, showing the social class distribution of parents, probands, and children. Findings were in good agreement with those reached earlier by Luxenburger on a larger material, and it was of interest that an illness as severe as recurrent manic-depressive psychosis occurring in more than one generation did not lower the social level of the families.

Apart from its basic data, the paper is of value for the discussion and application of different methods of correcting for the age structure of the sample observed — the conventional, empirical "shorter method" of Weinberg, Weinberg's full morbidity-table method, and the method pioneered by Strömgren and Slater himself which employs weights derived from the age structure of the general population and the observed age of onset of the disorder in a representative sample of patients. Since the publication of the provisional findings two years previously, the results of family studies by other investigators had become available for comparison. Particularly instructive is Slater's testing and rejection of the hypothesis of Rosanoff et al., a hypothesis which invoked an auxiliary sex-linked gene to account for the apparent excess of the disorder in females.

5

THE PARENTS AND CHILDREN OF MANIC-DEPRESSIVES

THE MATERIAL

SUMMARY (*by Editors*): As described in Paper 4, the sample consists of the following groups of recurrent manic-depressive probands: 114 without children; and 138 with children, divided into 84 typical cases ("A"-probands) and 54 cases with disturbing elements ("B"-probands). The sex and diagnostic distribution of the "A"-probands was given in the Case History section of the original paper and was as follows: pure mania, 2 m., 1 f.; pure depression, 5 m., 27 f.; circular, 20 m., 14 f.; mania with depressive elements, 4 m., 1 f.; depression with manic elements, 3 m., 7 f. The nature of the additional, atypical symptoms of the "B"-probands and the number of probands with each were as follows: epileptic, 1; congenital mental defect, 2; hysterical, 5; psychopathic, 10; organic, 14 (3 alcoholic, 4 clouding of consciousness, confusion etc., 7 arteriosclerotic); paranoid and schizophrenic-like, 22.

CALCULATION OF THE "BEZUGSZIFFER"
(CORRECTED DENOMINATOR)

We are not particularly concerned here with the advantages and disadvantages of the various methods of taking into consideration the age distribution of subjects in respect of a character with a limited period of risk. There are, so far as I know, only three methods, Weinberg's "shorter method", Strömgren's (1935) method[1] and the method which uses morbidity tables. None of these methods can be held to be

---

Abridged and translated by James Shields from: "Zur Erbpathologie des manisch-depressiven Irreseins. Die Eltern und Kinder von Manisch-Depressiven," *Zeitschrift für die gesamte Neurologie und Psychiatrie* 163: 1–47 (1938).

[1] In principle this is the same as the method which I recommended and applied to a population material in my paper "The incidence of mental disorder" (1).

absolutely correct; there is much to be said for and against each. The last, that employing the morbidity table, can only be used without reservation on a comparatively large material, and is of only very limited application to the present data.

Weinberg's shorter method, as he himself emphasizes, is only a comparatively crude procedure. A defined age period is taken as being the time of risk for the onset of the illness. All persons who have disappeared from observation before this time are omitted completely from the calculation. Those persons who disappear from observation during the period of risk are counted as one half. Those disappearing from observation after the end of the risk period are counted in full. In this way one obtains a *Bezugsziffer* (BZ) or corrected denominator, to which the actual number of sick persons is then related as numerator. In manic-depressive insanity the period of from 20 to 50 years of age has until now been taken as such a risk period in the works of the Genealogical Institute in Munich. The procedure would be unobjectionable if the following conditions were fulfilled. First, the risk period should correspond to the facts; and secondly, disappearance from observation and also the onset of the illness during the period of risk should either occur completely evenly or in such a way that any irregularities present cancel one another out. There is of course also the possibility that neither the first nor the second requirement is met but that the deviations from both of them nevertheless go in opposite directions so that the final result is approximately correct.

It is thus possible that, when taking a risk period of 20–50 (although indeed onsets may occur both before and after these ages) an approximately correct result will nevertheless be obtained; however, one can on no account be certain of this before discovering by more exact methods whether this is generally so. Thus Weinberg, who applied his shorter method to schizophrenia, in fact found, when he examined the question, that here the shorter method, assuming a risk period of from approximately 17–40, did give about the same result as was obtained from a morbidity table. Therefore, as will be seen below, I have not considered it to be in any way more correct to apply the shorter method by entering, e.g., a person aged 21 as 1/30th, one aged 22 as 2/30th, etc. I have thought it better to apply the method unaltered, as has been the practice in previous works from the Research Institute.

In applying the Strömgren method I proceeded as follows. All the manic-depressive cases from which I selected my original material were classified by age of onset. For this purpose I noted the age of first falling ill from the index cards of the Clinical Institute, even if the affected patient had not at that time been admitted to any clinic. The only criterion which was relevant for me was that the patient should then have shown clear symptoms of a (manic-depressive) psychosis. In the card index there were 759 male and 1773 female cases. These are shown in columns 2 and 6 of Table 5.1. As will be seen, their ages of onset fell within the age classes of

TABLE 5.1. DATA USED FOR DERIVATION OF STRÖMGREN-METHOD WEIGHTS

1	2	3	4	5	6	7	8	9†
Age		Men					Women	
13	1	216,498	0.4619	0.029	0	219,488		
14	1	218,498	0.4577	0.087	1	219,648	0.4533	0.016
15	4	216,874	1.8444	0.233	4	218,607	1.8298	0.093
16	3	213,546	1.4048	0.438	11	214,898	5.1187	0.327
17	3	207,370	1.4467	0.618	13	211,112	6.1567	0.706
18	7	195,310	3.5840	0.935	22	205,237	10.7193	1.277
19	8	168,472	4.7410	1.460	20	202,222	9.8901	1.973
20	9	154,369	5.8302	2.128	32	200,931	15.9259	2.842

TABLE 5-1. (Continued)

1	2	3	4	5	6	7	8	9 †
Age			Men				Women	
21	11	150,152	7.3259	2.958	27	195,843	13.7866	3.843
22	10	146,841	6.8101	3.850	34	192,474	17.6647	4.902
23	11	148,300	7.4174	4.748	40	191,524	20.8851	6.200
24	13	145,875	8.9117	5.779	37	186,980	19.7882	7.569
25	12	144,226	8.3203	6.866	38	185,275	20.5101	8.926
26	14	134,839	10.3828	8.047	42	175,579	23.9209	10.422
27	16	130,036	12.3043	9.479	44	172,343	25.5305	12.087
28	17	126,540	13.4345	11.103	42	169,909	24.7191	13.779
29	17	122,511	13.8763	12.827	44	167,702	26.2370	15.494
30	17	113,351	14.9977	14.649	43	156,940	27.3990	17.300
31	18	116,351	15.4704	16.572	48	158,130	30.3548	19.244
32	17	115,171	14.7607	18.480	38	155,501	24.4371	21.089
33	20	112,487	17.7798	20.533	43	150,474	28.5764	22.874
34	18	109,855	16.3858	22.690	46	146,892	31.3155	24.891
35	19	108,529	17.5068	24.829	41	143,052	28.6609	26.910
36	19	101,391	18.2008	27.089	47	138,342	33.9738	29.019
37	19	107,447	17.6831	29.347	47	140,838	33.3717	31.287
38	22	106,637	20.6307	31.765	46	138,444	33.2264	33.529
39	14	105,105	13.3200	33.908	43	135,385	31.7613	35.717
40	13	105,029	12.3775	35.529	44	132,789	33.1353	37.902
41	14	106,583	13.1353	37.139	39	132,590	29.4140	40.008
42	18	105,233	17.1065	39.048	41	128,805	31.8311	42.070
43	16	106,936	14.9622	41.073	35	125,093	27.9792	44.084
44	18	111,308	16.1713	43.038	35	122,947	28.4676	45.985
45	19	109,152	17.4069	45.157	40	117,298	34.1012	48.091
46	17	110,341	15.4068	47.228	44	118,567	37.1098	50.489
47	17	110,775	15.3464	49.169	40	118,374	33.7912	52.876
48	20	107,872	18.5405	51.307	39	112,904	34.5426	55.176
49	18	105,786	17.0155	53.551	40	112,305	35.6173	57.539
50	18	103,142	17.4517	55.726	40	108,354	36.9160	59.981
51	18	97,387	18.4830	57.994	38	104,078	36.5111	62.453
52	18	98,091	18.3503	60.319	34	103,479	32.8569	64.789
53	18	89,887	20.0251	62.741	33	97,578	33.8191	67.034
54	20	85,194	23.4758	65.487	33	91,304	36.1287	69.389
55	17	85,571	19.8665	68.222	31	91,225	33.9819	71.749
56	17	84,139	20.2047	70.751	25	92,643	26.9853	73.802
57	14	78,845	17.7564	73.147	26	86,249	30.1453	75.725
58	10	76,068	13.1461	75.097	28	83,677	33.4620	77.867
59	11	74,341	14.7967	76.861	27	82,286	32.8124	80.098
60	14	69,332	20.1927	79.069	21	76,074	27.6047	82.133
61	13	66,456	19.5618	81.578	20	74,352	26.8991	83.968
62	9	64,249	14.0080	83.697	15	71,561	20.9611	85.579
63	11	58,847	18.6925	85.761	19	65,254	29.1170	87.265
64	9	55,267	16.2846	87.968	13	63,312	20.5332	88.937
65	11	54,473	20.1935	90.270	15	62,745	23.9063	90.433
66	8	51,532	15.5243	92.525	10	60,357	16.5681	91.796
67	6	48,374	12.4034	94.287	14	56,173	24.9221	93.193
68	1	43,574	2.2949	95.215	11	52,185	21.0789	94.742
69	3	40,728	7.3659	95.824	6	47,351	12.6713	95.878
70	3	36,993	8.1096	96.801	4	43,226	9.2537	96.616
71	3	35,849	8.3684	97.841	8	43,374	18.4442	97.548
72	3	30,428	9.8593	98.992	5	36,342	13.7582	98.634
73	0	29,325	0.0000	99.614	4	34,861	11.4741	99.484
74*	5	163,355	3.0608	99.807	4	207,600	1.9268	99.935
				100.000				100.000

*74 and over
†For explanation of headings 2–9, see text.

13 and 74 or over. Next, in columns 3 and 7, the corresponding figures have been calculated from the census figures from Bavaria for the years 1905, 1916 and 1925. The 2,532 cases were admitted to the Kraepelin Clinic between 1903 and 1922; the figures calculated for the population correspond to the age distribution of the Bavarian population during this time, taking into consideration the changes in the male population caused by the war. Dividing the figures of columns 2 and 6 by those of columns 3 and 7, the figures of columns 4 and 8 are obtained (which have been multiplied by 100,000). They are thus an expression of the relative risk ("corrected frequency," "attack rate") for both sexes and for each year of life.

The figures of columns 4 and 8 are of interest in their own right. Represented graphically they result in the curves of Fig. 5.1. In order to exclude chance deviations, when drawing up the curves I have not used the calculated frequency for each year of age directly but for each year have calculated the mean value of the frequencies of the year in question and the four years above and below it. In this way the

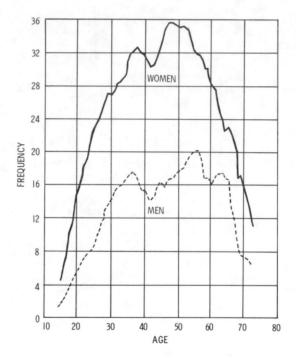

Figure 5.1. Attack rates for manic-depressive insanity in men and women and for each age group.

curve becomes smoother and the principal outlines stand out more clearly. The following facts can be seen. The frequency in women is nearly twice as great as that in men. In both sexes the curve is bimodal, in men with peaks at the ages of 36 and 54, in women at the ages of 38 and 48. The plateau of the curve appears to be somewhat longer in men than in women, and indeed reaches as far as age 65, while in women there is a rapid fall beginning at age 54. It is of interest that the main risk period in both sexes approximates more closely to a range of 30-60 than to the one of 20-50 which was previously assumed.

As control material I should like to present the data of Dahlberg and Stenberg (1931). The Dahlberg material of manic-depressives, when classified according to the Strömgren method in the same way as mine, gave the following figures which I compare with my own in Table 5.2.

TABLE 5.2. PERCENTAGE DISTRIBUTION OF MORBID RISK FOR
MANIC-DEPRESSIVE INSANITY

Age*	Material of Dahlberg and Stenberg		Present Material	
	Men	Women	Men	Women
5–9	0.49	—	—	—
10–14	1.92	—	0.35	0.15
15–19	5.13	8.99	2.15	3.23
20–24	5.25	8.13	4.89	6.24
25–29	4.09	10.22	8.21	8.60
30–34	4.08	8.49	10.33	9.66
35–39	7.29	9.99	10.38	11.14
40–44	5.00	8.59	9.95	10.22
45–49	9.76	10.52	8.37	9.50
50–54	13.84	11.91	14.85	14.15
55–59	14.33	7.57	10.86	10.17
60–64	11.18	4.41	11.21	8.18
65–69	14.15	6.24	5.76	5.69
70–74	2.90	1.49	2.69	3.07

*In Dahlberg and Stenberg age distribution is given as: 5–10, 10–15, etc.

From curves derived from this table it can be shown that in my data there is apparently no significant difference between men and women; the curves for both sexes are very similar to the female curve of Dahlberg and Stenberg. On the other hand, their curve for men is of a considerably different shape. In Dahlberg and Stenberg's men the period of greatest risk is shifted still further towards the higher age range. I believe that the differences between these various curves can mainly be regarded as due to chance. My curves, which are derived from a larger number of cases, occupy a position in between the two curves of Dahlberg and Stenberg.

Let us now turn to Table 5.1. The method of calculation is quite simple. The figures of columns 4 and 8 are summed cumulatively so that for every age a figure is obtained which corresponds to the risk, not for that age alone but for all earlier ages inclusive. Finally, one has a figure which expresses the total risk of becoming manic-depressive. This last, however, should be converted to 100%. Thus, dividing the figures by the final total, the result is the percentage risk for each year of age which has been accumulated up till then. These figures should then be reduced by half the increase of year to year, so that — as Strömgren showed in his paper — an expression is obtained for the risk lived through up to the middle of the corresponding year of life and not to the end of the year. The results of these calculations are shown in the figures of columns 5 and 9; the latter are used for calculating the BZ. From these columns it is seen, for example, that by the age of 35 only 26%, or 28% as the case may be, of the risk has been passed, while only by the age of 46–47 has half the risk of falling ill been passed. Accordingly, with this method the BZ will be smaller than with the shorter method of Weinberg and consequently a higher frequency of affected persons will be found among the relatives of manic-depressives.

THE FREQUENCY OF MENTAL ABNORMALITY IN
PARENTS AND CHILDREN OF OUR PROBANDS

We shall now comment upon Tables 5.4–5.7 which present the results of the research.[2] For calculating the frequency of manic-depressives among the relatives of the probands, I have used Weinberg's shorter method (W. in the Tables), in addition

TABLE 5.3. RISK PERIODS ADOPTED FOR WEINBERG'S "SHORTER METHOD"

Character	Age under which omitted	Ages between which counted half	Age above which wholly counted
Manic-depressive insanity	20	20–49	50
Schizophrenia	20	20–39	40
GPI	30	30–49	50
Arteriosclerotic psychoses	50		50
Senile dementia	60		60
Mental illness of unknown nature	30		30
Imbecility	10		10
Epilepsy	10		10
Hysteria	20		20
Criminality	20		20
Alcoholism	20		20
Emotionally labile personality	20		20
Psychopathy	20		20

TABLE 5.4. FREQUENCY OF VARIOUS DISORDERS IN THE PARENTS OF
DIFFERENT GROUPS OF PROBANDS

Disorder	114 childless probands			84 "A"-probands			54 "B"-probands		
	Cases	BZ	%	Cases	BZ	%	Cases	BZ	%
Hosp. manic-depression (St.)	14	193.30	7.2	7	141.59	4.9	4	83.44	4.8
Hosp. manic-depression (W.)	14	216.93	6.4	7	159.08	4.4	4	95.19	4.2
Manic-depression (St.)	28	193.30	14.5	13	141.59	9.2	7	83.44	8.4
Manic-depression (W.)	28	216.93	12.9	13	159.08	8.2	7	95.19	7.4
Man-dep., ?man-dep., suicide (St.)	35	193.30	18.1	26	141.59	18.4	12	83.44	14.4
Man-dep., ?man-dep., suicide (W.)	35	216.93	16.1	26	159.08	16.4	12	95.19	12.6
Emotionally labile personality	7	228.00	3.1	3	168.00	1.8	4	108.00	3.7
Schizophrenia (St.)	3	225.30	1.3	1	165.51	0.6	–	105.34	0.0
Schizophrenia (W.)	3	225.77	1.3	1	164.49	0.6	–	103.54	0.0
Epilepsy	3	228.00	1.3	–	168.00	0.0	–	108.00	0.0
GPI	–	216.93	0.0	1	158.09	0.6	1	95.19	1.0
Arteriosclerosis	–	205.97	0.0	1	148.16	0.7	–	83.37	0.0
Senile dementia	–	161.58	0.0	1	121.34	0.8	1	61.25	1.6
Mental illness of unknown nature	10	228.00	4.4	3	168.00	1.8	2	108.00	1.9
Alcoholism	11	228.00	4.8	12	168.00	7.2	5	108.00	4.6
Criminality	1	228.00	0.4	1	168.00	0.6	–	108.00	0.0
Psychopathy	10	228.00	4.4	4	168.00	2.4	1	108.00	0.9

BZ (Bezugsziffer): corrected total
St.: Strömgren method
W.: Weinberg shorter method

to the Strömgren (St.) method. For the frequency of manic-depressives in the parents it makes very little difference which method is used; in the children, however, there is a big difference between the results obtained by the two methods. Schulz (1937) has pointed out how comparatively frequently among the "manic-

[2] The figures in these tables should replace those of the provisional communication (4).

TABLE 5.5. FREQUENCY OF VARIOUS DISORDERS IN THE PARENTS OF ALL PROBANDS, ACCORDING TO SEX

Disorder	Fathers				Mothers				Total			
	Cases	BZ	%	σ	Cases	BZ	%	σ	Cases	BZ	%	σ
Hosp. manic-depression (St.)	9	209.40	4.3	1.4	16	208.93	7.7	1.8	25	418.33	6.0	1.2
Hosp. manic-depression (W.)	9	239.91	3.8	1.2	16	232.29	6.8	1.6	25	472.20	5.3	1.0
Manic-depression (St.)	20	209.40	9.6	2.0	28	208.93	13.4	2.3	48	418.33	11.5	1.6
Manic-depression (W.)	20	239.91	8.3	2.7	28	232.29	12.1	2.1	48	472.20	10.2	1.4
Man-dep., ?man-dep., suicide (St.)	35	209.40	16.7	2.6	38	208.93	18.2	2.7	73	418.33	17.5	1.9
Man-dep., ?man-dep., suicide (W.)	35	239.91	14.6	2.2	38	232.29	16.3	2.4	73	472.20	15.5	1.6
Emotionally labile personality	6	252.00	2.4	1.0	8	252.00	3.2	1.1	14	504.00	2.8	0.7
Schizophrenia (St.)	1	251.32	0.4	0.4	3	244.83	1.2	0.7	4	496.15	0.8	0.4
Schizophrenia (W.)	1	251.29	0.4	0.4	3	246.85	1.2	0.7	4	498.14	0.8	0.4
Epilepsy	–	252.00	0.0		3	252.00	1.2		3	504.00	0.6	
GPI	1	238.92	0.4		1	231.29	0.4		2	474.58	0.4	
Arteriosclerosis	–	225.89	0.0		1	210.61	0.5		1	436.50	0.2	
Senile dementia	1	172.01	0.6		1	172.16	0.6		2	344.17	0.6	
Mental illness of unknown nature	9	252.00	3.6		6	252.00	2.4		15	504.00	3.0	
Alcoholism	27	252.00	10.7		1	252.00	0.4		28	504.00	5.6	
Criminality	2	252.00	0.8		–	252.00	0.0		2	504.00	0.4	
Psychopathy	9	252.00	3.6	1.2	6	252.00	2.4	1.0	15	504.00	3.0	0.8

BZ (Bezugsziffer): corrected total
St.: Strömgren method
W.: Weinberg shorter method

TABLE 5.6. FREQUENCY OF VARIOUS DISORDERS IN THE CHILDREN OF "A"- AND "B"-PROBANDS

Disorder	65 "A"-probands			43 "B"-probands		
	Cases	BZ	%	Cases	BZ	%
Hosp. manic-depression (St.)	10	67.92	14.7	2	49.44	4.0
Hosp. manic-depression (W.)	10	116.50	8.6	2	87.50	2.3
Manic-depression (St.)	16	67.92	23.6	10	49.44	20.6
Manic-depression (W.)	16	116.50	13.7	10	87.50	11.4
Man-dep., ?man-dep., suicide (St.)	17	67.92	25.0	14	49.44	28.9
Man-dep., ?man-dep., suicide (W.)	17	116.50	14.6	14	87.50	16.0
Emotionally labile personality	30	194.00	15.5	18	151.00	11.9
Schizophrenia (St.)	2	151.38	1.3	6	115.14	5.2
Schizophrenia (W.)	2	147.13	1.4	6	108.01	5.6
Epilepsy	1	201.00	0.5	–	159.00	0.0
GPI	–	96.00	0.0	1	63.63	1.6
Imbecility	3	201.00	1.5	2	159.00	1.3
Hysteria	1	194.00	0.5	1	151.00	0.7
Criminality	1	194.00	0.5	1	151.00	0.7
Psychopathy	10	194.00	5.2	6	151.00	4.0

BZ (Bezugsziffer): corrected total
St.: Strömgren method
W.: Weinberg shorter method

depressives" which other investigators have found in the family of manic-depressives there are cases who have not been treated, either in the clinic or in the asylum. If one wishes to recognise only hospitalised cases as being certain manic-depressives, the frequency of manic-depressives will have to be estimated much lower. Therefore I have shown the number of "hospitalised" manic-depressives separately and calculated the corresponding frequencies. In addition, it will be clearly seen from the Tables how large the difference is between the figures given by the two methods (W. and St.), when it is a question of a fairly young material.

61

TABLE 5.7. FREQUENCY OF VARIOUS DISORDERS IN THE CHILDREN OF ALL PROBANDS, ACCORDING TO SEX

Disorder	Sons				Daughters				Total			
	Cases	BZ	%	σ	Cases	BZ	%	σ	Cases	BZ	%	σ
Hosp. manic-depression (St.)	2	51.58	3.9	2.6	10	65.78	15.2	4.4	12	117.36	10.2	2.7
Hosp. manic-depression (W.)	2	97.00	2.1	1.5	10	107.00	9.1	2.8	12	204.00	5.9	1.7
Manic-depression (St.)	9	51.58	17.4	5.1	17	65.78	25.8	5.4	26	117.36	22.2	3.8
Manic-depression (W.)	9	97.00	9.3	3.1	17	107.00	15.9	3.4	26	204.00	12.8	2.3
Man-dep., ?man-dep., suicide (St.)	11	51.58	21.3	5.6	20	65.78	30.4	5.5	31	117.36	26.4	4.0
Man-dep., ?man-dep., suicide (W.)	11	97.00	11.3	3.4	20	107.00	18.7	3.6	31	204.00	15.2	2.5
Emotionally labile personality	20	165.00	12.1	2.5	28	180.00	15.6	2.7	48	345.00	13.9	1.9
Schizophrenia (St.)	4	122.24	3.3	1.7	4	134.28	2.9	1.4	8	256.52	3.1	1.1
Schizophrenia (W.)	4	115.71	3.5	1.7	4	139.13	2.9	1.4	8	254.84	3.1	1.1
Epilepsy	–	174.00	0.0		1	186.00	0.5		1	360.00	0.3	
GPI	1	66.13	1.5		–	83.00	0.0		1	149.13	0.7	
Imbecility	4	174.00	2.3		1	186.00	0.5		5	350.00	1.4	
Hysteria	1	165.00	0.6		1	180.00	0.6		2	345.00	0.6	
Criminality	2	165.00	1.2		–	180.00	0.0		2	345.00	0.6	
Psychopathy	6	165.00	3.6	1.4	10	180.00	5.6	1.7	16	345.00	9.3	1.6

BZ (Bezugsziffer): corrected total
St.: Strömgren method
W.: Weinberg shorter method

For other than manic-depressives and schizophrenics I have used exclusively the shorter method in Tables 5.4–5.7, in the manner indicated in Table 5.3.

It is calculated that there are 11.5% manic-depressive psychoses in the parents and 22.2% in the children. There are certain differences here between the "A"- and "B"-probands. Manic-depressive insanity is more frequent and schizophrenia less frequent in the relatives of the "A"-probands than in the relatives of the "B"-probands. These differences I do not consider to be without significance. The manic-depressive psychoses of parents and children show only a limited resemblance to those of the probands. The difference consists mostly in the fact that the relatives fall ill only once, but partly also that their illnesses are not of such a severe character as those of the probands. This is quite understandable; for our probands represent a selection of clinic cases and furthermore such clinic cases as have had multiple illnesses.

The high frequency of manic-depressive insanity which is obtained in the children, using the Strömgren method, may seem somewhat doubtful. It is to be noted that the cases used by me for calculating the proportion of the risk period (Table 5.1) lived through were all hospitalised cases. It is just possible that cases who are hospitalised in the older age groups could have been diagnosed when younger; for this reason the control material used by me is perhaps little suited for calculating the frequency of non-hospitalised cases.

In order to examine this, I considered it appropriate to make a further calculation by means of the morbidity-table method. The results obtained are shown in Table 5.8.

From the Table the product of all the figures of column h can be calculated; it is 0.8030; accordingly, the probability of falling ill is 19.70%. This figure agrees not badly with that of 22.2% obtained by the Strömgren method. Certainly it may be objected that calculation by the morbidity-table method is not reliable either; for, as already mentioned, my material is far too small for this kind of calculation, particularly in the older age groups. If, for example, the two latest secondary cases to fall ill

TABLE 5.8. MORBIDITY TABLE: CHILDREN OF MANIC-DEPRESSIVES

a	b	c	d	e	f	g	h
0–14	491	134	–	134	424.0	424.0	1.0000
15–19	357	13	3	16	350.5	347.5	0.9913
20–24	341	39	6	45	321.5	315.5	0.9813
25–29	296	46	4	50	273.0	269.0	0.9854
30–34	246	54	3	57	219.0	216.0	0.9865
35–39	189	58	3	61	160.0	157.0	0.9813
40–44	128	37	3	40	109.5	106.5	0.9725
45–49	88	30	2	32	73.0	71.0	0.9727
50–54	56	26	–	26	43.0	43.0	1.0000
55–59	30	13	2	15	23.5	21.5	0.9147
over 59	13	13	–	13	6.5	6.5	1.0000

a = age
b = total non-manic-depressives remaining
c = disappeared from observation, or became schizophrenic*
d = onset of manic-depression
e = sum of c and d
f = observed for manic-depressive illness
g = remained well
h = proportion of those remaining well to those observed

*Among those disappearing from observation I have included persons who became schizophrenic as I consider it justified to assume that anyone who has become schizophrenic can no longer become manic-depressive and is consequently fully observed in respect of his becoming or not becoming manic-depressive.

had fallen ill 5 years earlier, the morbidity rate would have been 15.9% instead of 19.7%. In spite of this, the morbidity table agrees more closely with the Strömgren than with the shorter method.

COMPARISON WITH OTHER STUDIES OF
THE RELATIVES OF MANIC-DEPRESSIVES

I considered it of some interest to compare the findings of Röll and Entres (1936) with mine. For this purpose I have recalculated their findings according to the Strömgren method (Table 5.9).

With the aid of the formula

$$SD_{diff.} = \sqrt{SD_1{}^2 + SD_2{}^2}$$

we wish to see whether there are any statistically significant differences between the percentages found by me and by Röll and Entres. Only when the difference is twice as large as its standard error can it be concluded that there is a statistically significant difference. In the table there is apparently only one place where this could be the case, the frequency of schizophrenia in the female children; here the ratio is slightly larger than 2 and so not necessarily statistically significant. Accordingly the conclusion is justified that there is no essential difference between the two studies, either in the material or in the method of calculation (particularly in the method of assessing the secondary cases). Any actual differences in one or other respect should then balance one another. It must therefore be admitted that my attempt to pick out a genotypically especially pure and delimited group has completely failed. This argues that the probands selected by me from an especially strict point of view are entirely equivalent to the totality of manic-depressives in respect of their genetic constitution.

TABLE 5.9. COMPARISON OF PRESENT FINDINGS WITH THOSE OF RÖLL AND ENTRES

	Men				Women				Total			
	Cases	BZ	%	SD	Cases	BZ	%	SD	Cases	BZ	%	SD
			Manic-depressive insanity									
Parents:												
Röll and Entres (St.)	5	69.54	7.2	3.1	11	71.19	15.5	4.3	16	130.73	12.2	2.9
Slater (St.)	20	209.40	9.6	2.0	28	208.93	13.4	2.3	48	418.33	11.5	1.6
Röll and Entres (W.)											10.4	
Slater (W.)											10.2	
Sibs:												
Röll and Entres (St.)	11	120.92	9.1	2.6	15	114.50	13.1	3.2	26	235.42	11.1	2.0
Röll and Entres (W.)											9.1	
Nephews and nieces:												
Röll and Entres (St.)	5	119.20	4.2	1.8	4	130.28	3.1	1.5	9	249.49	3.6	1.2
Röll and Entres (W.)											2.3	
Children:												
Röll and Entres (St.)	4	29.30	13.7	6.3	4	24.01	16.7	7.6	8	53.31	15.0	4.9
Slater (St.)	9	51.58	17.4	5.1	17	65.78	25.8	5.4	26	117.36	22.2	3.8
Röll and Entres (W.)											9.5	
Slater (W.)											12.8	
			Schizophrenia									
Parents:												
Röll and Entres (St.)	–	62.22	0.0	0.0	1	61.98	1.6	1.6	1	124.20	0.8	0.8
Slater (St.)	1	251.32	0.4	0.4	3	244.83	1.2	0.7	4	496.15	0.8	0.4
Children:												
Röll and Entres (St.)	2	64.73	3.1	2.2	–	46.11	0.0	0.0	2	110.84	1.8	1.3
Slater (St.)	4	122.24	3.3	1.7	4	134.28	2.9	1.4	8	256.52	3.1	1.1

I should very much have liked to recalculate Hoffmann's (1921) manic-depressive material here. From the clinical statements of Hoffmann it is clear that he assessed secondary cases completely differently from Röll and Entres and myself. Hoffmann has included a whole lot of secondary cases as manic-depressive which I would have regarded at most as psychopaths with mood swings. It would therefore be essential to rediagnose these cases with the aid of the somewhat scanty clinical statements provided, which I did not feel able to do. The very interesting work of Weinberg and Lobstein (1936) reports data on Jewish patients which may not necessarily be comparable. According to the latter authors the corrected percentage of manic-depressives in the parents and children of their probands (shorter method) was 9.2% and 4.8% or 7.6%. These figures are not comparable with those of Röll and Entres and myself in regard to either the material or the statistical method. A corresponding recalculation on the basis of absolute figures did not appear to be justified on account of the different kind of tabular presentation in the work of Weinberg and Lobstein.

EXPECTANCY OF MANIC-DEPRESSIVE INSANITY
IN THE GENERAL POPULATION

The expectancy of manic-depressive psychosis in the general population has so far been calculated by the shorter method. I have therefore recalculated the material of the papers mentioned below according to the Strömgren method. In these papers a population totalling 4,368 men and 4,407 women is available, all over 10 years of age, including 5 male and 6 female manic-depressives. According to the Strömgren method the BZ is 1379.08 men and 1511.74 women. Accordingly, the frequency of manic-depressive insanity is:

Men	0.3626%	±	0.1619%
Women	0.3969%	±	0.1617%
Total	0.3805%	±	0.1145%

One can therefore say that the frequency of manic-depressive psychoses in the parents, sibs, and children is 30–60 times as great as in the general population. The authors of the papers from which the population material has been obtained, and the volumes of the *Zeitschrift für Neurologie* in which they appeared, are as follows:

Kattentidt, 103; Schulz, 109; Luxenburger, 112; Goeppel, 113; Wolf, 117; Magg, 119; Schulz, 136; Bleuler, 142; Brugger, 145; Klemperer, 146; Berlit, 152; Boeters, H., 153; Bleuler and Rapoport, 153; Panse, 154; Boeters, D., 155; Bormann, 159; and Dittel, *Zeitschrift für menschliche Vererbungslehre*, 20.

RELATIONSHIP BETWEEN MANIC-DEPRESSIVE INSANITY AND SCHIZOPHRENIA

From the present provisional results of family research, it can be said that manic-depressive insanity shows no statistical relationship to other psychoses or mental anomalies with the single exception of schizophrenia. The nature of the relationship to schizophrenia, if such exists at all, remains completely unclear. It has been maintained that schizophrenic ancestors, in particular schizophrenic parents, quite exceptionally rarely appear in the families of manic-depressives, while on the other hand schizophrenic children of manic-depressives are said not to be a rarity. The first supposition appears to be unjustified according to the present material. Among the parents of the probands of Röll and Entres there was one schizophrenic parent (frequency 0.8%), among the parents of my material 4 schizophrenics (frequency 0.8%). These figures correspond approximately to the frequency of schizophrenia in the general population (about 0.8%), and lie only slightly above the frequency among parents in the general population, which amounts to 0.5%. On the other hand, the frequency of schizophrenia in the children according to Röll and Entres is 1.8%, according to me 3.1%. These figures are somewhat high, but their statistical significance is slight. Weinberg and Lobstein have emphasized the frequency of schizophrenia in the nephews and nieces of their manic-depressives and discussed the whole-question of the connection between both psychoses. In their opinion the predisposition to manic-depressive psychoses is said to exercise an activating effect on the predisposition to schizophrenia. A similar opinion was expressed by me in an earlier paper (4). Such speculations, however, appear to me now to be unjustified; for in the first place the figures are too small to possess much statistical significance, and secondly it seems to me probable that faulty diagnosis may partly have had something to do with it. In other words, the possibility cannot be excluded that the true genotype and the phenotypical clinical picture do not completely coincide. In my material I found that the frequency of schizophrenia occurs much more rarely when the manic-depressive starting cases are so carefully checked that even the mildest atypical symptoms are excluded. Naturally this could also mean that the presence of a predisposition to schizophrenia could express itself in an atypical colouring of an actual manic-depressive psychosis.

In this connection we are also interested in the question how far schizophrenic psychoses which occur in the relatives of manic-depressives show an atypical colouring. On this point my material may not provide very much information. Among the parents and children I found a total of 13 schizophrenics.[3] Out of 4 schizophrenic parents of probands and 9 schizophrenic children, 3 parents and 5 children showed distinct manic-depressive features. Nevertheless, the diagnosis of schizophrenia was not in doubt.

ON THE MODE OF INHERITANCE OF
MANIC-DEPRESSIVE INSANITY

On the basis of my own and all other data published in the literature there is nothing that can be said with certainty about the mode of inheritance of manic-depressive insanity. I have discussed this problem in my earlier publications and assessed the reasons why I think it unjustified to exclude simple dominance. These reasons are a matter of course in present-day genetic research. Today we hardly any longer expect that family research will provide unambiguous Mendelian ratios. The part which environment and the genotypic milieu play along with the specific genetic factor needs no emphasis. It only remains to discover to what extent these factors are of importance in manic-depressive insanity. Only if we have established that environmental influences and those of the genotypic milieu are themselves insufficient to explain why the observed figures fall below the theoretically expected Mendelian figures need serious consideration be given to two- or three-gene or other such polymeric theories. It is of importance to keep in mind that with the existence of numerous statistical and practical sources of error over-complex hypotheses such as that of Rosanoff *et al.* (1935) are premature.

I mention Rosanoff here in particular because he and his colleagues have attempted to establish the theory of an additional sex-linked factor in order to account for the fact that the female sex is more often affected with the illness than the male. Rüdin (1923) long ago pointed out how frequently suicide in male relatives of manic-depressives seems to be a substitute for the psychosis. Weinberg and Lobstein have also discussed this question in detail and come to the conclusion that the excess of females is an artefact. In the general population material used here there is only a small and statistically non-significant difference shown between the frequencies of manic-depressives (not necessarily hospitalised) in the two sexes.

According to the theory of Rosanoff a dominant autosomal "cyclothymic" factor C must be combined with a dominant sex-linked "activating" factor A before the illness can appear. From the 6 different male and 9 different female genotypes, the results of 54 possible matings may be worked out, all of which are shown by Rosanoff. This theory naturally requires a doubled frequency of manic-depressive psychoses in women as opposed to men, which is not found empirically. However, the theory can be tested in another way. Under conditions of panmixia and an approximately equal frequency of the genes A and C, it can be calculated that the frequency of these genes must be in the neighborhood of 0.03–0.04 in order to give a frequency of 0.0036–0.0039 manic-depressives in the general population. Accordingly all homozygotes will be very rare. Of the matings producing manic-depressives, only Rosanoff's types 24, 26, 27, 28, 32, 41, 47, 49 and 50 will be

---

[3] Case descriptions of the illnesses in these families which appeared in the original publication have been omitted. – *Editors*.

comparatively frequent. It would also be expected that male probands could have affected mothers but hardly ever affected fathers, and female probands affected fathers and mothers in approximately equal proportions. Similarly, male probands would mainly produce affected daughters, female probands affected sons as well as daughters with perhaps a slight excess of affected daughters. In other words, the findings would resemble those of simple sex-linked dominance. My material provides the following data (Table 5.10):

TABLE 5.10. SEX OF PROBAND AND SEX OF AFFECTED RELATIVE

	Parents		Children	
	Male	Female	Male	Female
Probands:				
Male	10	7	4	4
Female	14	19	4	13

From this it can be seen how little my data fit such a hypothesis.

SUMMARY

1. A special group of recurrent manic-depressives was selected and an investigation made into the mental attributes of their parents and children.

2.[4] The causes of death in these families show a clearly raised frequency of arteriopathic diseases.

3.[4] The occupations and social class of the three generations show no clear drop.

4. The *Bezugsziffer* (BZ) has been calculated by the Strömgren method in addition to the "shorter method" of Weinberg. The main period of risk for falling ill with manic-depressive insanity is shown to lie between the ages of 30 and 60.

5. The frequency of manic-depressives in the parents and children of the probands is found to be 11.5% and 22.2% respectively. When doubtful manic-depressives and suicides are included, the figures are raised, calculated according to the Strömgren method, to 17.5% for the parents and 26.4% for the children. The corresponding figures for schizophrenia are 0.8% and 3.1%. A morbidity table for the children gives a manic-depressive frequency of 19.7%. The figures are comparable with those of Röll and Entres.

6. Data on the general population collected from the literature gives a frequency according to the Strömgren method of 0.36% manic-depressives in men, 0.40% in women, 0.38% in both sexes together.

7. Various hypotheses as to the relation of the psychosis to schizophrenia, the mode of inheritance, etc., are briefly discussed. The theory of an additional sex-linked factor can be excluded with a fair degree of certainty.

---

[4] Section omitted. See editorial comment, p. 54. — *Editors*.

EDITORS' COMMENTS: Two theoretical papers in German stemmed indirectly from the above work. In 1939 Shrimpton and Slater (15) addressed themselves to the problem of calculating the standard error of the morbid risk obtained by Weinberg's morbidity-table method. A formula was devised and applied to the recently published data of Kallmann (1938) on the children of schizophrenics. A drawback to the method is that a large material is required, in which the smallest age groups in which the condition occurs with any appreciable frequency are adequately represented, before the method can be properly applied. As was noted, this was unfortunately not the case in Slater's manic-depressive material, relatively large though it was.

The other German paper (13), though not directly connected with his manic-depressive study, may be mentioned here. This was Slater's contribution to a volume in honour of Ernst Rüdin, director of the Munich Institute, and it took the form of a critique of the concept of the "probability of manifestation" of a gene and its application. He stressed its dependence on hereditary and environmental influences which will differ from one group to another, and was particularly critical of the use of a theoretical estimate of manifestation probability derived from the provisional results in series of MZ twins, applied as if it was a universal attribute of the gene.

When Slater himself returned to the problem of the genetics of the affective disorders, it was in the context of his own twin study (63). Twin probands with affective illnesses were rare in his sample. As will be seen later (Paper 9) there were only 38 cases of which only 23 were typical manic-depressives. In the total group of affective disorders about 14% of the parents, 9% of the sibs, 29% of the 30 DZ co-twins and 57% of the 8 MZ co-twins were affected (shorter Weinberg method). No opinion was expressed in the monograph on mode of inheritance, manifestation rate or possible heterogeneity. There was no excess of schizophrenia in the relatives of the affectively ill probands. However, Slater found an incidence of affective illness of around 5% in the first degree relatives of his schizophrenic probands. These were not as a rule typical manic-depressives but tended rather to be cases of involutional depression.

Current trends in diagnosis and the readier recognition of milder forms of endogenous affective disorders, some of them probably related to the older Kraepelinian concept of manic-depressive insanity, led to higher estimates of incidence in the population than that of 0.4% by Slater and other pre-war workers. Stenstedt (1959) places it at around 1% for manic-depressive illness and 3% for all endogenous affective disorders. Theories involving some degree of polygenic inheritance or heterogeneity of one kind or another have been put forward. As he states in the *Retrospect* (page 378), Slater himself no longer considers it likely that a single dominant gene accounts for all endogenous affective disorder. Nevertheless, Slater's pioneer work is still much cited; and a general order of morbid risk of around 15%, depending on the nature of the starting cases and the risk period used in correcting for age, is still found for first degree relatives by most recent investigators in this field. Some still believe that, whatever else may be involved, there is at least a nucleus of cases, perhaps the bipolar psychoses, in which there is a strong element of dominant transmission from parent to child.

III

SCHIZOPHRENIA

EDITORS' COMMENTS: In this — the longest — section of the book all nine papers are devoted to one or another of the genetic aspects of schizophrenia. They are presented in chronological order. The following comments relate the papers to one another and to the rest of Slater's work.

It is appropriate that before tackling aetiology *per se* Slater should first have written about the frequency and natural history of the disorder. In 1935, his first published paper (1) grappled with the task of estimating the incidence of various forms of mental disorder in the general population. Slater was forced to rely on mental hospital statistics couched in such antiquated terms as contusional insanity, non-systematised delusional insanity, and primary dementia. His final figures for the incidence (life-time expectancy) of schizophrenia were 0.53% in men and 0.48% in women; these he considered were probably under-estimates. In 1939 (14) he collaborated with Guttmann and Mayer-Gross in a three-year follow-up study of an untreated but prognostically favourable group of 188 schizophrenics from the Maudsley Hospital in order to obtain a baseline for the assessment of the results of physical methods of treatment such as insulin and ECT, which were then coming into use. Of this group 41% were in mental hospital at the end of the period and 50% were invalids either at home or in hospital. Over one-third had made total or social recoveries. Outcome was generally better in women than men. This study proved useful when later workers at the Maudsley came to assess the results of treatment (Hoenig, 1967). Not only did patients treated in 1949–50 with physical methods do better than the 1934–35 cohort of Guttmann *et al.*, but patients who did not have these treatments did better too.

Slater's first project on the genetics of schizophrenia was, as described in his autobiographical sketch, his now classical twin study (63), which eventually appeared in 1953. The first to be published, however, was the frequently cited case report of schizophrenia in uniovular (i.e. monozygotic) twins reared apart (Paper 6). The co-author of this paper, W. H. Craike, at present at Paddington Clinic and Day Hospital in London, has subsequently worked mostly as a consultant in child psychiatry and juvenile delinquency. They were assisted by George Burden, psychiatric social worker, who is now Secretary General of the International Bureau for Epilepsy. We have not suggested altering the term *folie à deux* in the title, although it is nowadays usually restricted to persons who are not genetically related. The case was certainly of sufficient interest to merit publication. One could not be sure at the time whether the conclusions suggested would hold in a representative series. However, subsequent findings in series of MZ twins not selected for concordance or for having been reared apart show that this pair is not exceptional (121, 131). Furthermore, foster child studies (Heston, 1966; Kety *et al.*, 1968; and Rosenthal *et al.*, 1968) reveal no tendency for the absence of schizophrenia in the rearing family to decrease the already high probability of the biological relative of a schizophrenic becoming psychiatrically abnormal.

If genetic factors contribute to the aetiology of a psychiatric disorder, one of the tasks of genetics is, as Slater put it in 1936 (5), to come to the aid of clinical psychiatry by "the clearing up of the clinical picture into the essential features which are directly dependent on the hereditary factor in question, and the inessential features as they are introduced into the picture either as the manifestation of other accidentally present hereditary factors or as a result of the influence of the environment." His analyses of Zehnder's data (Paper 7), of Bleuler's data in his 1944 review (26), and of his own data (Paper 9) were largely devoted to this latter task in respect of schizophrenia. Ødegaard (1963) and Tsuang (1967) have also tried to throw light on this still intractable problem.

The 1953 twin study, or at least that part of it which deals with schizophrenia, has been discussed in detail and from various points of view, by Jackson, Rosenthal, and ourselves among others. (Jackson, 1960; Rosenthal, 1959, 1962a; and Gottesman and Shields, 1966a). One major advantage of the study was that it presented its findings in such a way as to make re-analysis possible. Another advantage was that it included all twins in a particular sample, whatever their diagnosis, and not just those with typical textbook diagnoses of particular kinds. Rather more than half the 297 probands were schizophrenic. The report consists of 385 pages, 24 of which are appendices and 271 pages of case history material. Inevitably, if regrettably, we can only include an abridged version, but consider this preferable to omitting it altogether since the monograph is not readily available. We present an edited version of the section which describes the methods of investigation and some general results from the study as a whole. The section on the schizophrenic twins is reproduced virtually in full. The sections on the smaller groups with affective, organic, and psychopathic or neurotic diagnoses are in effect restricted to the Summary and Conclusions. Appendices and case histories have had to be omitted, together with the introductory section on twin investigations in psychiatry up to that time.

The 1953 report concluded that *genetic causes provided a potentiality for schizophrenia, perhaps an essential one.* It did not discuss the mode of inheritance. Paper 8 gives Slater's opinion on this subject as he then saw it. The likelihood of aetiological heterogeneity is stressed both here and in a paper on the offspring of consanguineous marriages (79). In subsequent papers he attempted to isolate some of the distinct causes of schizophrenic symptomatology. Those that could be identified with varying degrees of certainty were either rare, such as the schizophrenic-like psychoses associated with epilepsy (Paper 12) or very rare (Paper 11). The co-authors of these papers were colleagues at the National Hospital. Dr. Beard is currently a consultant psychiatrist at the Middlesex Hospital, London. Mr. Glithero, a psychiatric social worker, is now Deputy Chief Social Work Officer in the Department of Health and Social Security, and Dr. Zilkha a consultant neurologist at King's College Hospital. The so-called psychogenic schizophrenias (Paper 13) Slater also considered to be rare. A heterogeneity theory, with an unspecified number and distribution of subtypes for schizophrenia is, however, an unsatisfactory conception in many ways. In 1958 in an important paper he put forward the hypothesis of a single partially dominant gene as the essential cause of most schizophrenias (Paper 10). He has since applied the theory in different ways (137, 140, 142), either assuming a higher estimate of the frequency in the general population or using pooled data for the frequency of schizophrenia in relatives, and extending the theory to include second-degree relatives. The effect of these modifications has been to reduce even further the proportion of heterozygotes who will manifest schizophrenia (26% according to the original version) to 13% or even lower. Since 1958 a theory of polygenic inheritance with a threshold effect (Edwards, 1960; and Gottesman and Shields, 1967) has become a serious contender for anyone who wishes to put forward a unifying hypothesis, and in a forthcoming chapter on schizophrenia (142) Slater is concerned with methods of deciding which of the two theories predicts consequences which are closest to the best currently available data. Paper 24 presents one such method and on page 260 we refer to his first attempts to apply it.

As editor of the *British Journal of Psychiatry* Slater commissioned from Hans Kind, a colleague of Manfred Bleuler, a review of the literature on the *psycho*genesis of schizophrenia. This was published in the *Journal* in 1966 and was later selected to appear in the *International Journal of Psychiatry* where it was discussed by Slater among others; that discussion forms the final chapter in this Section. As in a previous discussion of Bleuler's views (110), Slater, while agreeing with Kind that we should abandon a "one-sided and barren either-or" view of schizophrenia, strongly deprecated any playing down of the positive conclusions drawn from genetical research. He could see no reason why in future we should abandon investigations conducted along specifically genetical *or* environmental lines.

6

FOLIE À DEUX IN UNIOVULAR TWINS
REARED APART

INTRODUCTION

Uniovular twins who have been separated in the earliest years of infancy and have been brought up apart from one another are phenomena of great scientific interest. Owing to their uniovularity, both members of such a pair have identical hereditary equipment, and any differences between them must be attributed to environmental influences. Most twins are brought up in the same home, and thereby come under the same sort of education and training, and under very similar influences from parents, brothers and sisters, and comrades. They are therefore likely to be more like one another than hereditary factors alone would ensure. Furthermore, the psychological relationship of one uniovular twin to the other is of a peculiarly intimate and, as a rule, affectionate kind; so that when they are brought up together they are likely each to influence the development of the other. The mutual relationship and the similarities of environmental influence do not hold in cases where the twins have been separated in early years, and we then see a controlled experiment of nature in an almost pure form. Unfortunately, uniovular twins who have been separated in infancy are exceedingly rare. After intensive search extending over many years, Newman, Freeman, and Holzinger were only able to discover in the whole of the U.S.A. nineteen such pairs, which they have reported at length (1937). None of their pairs had any mental illness and, as far as we know, the case here reported is unique in the literature.

The twins here described were separated at the age of 9 months, were brought up in different families in different parts of the country, met each other for the first time at the age of 24, never lived together or had any close contact with one another, but each in due course developed a paranoid psychosis, each involving the other in her own system of delusional ideas. It is this mutual involvement in a

By W. H. Craike and E. Slater, with the assistance of George Burden. Originally published in *Brain* 68: 213–21 (1945).

paranoid system which suggested the title of "folie à deux," although the possibility that the psychosis of either "induced" that of the other has, we think, to be rejected.

The first member of the pair to appear was Florence. She was referred to the Maudsley Hospital Out-Patient Department from the Observation Ward of Fulham Hospital by Dr. Alexander Walk, to whom our thanks are due. She was there examined by both of us, and her twin was eventually contacted and examined in her own home (by W. H. C.). Attempts were made to get information from external sources about the twins. All the relatives are dead, and the Children's Home, where Edith was brought up, was closed years ago. Contact was, however, made with Edith's employers, as will later appear.

HISTORY

The father of the twins was a farmer in South Wales, but after the death of the mother he sold the farm and became a coal-miner, and later married again. He was at first an irreligious man, but was converted by his second wife. They used to "live in church" on Sundays, and he became a Sunday-school teacher. Edith says he was a very violent man and drank heavily. She lived with him until she was 8½, and was terrified of him. There were always family scenes, and she still bears on her head a scar where he cut her with a razor. Of the mother nothing is known except that she died about the age of 35, nine months after the birth of the twins. There was a boy born previously, who was about 5 at the birth of the twins, but he is said to have run away from home and to have died in 1914, when he would have been 27.

Immediately after the death of the mother, Florence was adopted by an unmarried maternal aunt and went to live in her home. Edith stayed on with her father, to lead a miserable childhood. She walked in her sleep, as a child, and before her first confession, which she dreaded, had nightmares of being flogged. About the age of 8½, her father put her into a Children's Home, where she lived until she was 19. She did quite well at school, and says she reached the top standard (VII) two years before leaving school at 15½. She then started working on a farm, but developed "nervous dyspepsia and anaemia," and was in Cardiff Workhouse at 20. Her father took her back into his home from the workhouse, but soon told her to get out, and she ran away to live with an uncle. During all this time she had known of the existence of her twin, but had never met her or corresponded with her. She says, however, that even when she was living with her father, Florence was making trouble for her by writing to her father and telling him Edith had told her that he was a drunkard. From Wales Edith came to London to seek employment. Her uncle paid her fare, but Edith says Florence claims that she paid it and that Edith is under an obligation to her. Edith first met her sister when they were 24. A little money had been left them by an aunt, and the solicitor got in touch with both of them. Even at this first meeting Florence accused her of stealing a ten-shilling note from her purse, quite untruly; the only money Edith ever stole was from her father when she was living with him. The sisters saw a little of one another, but could not get on. Florence used to spy on her and write anonymous letters to her employers. About this time Edith saw Florence in the street on a bicycle with a man; she recognized her, because she was wearing a yellow velour hat, and knew she was spying on her.

Edith continued to live in London, working as a domestic. She has excellent references from her employers, and seems to have been of quiet, reserved disposition, with few friends, but hard-working and of stable mood. She has always been keenly religious and an Anglo-Catholic. Her last employer, who kept her for eleven years until 1940, reports that she had to get rid of her in the end because of her delusionary ideas, "which led her to believe that not only her own friends and relations but practically everyone who visited the house accused her of wrong doing. Apart from these ideas she was an excellent woman in the house, perfectly honest, willing, trustworthy and possessed of a kindly disposition. . . . The two sisters did not see much of each other and when they did meet they could never agree. Edith always gave me to understand that when Florence did call to see her it was to seek financial help." After this, Edith was directed to a glass factory. The Welfare Officer there says that she is very good at her work, and though the firm is cutting down staff, she would be kept as long as she wanted to stay. She seems quite happy there, but has lately suggested that she would like her release to become a nun. The only thing odd about her is that from time to time she asks to see him and inquires whether people are talking about her, and whether she is causing any trouble.

During these latter years, Edith has continued to have reason to complain of Florence's behaviour. As recently as November, 1944, she has seen Florence watching her house. She thinks she must be jealous. She has had a very hard struggle, everybody has been against her, and she has lost many good jobs in domestic service. All this is entirely due to the influence of Florence.

Florence was brought up by her mother's sister, and made her home with her until her death in 1944 at 85. She was very happy with her. Her childhood was happy, though she was rather nervous and frightened of the dark; she did not walk in her sleep and remembers no nightmares. She attended an ordinary elementary school where she was rather backward, leaving at 14 from the third standard from the top (IV). This was partly due to missing a lot of schooling because of fainting attacks. She says she has picked up a lot afterwards from reading. After school she got a post as a children's nursemaid. She took some of her employer's soap, and was charged with the theft and put into a convent for two years. While there she was happy. Ever since then she has worked as a domestic, and has risen as high as head housemaid. She has had regular employment, and in intervals between jobs has stayed with her aunt. About the age of 18 she had an attack of "nervous debility," with symptoms of abdominal pain, vomiting and nerviness. She went to stay with another aunt in Wales and recovered. Apart from that she has had no nervous trouble in the past. She describes herself as of quiet but cheerful disposition, always of much the same mood, not inclined to be suspicious, and with many friends. She was very religious in her youth, especially at the time of her confirmation at 16; she kept up going to Communion for many years, but has been less regular and interested "since I've been like this." In 1916 her aunt died, from whom the money came, and in 1917 the money was divided between her and Edith, whom she then met for the first time. She noticed at once how like they were, and rather took a fancy to her. She met her sister twice more, and then the letters began. Out of the blue, Edith wrote her several letters accusing her of spying. About that time a fellow servant at her place of employment, who had been reproved by Florence, said to her, "You think a lot of yourself, but you've been to prison." Florence thinks that it must have been through Edith that knowledge of her being charged for theft in the past had got around. It was about that time that Edith wrote to her, "Why do you come down on the back of Alf's bike spying on me? I know it's you because of your lemon hat and brown coat." There was no more trouble until years later. About three-and-half years ago, "people said they knew all about me. They (the staff) said, 'Why don't you get married? That's what's the matter with you.' " "There was a general undercurrent." "It was after I knew her that all this started, and I began to wonder whether it was her. She must have been spreading rumours about me. But you can't accuse people unless you're absolutely sure." About a year ago Florence met Edith again. "We spent one or two nice week-ends. I mentioned I had a chance of two rooms and should we take them. She said no, she wanted me to keep away. She accused me that Sunday of going to neighbours saying she was mental."

On 27.12.44 Florence was admitted to the Observation Ward. The notes there read:

> Admitted. Physically n.a.d. Mentally very depressed, weeps and sobs copiously as she tells of all the undercurrent against her. People say she is mad, she is mental, they throw up at her all her past life. She is determined to get at the bottom of it. Only once did she actually catch a voice, a man's voice, saying horrible things. 29.12.44: Seen by magistrate. Continues to complain of some undercurrent going on against her. 6.1.45: Improved, still some depression but not so worried by delusional ideas. Seen by Dr. Walk who notes: depressed and preoccupied, although she says she feels much happier under care. Only one remark has been passed about her since admission, but there were plenty before. . . . She says that among other things the voices have told her that she is mental, they have accused her of having been in prison.

Florence continued to improve, and shortly after having been sent for examination to the Maudsley Hospital she was sufficiently well to be allowed home.

FINDINGS ON EXAMINATION

Physically: The twins had to be examined separately, as they could not be induced to meet. Edith was interviewed in her own home, Florence at the Maudsley. Physically, there were no abnormal findings other than a slight degree of deafness, probably due to otosclerosis. Florence stated that she began to go deaf about three years ago, and had been examined at the West London Hospital. Inquiries at that hospital showed that no one of her name had attended in the E.N.T. Department during that time. As Edith refused under any circumstances to have her ears examined, it was not thought worth while pursuing the matter. Florence states that her twin is not the least deaf, and that Edith has accused her of not being deaf herself but pretending it. Actually both twins are of about the same degree of deafness, needing no instrument but hearing well with some raising of the voice.

Both twins are of middle height, and of dumpy pyknic build, with broad face and slightly cleft chin, broad-based retroussé nose, and a suggestion of widow's peak in the hair-line over a high rounded forehead. In both hair is abundant, a dark brown with streaks of grey, eyes grey with some brownish flecks. The voices are extremely alike, and listening to either one might imagine the other was speaking.

Comparison of the finger-prints shows the following pattern types and ridge counts (count to radial triradius given first; W, whorl; DL, double loop; UL, ulnar loop):

Florence:	R. 1. W	18, 25	2. UL	15	3. UL	18	4. UL 17	5. UL 19
	L. 1. DL	13,21	2. UL	14	3. UL	16	4. UL 17	5. UL 15
Edith:	R. 1. W	18,24	2. W	14, 13	3. UL	16	4. UL 13	5. UL 17
	L. 1. W	16,20	2. UL	13	3. UL	14	4. W 20,6	5. UL 15.

These prints show a closer similarity between the twins than between their right and left sides. The Florence-Edith product-moment correlation coefficient is +0.84, the right- left correlation coefficient is +0.82.

General appearance and bodily constitution are in favour of uniovularity; there is a striking facial resemblance between the twins, in addition to general conformity of build and colouring. There are no points of physical discrepancy. The degree of similarity of the finger-prints is practically conclusive of uniovularity.

Mentally: When seen at the Maudsley Hospital on 8.1.45, Florence still had feelings of an undercurrent against her, and said she had heard opprobrious remarks being passed, but was unwilling to go into detail. She thought the undercurrent was Edith's work; Edith had been accusing her for many years. She was slightly suspicious and reserved, but there was no marked degree of depression and affective rapport was good. There was no evidence of any shallowness of affect or of any bizarre quality, nor of any schizophrenic features in attitude, expression or motor behaviour. She did not appear to be hallucinated. Intellectually she was well preserved. She was seen for a second time on 29.1.45. She was then back at work and feeling very well, which she attributed to taking a course of "sanatogen." She said she had neither seen nor heard further sign of the "undercurrent." She was seen for a third time on 16.7.45, and then showed no abnormal sign at all. She was working at a hospital as a domestic, but did not like it and did not feel she could go on doing it, although she got on all right with the others. She had met Edith the week before Easter, and remarked that her sister seemed nervous of her.

Edith was examined in January, 1945, at home. She was found to be living in one room in an old Victorian house converted into flatlets. She gave the history in quite co-operative manner, but during the interview became very emotional and tearful. She was seen again on 18.2.45, when the finger-prints were taken. She was very suspicious of these proceedings. She said that when she first came to her flat the other boarders in the house avoided her; they had since become more friendly, but now they avoided her again, because she is no good. One of the men in the house had told her to get away, because the police were after her. The police are checking up on how much she earns and spends, although she has done no wrong. The police car stops outside her house every night, and they are watching her. Last year someone in the house next door committed suicide, and that house and the one in which she lives were full of police, and there was a policeman stationed outside. They were watching her. Her sister may be connected with all this, because she has told Edith's employers that Edith is immoral and has an illegitimate child, which is not true. Edith was seen for a third time on 16.6.45. She said she had seen Florence in March, meeting her by chance in a Boots in Ealing on the way to Church. At first she did not recognize her, she looked so well. Florence was very annoyed with her, and accused her of having said she was mad; this, Florence said, was not true, because she had been discharged from hospital on 12.1.45 and had not returned again. The whole of this was news to Edith. The two sisters went to Church together, but Florence took no part in the Service, did not speak again, and "took to her heels" on leaving. Edith does not know what she was doing in Ealing, and presumes she was spying again. The general undercurrent against Edith continues; someone is prying into her affairs, and she suspects it is Florence. She has never seen any of the letters about her, but has learned of them in roundabout ways. She recently went to St. Bernard's Hospital to apply for a job, but declined it because she was upset by the patients she saw. Now people are saying she has been a patient in the Asylum. Edith also complains she has been having "very severe turns" in which she falls like a log. They began on Easter Monday, are becoming more frequent, and are leading to absence from work. This has aroused a lot of comment. In these later interviews Edith was inclined to be suspicious and reserved, but there were no characteristic schizophrenic symptoms. Intellectually she was well preserved, but probably of low average intelligence.

COMMENT

These uniovular twins were brought up along entirely different lines. Florence had a stable home with an affectionate maternal aunt, and has lived with her all her life until a year ago. Edith lived with a drunken and violent father of whom she was terrified, and was put into an institution from 8½ till 19, and since 20 has lived on her own. Nevertheless their careers bear very striking resemblances. Both were nervous as children; Edith walked in her sleep and had nightmares, Florence had fainting attacks and was nervous of the dark. Both stole as children or adolescents, Edith from her father, Florence from her employer; in the paranoid state which each subsequently developed, stealing enters into the delusional content. The school careers are said to be very different, Edith reaching the top standard, Florence only the fourth. But the intelligences of the twins when adult are probably about the same, and the different success at school is probably due to adventitious circumstances. Edith at the age of 19 and Florence at 18 had some form of gastric disturbance, accompanied by indications of a neurotic aspect, which in each case passed off rapidly. Both went into domestic service. Neither married, though Florence says Edith was once engaged. A sexual element enters later into the delusions of both; Edith thinks she is accused of having an illegitimate child, Florence says people have hinted she is sex-starved. Their personalities are very similar, although on the whole Florence is the more open, sociable and conciliatory of the two; both are religious, Edith the more so. Both have got gradually deaf, and both imply that the other merely pretends it. Paranoid symptoms appear in each about the same time, soon after their first meeting. In the case of Edith, there is a suggestion of a still earlier onset, but this may be due to a falsification of memory. From the first Edith directs her suspicions against her sister, Florence however against her fellow employees. Apparently Florence does not begin to believe evil of Edith until the latter's accusations have begun. It seems improbable that the onset of the psychosis was in either case associated with deafness; the deafness even now is slight in both, and it can hardly have existed to an effective extent in the twenties. The development of the paranoid state was in Edith quiet and insidiously progressive, with good preservation of personality and without social decline. With Florence, too, the personality remains well preserved, and symptoms appear only episodically at times of stress, and eventually more floridly in the involutional period. At the height of this episode, which is quite short-lived, appear auditory hallucinations and a severe depressive reaction, which are never shown by Edith. On the whole, however, Edith's state is the graver one. It is tempting to relate the different degrees of severity to the more fortunate upbringing and early life enjoyed by Florence. The psychotic symptoms, as already remarked, show many resemblances, even in the content of the delusions. It is rather remarkable that, despite the religious interests of the twins, neither shows a religious colouring to the mental content.

In the opinion of the authors, the diagnosis in each case must be one of an endogenously determined chronic paranoid state, probably basically schizophrenic in nature. The illnesses at 18 and 19 may in each case have been mild schizophrenic attacks, though there is no positive evidence to support this. The mild degree of deafness, from which both twins suffered, probably did scarcely more than favour the paranoid development. The possibility that Florence's illness was induced by that of Edith, and is psychogenic in nature, and that we have a case of *folie à deux* in the classical sense, must be rejected. Florence's acute episode was in no way related to any action on Edith's part, and the other occasions on which she became more openly paranoid are equally unrelated to Edith's behaviour. Edith's report of recent falling attacks remains an unexplained feature. A late symptomatic epilepsy cannot be excluded, but equally cannot be confirmed, as nothing will bring Edith to go to hospital. The possibility of a constitutional tendency to manifestations of the epileptic type is also suggested by Florence's fainting attacks in childhood.

The development of the inter-twin relationship is unusual and interesting. Unlike the extremely affectionate bond which usually unites uniovular twins, the relationship here is one of suspicion and dislike. Florence says that when they first met, she took a fancy to her sister, and hints that more than once since then she has made gestures of reconciliation; her attitude throughout is much the less unfriendly of the two. Edith, however, was hostile from the first. It seems possible that this was caused in the first place by resentment at her own less fortunate lot; but that the attitude once set up caused its own perpetuation and aggravation. Each twin occupies for the other an over-valued position; to each the other is supremely important, although the circumstances of their lives touch at few points. Edith at first sight places Florence in the centre of her persecutors; Florence, with her own inborn tendency to paranoia, reacts to this by coming in her turn to regard Edith as her chief enemy.

SUMMARY

Two uniovular twin sisters of 52 are described, who were separated at the age of 9 months, but each in due course developed a paranoid psychosis. Concordance of childhood neurosis, of life story, of personality, and of eventual symptomatology are shown, despite very different upbringings. The principal difference between the psychoses is that while one shows a chronic insidiously progressive paranoia, the other shows paranoid symptoms only episodically. Each sister centres her delusions around the other; this appears in one of them to be reactive to the accusations of the other. Both are regarded as being the subjects of a basically schizophrenic illness.

7

GENETICAL CAUSES OF SCHIZOPHRENIC SYMPTOMS

In a work that came out early in the war, M. Zehnder (1940) gave an account of 92 schizophrenic brothers and sisters. The account is of more than common interest, because the writer gives us details of the illness in every one of these men and women. With the help of these data, and of present-day statistical methods, one is able to go further than Zehnder in obtaining information of interest. She did no more than divide the 92 persons into two groups of families, one in which the clinical picture in the separate siblings was similar, and one in which it was not. In this way Zehnder reached certain conclusions. It is not my purpose to express any personal opinion on Zehnder's views, but instead to make a wider use of her observations.

Zehnder's material is made up of 5 families of 4 siblings, 6 families of 3, and 24 families of 2. There are in addition 3 pairs of twins. Of the latter, the twins in one pair were two-egg; of the other 2 pairs we have no knowledge. So, if we omit these last two twin pairs, we have 36 families which consist of 73 pairs of siblings; for each family of three makes 3 separate pairs, and each family of four makes 6 separate pairs. In what follows, leaving out the possibly one-egg twins, we shall deal with these 73 pairs of affected siblings.

DIVISION BY SEX

Omitting the opposite sex twins, we have 72 pairs: 13 MM, 29 MW and 30 WW, for there are 89 women to 55 men, i.e. there are 43 pairs of like sex to 29 pairs of

Originally published in *Monatsschrift für Psychiatrie und Neurologie* 113: 50–58 (1947). The paper was originally written in Basic English, a "universal language" of 850 basic words. In the interests of clarity it has, with the author's permission, been "translated" into standard English. A German quote from B. Schulz has also been translated. A 16 X 16 table has been omitted, showing the significance levels for the correlations between clinical features. The original publication catalogues the individual cases identified as having catatonia and other features analysed. These lists of case numbers have been omitted, since present readers will not have the same ready access to Zehnder's case material as did the original readers of the *Monatsschrift*.

opposite sex. The excess of like-sexed over opposite-sexed is probably no more than we can account for by chance ($\chi^2 = 2.01$; P $<$ 0.05). But the tendency is the same as in the observations of L.S. Penrose (1942). The tendency in psychiatry is for affected relatives of any degree of relationship to be more frequently of the same than of opposite sex.

SIBLING RESEMBLANCE IN CLINICAL FEATURES

In age at *onset of the illness* we have something which can be measured, which is far from frequent in psychiatry. In schizophrenia one is frequently not able to say within wide limits of error when a man falls ill for the first time; but against that, one is able to state without error the time when he first came into hospital. Zehnder has recorded this in every one of her cases. The ages on admission may, with two brothers, be the same, or similar, or widely different; and we can measure the tendency for the ages to be similar or different. If in every one of the 73 pairs we plot against one another, two by two, the age on admission, this measure of resemblance will be given by the correlation coefficient r.

In this material $r = +0.55 \pm .08$. It is of great interest that r is as high as +0.5, for this is about the value of r in the comparison of siblings in such things as weight and height; and it is the value to be looked for in the comparison of siblings in features dependent on a great number of genes. For siblings will normally have half their genes the same and half different. A natural conclusion, then, would be that the time of onset in schizophrenia depends for the greater part on a number of genes working together. To test this theory, the calculation of the values of r with other kinds of relatives, such as nephews and nieces, would be a help.

In most of the cases Zehnder has given a diagnosis of *Kraepelinian type* and we may note cases in which catatonia is to be found (in 53 cases in all), in which hebephrenia (18) and in which paranoid schizophrenia (18). For catatonia we have the groups C-C 36, C-not C 18, not C-notC 19 ($\chi^2 = 16.9$; P $<$ 0.001), and for hebephrenia H-H 11, H-not H 7, not H-not H 55 ($\chi^2 = 28.5$; P $<$ 0.001). So for all three types there is a strong tendency for like to go with like, a strong positive correlation. The material may be compared with that of other workers. Thus B. Schulz (1932) says of his material of schizophrenic siblings, given in his Table 20: "If in this Table we consider only the 3 pure groups, we do indeed find a clear correlation. But this correlation is no longer found when the mixed proband groups and mixed secondary cases are also included." His material is smaller than Zehnder's, and certainly such positive correlation as there is might be caused by chance. F. J. Kallmann (1938) gives figures that are of interest here:

	Relatives		
	H	C	P
Hebephrenics	49	10	21
Catatonics	6	31	15
Paranoid	5	10	13

Kallmann says about this table:

In this way we are able to show that only about half the schizophrenias in the children and grandchildren of our probands correspond to the disease form of the related probands (53.2

81

per cent and 58.3 per cent respectively) .... We may conclude that the individual form of schizophrenia must be determined not solely by the special nature of the hereditary predisposition, but by a series of other factors.

But Kallmann has overlooked that, if there were not positive correlation, the association of similar types would be even less frequent. From his table it may be calculated that instead of the numbers 49, 31, and 13, the numbers probable by chance are 30.0, 16.6, and 8.6. So that in place of 93/160 = 58%, chance would give us 55.2/160 = 34%. The difference is a great one (χ^2 = 39.6; P < 0.001). Though this is not Kallmann's opinion, his numbers make it very probable that the type of illness is at least partly dependent on the genes, which is in agreement with the suggestion given by Zehnder's material.

In every one of her cases, Zehnder gives her opinion on the *outcome of the illness* — dementia (51), chronicity (14), or remission (27). They may be grouped D-D 33, D-not D 25, not D-not D 14 (χ^2 = 4.2; P < 0.05). So there is a more than chance positive correlation between the siblings in this respect.

In only 51 persons has Zehnder given details of *body build*, pyknic, athletic, or asthenic. Testing the numbers gives no sign of a more than chance similarity between the siblings. However, no measurements are given.

The material for the above discussion has been taken from what Zehnder herself has said. But there are other details in her case histories which can be used.

From Zehnder's accounts of *hallucinations* we may take it that auditory hallucinations were present in 43 specified cases, visual hallucinations in 12, and hallucinations of other senses in 20. There is no sign of any correlation between the siblings in this respect.

Destruction of thought processes is to be seen in 33 cases. There is no correlation between siblings.

Affect was poor and feeble in 38 cases. There is here a positive correlation (χ^2 = 4.4; P < 0.05).

Signs of *catatonia*, stupor, negativism, etc., were seen in 21 cases. The small positive correlation might be caused by chance.

Excitement (Erregungszustände) is noted in 45 cases. The correlation is quite strong (χ^2 = 6.2; P < 0.02).

Depressive colouring is noted in 33 cases. The positive correlation is a strong one (χ^2 = 29.8; P < 0.001).

A *paranoid* way of looking at the environment, false beliefs of ill-doing by others, etc., are specially noted in 50 cases. The positive correlation is quite strong (χ^2 = 5.7; P < 0.02).

From our observations we may say, then, that in clinical features such as age on onset, outcome, Kraepelinian type, affective dilapidation, catatonia, excitement, depressive colouring, and paranoid behavior, siblings are more like one another than may be accounted for by chance. The natural conclusion is that the cause is to be looked for in the genes, not the gene of schizophrenia itself, but the great number of genes of small effect, half of which are common to any two siblings.

CORRELATIONS BETWEEN CLINICAL FEATURES

It is probable that the observations we have looked at are dependent to some degree either on one another or on some common tendency. For example, a man's age may have an effect on more than one of the clinical features of the illness. One may note the correlations between separate observations, i.e. how strong the tendency is for two observations to be made on one and the same person. When these are tabulated, we see that catatonia is more frequent in the young and in the asthenic, and shows a tendency to excitement but none to paranoid development. Hebephrenia is seen in young and old, has no special correlations with other observations, but is negatively correlated with auditory hallucinations. Paranoid schizophrenia is more frequent in the old and those of pyknic build; it has a strong tendency to chronicity but not to dementia or depressive colouring. If the outcome is towards dementia, damage of thought processes and affective dilapidation will be seen, but not depressive colouring or excitement. Chronicity of the disease process makes auditory hallucinations probable, but affective dilapidation does not do so. A tendency to remissions is seen frequently with depressive colouring, far from frequently with affective dilapidation and paranoid tendency. Persons of pyknic build have strong tendencies to a paranoid subtype, less so to hallucinations of hearing, and frequently are without damage to thought processes. Asthenics have a tendency to catatonia, to excitement, and to depressive colouring, but very little to paranoid schizophrenia. In younger persons catatonia and excitement are frequent, in the older paranoid schizophrenia and chronicity.

SUMMARY

The data provided in an earlier work of M. Zehnder have been analyzed statistically. The material consisted of 92 schizophrenic siblings. Analysis shows that there are family resemblances too great to be accounted for by chance in age of onset, Kraepelinian type, course and outcome of the disease, degree of affective dilapidation, presence of catatonic signs, occurrence of states of excitement, of a depressive colouring, and of paranoid development. It is suggested that individual differences of these kinds, though not determined by the presence or absence of the specific schizophrenic gene, are genetically caused and are to be attributed to the action of modifying genes. In addition, the material suggests that various features of the illness are correlated among themselves. Thus particular symptoms are found to be associated with an early and a late onset, with pyknic and with asthenic habitus, with a psychosis that runs a remitting, chronic, or a dementing course.

8

SCHIZOPHRENIA: PROBLEMS OF HETEROGENEITY

Since Rüdin (1916) first showed that among the sibs of schizophrenics there was an excess of schizophrenic illness, the question of the mode of inheritance has been debated with a vigour and enthusiasm unmatched elsewhere in psychiatric genetics. Weinberg, the statistician who handled Rüdin's data, proposed a complex theory involving more than one gene. A later expert, Luxenburger (1928, 1930, 1935b), who carried out the first systematic twin survey in psychiatry, on schizophrenic propositi, was inclined to support a hypothesis attributing the disorder to a recessive autosomal gene. Lenz (1937), whose interests embraced the whole range of human genetics, supported the notion of dominance. The latest in the field to take a definite standpoint is Kallmann (1938, 1946), and he bases his opinion on the widest experience of actual investigation. He is strongly in favour of the hypothesis of recessivity.

KALLMANN'S DATA FOR MONOFACTORIAL RECESSIVE INHERITANCE

Kallmann's contributions of a major kind are twofold. He made a very extensive family survey (1938) covering the sibs, half-sibs, children and grandchildren of 1,087 schizophrenic propositi, the study differing in a significant particular from similar studies which had been made before. In earlier studies of the children of schizophrenics, families were almost automatically taken in which there were known to be one or more children. This involved a degree of biased selection of the parents, parents being automatically overrepresented whose illness came on late or was so mild that reproduction could still occur after the illness had begun. Kallmann started from a hospital population, without selection, and without knowledge whether there were children or not. His material contained a fairer selection of the graver forms of psychosis than had been obtained before. His second major contribution has been the collection and examination of a very large series of twins from the New York

Extracted from Chapter 18, "Psychiatry," in *Clinical Genetics* ed. A. Sorsby, pp. 345–49 (London: Butterworth, 1953). Title and references added.

State mental hospitals. This series includes 953 schizophrenic propositi, as well as much smaller numbers of manic-depressive, involutional, and senile psychoses. A detailed statistical study of the first 794 schizophrenic pairs appeared in 1946, when 2,741 sibs as well as parents, consorts, and other relatives had been investigated. The material was gathered by a systematic attempt to discover all the twins in a total mental hospital population of some 85,000 persons. From these studies the follow-ing percentage figures relating to the incidence of schizophrenia among various classes of relatives are of interest: (1) unrelated: general population, 0.85; stepsibs, 1.8; husbands and wives, 2.1; (2) relatives: first cousins, 2.6; nephews and nieces, 3.9; grandchildren, 4.3; half-sibs, 7.0–7.6; parents, 9.2–10.3; full sibs, 11.5–14.3; dizygotic co-twins, 12.5; children, 16.4; children of two schizophrenic parents, 68.1; same-sexed dizygotic twins, 17.6; monozygotic twins who have been separated for five years or more, 77.6; monozygotic twins who have not been so separated, 91.5. The increasing likelihood of schizophrenia with increasing nearness of blood rela-tionship to a schizophrenic is very striking.

Kallmann considers that his findings and the findings that have been made by others support the hypothesis of single-factor inheritance of a recessive type, but with a lower than 100 per cent rate of manifestation, that is, some homozygotes never develop schizophrenia but will nearly always be schizoid personalities. Mani-festation in the heterozygotic state is not entirely suppressed, but may also be shown in some schizoid traits of personality. Nonspecific genetical factors are postu-lated to account for variation in the clinical form of the disease and its degree of malignancy. Kallmann and his co-workers have found that a robust bodily physique tends to mitigate the severity of the disease, or to protect against it, while loss of weight and an asthenic physique have the opposite tendency.

Some Difficulties

The hypothesis of recessivity has been criticized by Koller (1939), and his argu-ment is an important one. Although in the detail in which he presented it, it is complex, it can be quite simply presented. If the schizophrenic is homozygous for gene s, he will only produce schizophrenic children by mating with a heterozygote, or with another individual homozygous like himself. Schizophrenics compose ap-proximately 1 per cent of the population, so that the frequency of s in the popula-tion is approximately 0.1, and the frequency of heterozygotes approximately 0.18, if one assumes that mating is at random. The frequency of persons homozygotic for s among the children of schizophrenics should be, accordingly, and again assuming random mating, $0.5 \times 0.18 + 0.01 = 0.10$. The frequency of homozygotes among the sibs of schizophrenics, which is not affected to the same degree by the gene frequency, may be taken as 0.25. If s is recessive the frequency of homozy-gosity for s, and therefore the frequency of schizophrenia, should be higher among the sibs of schizophrenics than among their children. Assortative mating would only equalize the two frequencies, or lead one to expect a higher frequency of schizo-phrenia in the children than in the sibs, if it was of a very extreme degree, if in fact a very large proportion of schizophrenics married others also homozygotic for s. Sev-eral studies of the consorts of schizophrenics and their families have been published and it is clear that in them the incidence of schizophrenia is only very slightly greater than in the general population. The incidence of schizophrenia in the con-sorts themselves has, for instance, been found to be 2 per cent. Assortative mating therefore can be neglected for this purpose.

The actual observations, however, do not fit these expectations. The incidence of schizophrenia has been found by Kallmann to be higher in the children than in the sibs. This is therefore a strong indication of dominance. On the dominance hypothesis one would of course expect an equal incidence in children and sibs, but a difference of the extent which actually exists would not be a serious objection to the theory as it may result from a sampling error or be explicable in other ways.

One of the findings which Kallmann has adduced as evidence in favour of recessivity is that approximately 5.7 per cent of schizophrenics have been found to be the children of consanguineous matings. The relation between gene frequency (p), the incidence of cousin-marriage in the general population (a) and the incidence of cousin-marriage between the parents of recessive homozygotes (c) is given by Dahlberg's formula, which may be written $p = a(1-c)/16c$. If for a we write 0.006, which is Bell's estimate of the frequency of cousin-marriage in England and Wales (the incidence in the United States of America is unknown to the writer), and if we assume that about two-thirds of Kallmann's consanguineous matings were first-cousin marriages and give the value of 0.042 for c, the value of p proves to be 0.008554, and the value of p^2 0.000073. However, the expectation of schizophrenia for a member of the general population, and the frequency of hypothetical homozygotes is about 0.009. The theory therefore leads us to the supposition that some 125 distinct autosomal recessive genes are involved.

This number is not, perhaps, quite such an unlikely one as it would seem to be at a first glance. There might well be a large number of different genotypes in schizophrenia, just as there almost certainly are in the hodge-podge of clinically inadequately differentiated imbecilities and idiocies. There are, however, factual grounds for considering this consequence of the recessivity hypothesis improbable. A fair number of families have now been collected in which two schizophrenic parents produced children. The incidence of schizophrenia among these children has been estimated by Schulz (1940) as 38 per cent, or 45 per cent if doubtful cases were included. An earlier estimate made by Luxenburger was 66 per cent, and Kallmann's (1938) estimate is 68 per cent. Whatever the true figure, it is quite a high one: but if there are 125 different genes involved, it would be extremely unlikely for any two schizophrenic parents to be of the same genotype, and the incidence of schizophrenia in their children should be little higher than the incidence of schizophrenia in the children of one schizophrenic and one normal parent.

The incidence of schizophrenia in the children of schizophrenics is rather more easy to reconcile with the dominance hypothesis. If dominant genes are involved, we must calculate their manifestation rates as approximating to 0.3. The children of two parents both of whom carry a dominant gene, but at different loci, should contain equal proportions of persons carrying one gene, carrying the other, carrying both, and carrying neither. The expectation of normality should therefore be $(0.7 + 0.7 + 0.49 + 1)/4 = 0.72$, and we should expect an incidence of schizophrenia of 0.28. If, however, the genes were at the same loci, the homozygous dominant would almost certainly be abnormal and, unless the double dose proved lethal, the incidence of schizophrenia would be 0.40.

The Possibility of Heterogeneity

None the less, Kallmann's finding of a greatly increased rate of consanguineous marriage among the parents of schizophrenics would seem to be a direct proof of the operation of recessive genes. The only reasonable way in which to reconcile all the conflicting evidence is on the supposition of heterogeneity. In view of the fact that schizophrenia is a great deal more common than any single genetically determined disorder is otherwise known to be, heterogeneity is inherently probable. As far as the writer is aware, there is no evidence to the contrary which should be allowed great weight. The principal objection to the hypothesis of heterogeneity is that so far it has proved impossible to identify genetically distinct forms of the disorder. A brief glance at the work which has been done on this aspect may be allowed.

If schizophrenia is genetically heterogeneous, we may expect to find some forms which are not genetically determined at all. There is some evidence that they exist. It is an accepted finding of clinical psychiatry, since the work of Kretschmer, that schizophreniform reactions may occur, that is, states of mental disturbance clinically resembling schizophrenia, but produced by some form of physical or mental stress, accessible to treatment by psychological means and by adjustment of the environment, and likely to recover without, as in the great majority of cases of schizophrenia, leaving some sequelae behind. Schulz (1932) found in his investigation into the sibs of schizophrenics that, if he singled out a group of propositi whose illness came on after a head injury, the incidence of schizophrenia in their sibs was much lower than in the families of the remaining propositi. The work of Leonhard (1934) showed that in some rare families a clinically distinct form of psychosis, with many schizophrenic-like features, may be identified with possession of a dominant gene. Leonhard, following Kleist (1921), believes that it is possible to distinguish between "typical" forms of schizophrenia, which take a progressive and malignant course, and "atypical" forms with a better prognosis. An experiment was staged in which the clinical differentiation was done by Leonhard, without knowledge of family relationships, and the familial investigation was done by Schulz without knowledge of the clinical findings in the propositi. One of the interesting findings that emerged was that the incidence of schizophrenia in the parents of the propositi was in the typical group 1 per cent, in the parents of the atypical group 6 per cent (Schulz and Leonhard, 1940). This does suggest a preponderance of recessive types in the former, and a proportion of disorders due to a dominant gene in the latter.

On the other hand the attempt to identify the clinically recognized subforms of schizophrenia — catatonia, hebephrenia, paranoid schizophrenia and schizophrenia simplex — with distinct genotypes has failed. Some suggestive points have emerged, but do not take us far. Kallmann's figures, derived from his investigation of the children of schizophrenics, show, though he did not observe the point himself, a noteworthy correlation between the form taken by the illness in the propositus and in the relative. Furthermore, he found that the incidence of schizophrenia was more than twice as high in the children of catatonic and hebephrenic propositi as in the children of paranoid and simplex cases.

The matter must be left here, with the important questions still all unanswered, although the available evidence has been far from exhaustively discussed.

9

PSYCHOTIC AND NEUROTIC ILLNESSES IN TWINS

PREFACE BY THE MEDICAL RESEARCH COUNCIL. One of the fundamental problems in any analysis of human behaviour is to weigh the relative effects of heredity and environment, and to decide how far man's nature is the inescapable corollary of his genetical inheritance and how far it is the result of the varied experiences which he has undergone since birth. It was Galton, the founder of scientific genetics, who first saw that a step towards solving this problem would be to examine a series of twins of both the binovular and uniovular kind. The rationale for this type of work, which has been greatly developed since Galton's time, rests on the fact that a pair of so-called "identical" twins develop from a single fertilized ovum and therefore share a common set of genes. This identical genetical inheritance must necessarily make them more alike, in all ways in which genes play a part, than are binovular twins, who need resemble one another genetically no more than do ordinary brothers and sisters. Where differences do occur between the two members of an "identical" twin pair, it is the environment which is responsible. Studies on twins thus provide unique opportunities for conducting controlled investigations on man, and of weighing, as Galton said, "in just scales the effects of Nature and Nurture". The present report takes full advantage of the opportunities which work on a series of twins can provide.

In 1935, a grant from the Medical Research Council enabled Dr. Slater to start an investigation of mental abnormality in twins. During the war the investigation virtually came to a halt but, although this interruption caused some difficulties, the lapse of time enabled a valuable and informative follow-up to be carried out in 1947–49. This survey was made by Mr. Shields with a grant from the Council, and he has also collaborated in the heavy task of preparing the material for publication. The results of the whole investigation, which covered a period of thirteen years, are given in this monograph, which the Council are glad to include in their series.

London, S.W.1
20th April, 1953

With the assistance of James Shields. Originally published under same title as *Medical Research Council Special Report Series No. 278* (London: Her Majesty's Stationery Office, 1953). Abridged.

TWIN INVESTIGATIONS IN PSYCHIATRY

EDITORS' COMMENTS: In the opening section of this report, Slater discusses the history, rationale, and validity of the twin method and reviews previous work on unselected series of psychiatric twins. We commence our selection with his conclusions.

In abbreviating the subsequent sections on the lines mentioned on p. 70, we have omitted those parts so indicated in the unabridged Summary and Conclusions (p. 118ff.) and we have considerably shortened two sections (pages 97 and 99). We have omitted most references to case numbers, since without the case histories many are unnecessary. Three tables have been deleted where the data shown were summarized in the text. The omitted appendices consist mostly of age correction tables and of fingerprint data and analyses. Part II, devoted to case history material, gave for each diagnostic group clinical histories of all uniovular pairs, of all concordant binovular pairs and of selected binovular pairs of special interest. Short summaries were given of psychiatric illnesses in pairs of relatives, not recorded elsewhere. Data were tabulated for all discordant binovular pairs. The present abridged version does not claim to be a substitute for the complete monograph.

If therefore we look back over the development of investigations into psychiatric twin material, we see a progressive improvement in technique and range. Such studies have been conducted on a much greater scale in the field of mental disorder than in any other realm of human biology, and in spite of the difficulties of the work much has been learned that otherwise would have been unascertainable. Progress, however, has revealed as many new problems as it has supplied partial solutions to old ones, and these must be solved, for one of the most important justifications for work of this kind is that it is a contribution to fundamental theory. We cannot come to any conclusion about the basic pathology of mental illness without taking genetical aspects into account; and the genetics of mental disorder may well in time provide the foundation for a reliable nosology.

THE PRESENT INVESTIGATION: GENERAL

Planning

The investigation was begun in 1936 and concerned itself in the first place with the standing population of ten hospitals of the London County Council Mental Health Services: Banstead, Bexley, Cane Hill, Claybury, Friern, Horton, Long Grove, St. Bernard's, St. Ebba's and West Park. All of these were hospitals for the adult psychotic patient, and hospitals for mental deficiency were not included. The standing population of these hospitals was at this time approximately 20,640 patients; requests for information were circularized to 16,632 relatives, and in the case of 364 patients we discovered that there had been a twin.

These figures would give an incidence of twinning of 2.2 per cent, but unfortunately this estimate is unreliable: part of the records, including many of the returned postcards bearing "no" answers, were lost during the war, so that no check can be made. However, the proportion of twins is about what might be expected. In England and Wales in the year 1948, out of a total of 975,306 live births there were 17,655 individuals live-born from a multiple birth with a surviving partner, a proportion of 2.28 per cent. Even if persons are included who have no surviving partner, the figure only rises to 2.37 per cent. There are, therefore, no grounds for thinking that in our material there was any excess of twins, such as was found by Conrad (1935, 1936) in a population of epileptics and by Juda (1939) in one of mental defectives.

The relatives of the 364 twins who were ascertained in this way were asked by letter whether the twin was alive or dead, and they were also asked for some further particulars. It was found that in 167 cases the patient's twin partner had died young, most usually in infancy, and that 155 twins had survived to adult life; in the remaining 42 cases no answer was received.

A second source, which yielded material of a very different kind, was provided by the Maudsley Hospital. Whenever there was an admission to their In-patient, Out-patient or Children's Departments from 1936–39, the Admission Clerk on duty at the time inquired whether the patient had a surviving twin; 86 twin pairs were discovered in this way.

The third source of material was the admissions to the ten mental hospitals which took place while the investigation was in progress, 1936–39; this provided 38 twin pairs. An arrangement was made by which a numbered tear-off strip was attached to the History Sheet sent by the Hospital to relatives of patients admitted. This slip inquired whether or not the patient was born a twin. The twin slips were collected by the hospital clerical officers and forwarded in batches to the writer. Some hospitals, notably Long Grove Hospital, continued to do this even during the war, when matters became difficult, but most hospitals soon ceased to carry out the arrangement. In this way 16 twin cases were ascertained.

Altogether, therefore, 295 persons born in a multiple birth were collected. These included nine cases where both members of the same twin pair were notified. There were also two sets of triplets, in which all three of the triplets had survived.[1] As each set of triplets provides two twins for comparison with the propositus,[2] we had a total of 297 twin pairs for statistical analysis. It may fairly be claimed that the selection was unbiased, even when, as during the war, it became rather haphazard.

For two years, 1935–37, the present writer was able to give his entire time to the investigation, with the assistance of a clerk, Mr. C. J. Martin, who was responsible for sending out the routine inquiries. During this time the author moved from hospital to hospital, investigating the patients, getting in touch with relatives and, if possible, seeing and examining the twins. In addition, full copies or personally prepared abstracts of all available hospital records, both of propositi and of near relatives, including twins, were made. After 1937 the writer had to return to normal clinical work and continued the investigation in a part time capacity, getting help, however, from Miss Marjorie Brown, who was then Research Psychiatric Social Worker attached to the Maudsley Hospital and took some 80 family histories, mostly supplementing family histories already obtained which were in one way or another inadequate. At the outbreak of the war the investigation had perforce to be interrupted and circumstances were unfavourable to its reopening until 1947. Then a full-time Psychiatric Social Worker, Mr. J. Shields, was appointed to follow-up all cases and bring those in which inquiries were unfinished to completion.

---

[1] Where both members of the twin pair are propositi the case is numbered thus, 26/27. In statistical analysis such a pair has to be counted as two separate cases. Where the propositus is one of triplets with two surviving twins for comparison the case is numbered thus, 41 (a) and (b).

[2] *Propositus*: The "proposed" case, "proband" or "index-case", the case which provides the starting point from which the investigation begins. In subsequent statistical operations the propositi have a special place, as they have to be omitted from many calculations (e.g., in estimating the frequency of schizophrenia among the sibs of schizophrenics).

The plan in every case was to obtain a family history as complete as possible about parents, sibs, children, and children of sibs; to obtain also a personal history about the patient and his twin including the history of any illness either or both might have had; and to make an anthropometric and a psychiatric examination of both twins.

The anthropometric examination, which was only made in the case of same-sexed twins, included measurement of the height, of the hair colour (against a standardized range of human hair samples), eye colour (against a standardized scale of glass eyes), four skull measurements (length and breadth of cranium, maxillary breadth and height of face), and the taking of finger-prints. Early on in the investigation blood samples were taken for grouping, but difficulties appeared in practice with this procedure, and it had to be dropped. The material for comparison which was supplied by these methods was, however, taken in conjunction with the personal history of similarity or otherwise, such as to leave doubt of the ovularity diagnosis in very few cases.

As in all such investigations it is with a sieve rather than a scoop that the human material is gathered. Patients are discharged from hospital before they can be seen, relatives refuse their co-operation, and other impediments appear. The thoroughness with which the material was examined is given in Table 9.1. It is probable that these figures would have been much improved but for the interruption of the war.

TABLE 9.1. NATURE AND EXTENT OF EXAMINATION OF TWIN PAIRS

	Propositi		Twin partners	
Personally examined	266		156	
Examined by P. S. W. only	5		46	
Total examined		271		202
Died before examination	11		49	
Abroad or untraced	10		?1	
Unco-operative	5		25	
Total not examined		26		95
Total		297		297

The war, though it had dealt the investigation a blow in some respects, also gave rise to a valuable opportunity for follow-up. Admittedly a follow-up engaged in so many years later might run into difficulties but it might also bring in much new and valuable information, especially about those patients and twins whose mental state was capable of change and development. Mr. Shields, who was appointed to carry out this work, found that in the material already to hand at the outbreak of the war there were 14 cases in which no information whatever had yet been obtained and in addition there were the 16 cases notified during the war. During 1947–49 these cases were investigated; gaps in old cases were filled, and in about 46 cases we were able to obtain additional information about earlier history; all outstanding cases where there was a hospital record obtainable from other than L.C.C. hospitals were completed. As many cases as possible were followed up, though in 21 cases the follow-up did no more than obtain up-to-date mental hospital records, mostly of those cases where the twin partner was already dead by 1939. In 27 cases twins and relatives could not be traced, and in 5 cases the relatives proved unco-operative. Concerning all the remainder, information, sometimes scanty, at other times of the greatest value, was obtained.

91

Sex and Ovularity Distribution of Twin Pairs

This distribution is given in Table 9.2. From the table it may easily be read that we had a total of 104 male and 193 female propositi, with 128 male and 169 female twin partners. It also shows that there were 195 same-sexed pairs and 102 opposite-sexed pairs; and finally that there were 66 uniovular and 225 binovular pairs and 6 pairs of doubtful ovularity.

TABLE 9.2. SEX AND OVULARITY DISTRIBUTION OF TWIN PAIRS

Propositi	Twin partners		
	Male	Female	Total
Male			
Uniovular pairs	18	–	18
Pairs, ? ovularity	4	–	4
Binovular pairs	43	39	82
Total males	65	39	104
Female			
Uniovular pairs	–	49	49
Pairs, ? ovularity	–	2	2
Binovular pairs	63	79	142
Total females	63	130	193
Total	128	169	297

The two female same-sexed pairs of doubtful ovularity were probably uniovular. There is no information about the 4 male same-sexed pairs of doubtful ovularity. If we allot 2 of them to the uniovular group, as well as the 2 female pairs, and the other 2 to the binovular group we have a total of 70 uniovular to 227 binovular pairs, and the uniovular pairs constitute 24 per cent of the total. It will be remembered that Kallmann's (1946) figure was 25 per cent, and was in accordance with expectations based on the general American population. The figures for Britain are very similar: according to the Registrar-General's Statistical Review for England and Wales (1948) there were in that year 9,597 twin births, both twins being born alive. Of these 3,173 consisted of two males, 3,486 of a male and female, 2,938 of two females. Using Weinberg's differential formula uncorrected this gives a proportion of 27 per cent uniovular twins. Our figure of 24 per cent is not significantly lower: we should have expected 81 uniovular pairs instead of the 70 we found.

The sex ratio in the binovular propositi is different from the sex ratio in their twins by a margin which exceeds the 5 per cent level of significance. We may therefore apply a correction to Weinberg's formula in order to get the most exact estimate of the expected number of uniovular twins. We can write:

$$p + (1 - p)(\lambda\lambda' + \mu\mu') = 195/227$$

where p = the proportion of all pairs which are uniovular
λ = the proportion of males in the binovular propositi
λ' = the proportion of males in the binovular twins
μ = the proportion of females in the binovular propositi
μ' = the proportion of females in the binovular twins

$\lambda = 84/227 = 0.3700$ $\lambda' = 108/227 = 0.4758$
$\mu = 143/227 = 0.6300$ $\mu' = 119/227 = 0.5242$
from which $p = 90.4/297$

But the margin by which this expectation differs from the observation of 70 (x^2 = 4.60) is significant at the 5 per cent level. It is therefore possible that our material contains an excess of binovular twins. If this is so, the most likely explanation would be the fact that a binovular pair of twins are more likely both to survive birth and infancy than a uniovular pair. Karn (1952) shows that in only 68 per cent of same-sexed twin births did both babies survive; the percentage of opposite-sexed pairs surviving was 80.

Clinical Diagnosis of Propositi

Our material divides itself conveniently into four main diagnostic groups. By far the largest of these is formed by the schizophrenic psychoses as can be seen from Table 9.3. Out of 297 pairs the propositus was schizophrenic in 158 cases.[3] This is understandable when it is remembered that most of our twins were selected from the standing mental hospital population. The second group, that of the affective disorders, accounts for 38 cases. Twenty-three of these had manic-depressive psychoses or primarily endogenous depressions; there was 1 case of probably recurrent mania in a man of low intelligence; 11 involutional depressions; and 3 reactive depressions. The third group is less homogeneous and consists of epilepsy and the organic psychoses, 49 cases in all.[4] The psychopathic and neurotic group of 52 includes cases of psychogenic behaviour disorders in children and psychopathic reactions occurring in mental defectives, besides other neurotic and psychopathic states, many of them referred in the first instance to the Maudsley Hospital.[5]

Before discussing these groups separately, it will be of interest to compare them in a few particulars.

Size of Family

The affective propositi come from the largest sibships (average number of sibs of known sex, including stillbirths and premature births = 5.18) and following them the organics (4.37) and the schizophrenics (4.31), the psychopaths and neurotics having the smallest average number of sibs (3.50). The last group, however, were on the average younger than the others and so were born in an age when the fashion for smaller families was spreading. It is worth noting that the rate of miscarriage, or death before the age of 5 was found to be higher in the organic group, taken as a whole (60 miscarriages or early deaths in 49 families), than in any other clinical group; but the difference just fails to reach statistical significance (x^2 = 3.58, p > 0.05).

Abnormality in Family

Table 9.4 shows the incidence per cent of mental abnormality which was found among the different degrees of relatives in the four clinical groups. In correcting for

[3] 156 propositi, 2 of whom had surviving triplets for comparison. In 4 uniovular and 3 binovular pairs, both twins were propositi in the schizophrenic group. — Editors.

[4] Epilepsy, 14; arteriopathic and organic paranoid psychoses, 9; presenile and senile psychoses, 5; other abnormalities with possible constitutional basis, 5; general paresis, 7; symptomatic psychoses and other conditions, 9. — Editors.

[5] Predominantly psychogenic behaviour disorders in children, 10; neurotic reactions in adolescents and adults (including psychopaths and defectives), 16; psychopathic disturbances in mental defectives, 8; other psychopathic states, 18. — Editors.

TABLE 9.3. SEX, OVULARITY AND CLINICAL DIAGNOSIS OF ALL TWIN PAIRS

	Uniovular pairs			Pairs of doubtful ovularity			Binovular pairs					All pairs				
	m*m	f f	Total	m m	f f	Total	m m	m f	f m	f f	Total	m m	m f	f m	f f	Total
Schizophrenic propositus																
Co-twin Schizophrenic	6	22	28	–	–	–	2	–	2	9	13	8	–	2	31	41
Co-twin Affective	–	1	1	–	–	–	–	1	1	3	5	–	1	1	4	6
Co-twin Organic	–	–	–	–	–	–	–	1	1	–	2	–	1	1	–	2
Co-twin Pp./neurotic	2	2	4	–	–	–	7	4	11	5	27	9	4	11	7	31
Co-twin Normal	4	4	8	2	–	2	12	13	20	23	68	18	13	20	27	78
Total	12	29	41	2	–	2	21	19	35	40	115	35	19	35	69	158
Affectively ill propositus																
Co-twin Affective	–	4	4	–	–	–	1	1	3	2	7	1	1	3	6	11
Co-twin Schizophrenic	–	–	–	–	–	–	–	–	–	–	–	–	–	–	–	–
Co-twin Organic	–	–	–	–	–	–	–	–	–	–	–	–	–	–	–	–
Co-twin Pp./neurotic	–	1	1	–	–	–	1	–	1	2	4	1	–	1	3	5
Co-twin Normal	–	3	3	–	–	–	4	5	5	5	19	4	5	5	8	22
Total	–	8	8	–	–	–	6	6	9	9	30	6	6	9	17	38
Propositus with epilepsy or organic mental illness																
Co-twin Organic	–	4	4	–	–	–	1	–	1	–	2	1	–	1	4	6
Co-twin Schizophrenic	–	–	–	–	–	–	–	–	–	–	–	–	–	–	–	–
Co-twin Affective	–	–	–	–	–	–	–	–	1	–	1	–	–	1	–	1
Co-twin Pp./neurotic	–	–	–	–	–	–	1	1	3	3	8	1	1	3	3	8
Co-twin Normal	2	3	5	1	2	3	5	7	6	8	26	8	7	6	13	34
Total	2	7	9	1	2	3	7	8	11	11	37	10	8	11	20	49
Psychopathic or neurotic propositus																
Co-twin Pp./neurotic	2	–	2	–	–	–	3	–	1	1	5	5	–	1	1	7
Co-twin Schizophrenic	–	–	–	–	–	–	–	–	–	–	–	–	–	–	–	–
Co-twin Affective	–	–	–	–	–	–	1	–	–	1	2	1	–	–	1	2
Co-twin Organic	–	–	–	–	–	–	–	1	–	–	1	–	1	–	–	1
Co-twin Normal	2	4	6	1	–	1	5	5	7	18	35	8	5	7	22	42
Total	4	4	8	1	–	1	9	6	8	20	43	14	6	8	24	52
Grand total	18	48	66	4	2	6	43	39	63	80	225	65	39	63	130	297

*Propositus italicized.

TABLE 9.4. PERCENT INCIDENCE OF MENTAL ABNORMALITY AMONG RELATIVES OVER 14
(Figures corrected for age in brackets)

	Schizophrenic propositi (156)				Affective propositi (38)				Organic propositi (49)				Psychopathic or neurotic propositi (52)			
	Uniovular twins	Binovular twins	Sibs	Parents	Uniovular twins	Binovular twins	Sibs	Parents	Uniovular twins	Binovular twins	Sibs	Parents	Uniovular twins	Binovular twins	Sibs	Parents
No. of relatives diagnosed	41	115	568	304	8	30	171	75	9	37	156	96	8	43	134	100
Percentage:																
Schizophrenia	68.3 (76.3)	11.3 (14.4)	4.6 (5.4)	3.9 (4.1)	—	—	0.6 (0.7)	—	—	—	0.6 (0.8)	1.0 (1.1)	—	—	0.7 (1.0)	1.0 (1.0)
Affective illness	2.4 —	4.3 (6.6)	2.6 (3.7)	5.3 (5.8)	50.0 —	23.3 (28.6)	7.0 (8.8)	12.0 (13.6)	—	2.7 (3.8)	1.9 (2.7)	3.1 (3.6)	—	4.8 (10.7)	0.7 (1.3)	3.0 (3.5)
Organic mental illness (incl. epilepsy)	—	1.7	1.1	3.1	—	—	1.2	—	44.4	5.4	5.1	3.1	—	2.4	2.1	55.0
Psychopathy or neurosis	9.8 —	23.5 (30.0)	11.0 (13.2)	21.1 (21.9)	12.5 —	13.3 (14.8)	11.7 (13.2)	16.0 (16.9)	—	21.6 (25.5)	10.9 (13.0)	18.7 (21.9)	25.0	11.6 (21.2)	17.9 (26.2)	31.0 (32.5)
All abnormalities	80.5	40.8	19.3	33.4	62.5	36.6	20.5	28.0	44.4	29.7	18.5	25.9	25.0	18.7	21.4	40.0
Normal	19.5	59.2	80.7	66.6	37.5	63.4	79.5	72.0	55.6	70.3	81.5	74.1	75.0	81.3	78.6	60.0

TABLE 9.5. PERCENT INCIDENCE OF ABNORMALITY AMONG SIBS

Diagnosis of propositi	Incidence among sibs (to nearest per cent) of			
	Schizophrenia	Affective illness	Organic states	Psychopathy, neurosis
Schizophrenia	5	4	1	13
Affective illness	1	9	1	13
Organic states	1	3	5	13
Psychopathy/neurosis	1	1	2	26

age, Weinberg's shorter method was used.[6] In general, schizophrenia is highest in the relatives of schizophrenics, affective mental illness in the families of the affective group, and so on. To take one example, Table 9.5 shows the incidence of abnormality among the sibs.

In the affective group there is a comparatively large number of families with many affectively ill members. Excluding the illnesses of the propositi and their uniovular twin partners, there are, in 38 families, 1 family with 5 other concordant illnesses, 1 family with 3 others, 5 families with 2 others, and 9 families with 1 other. In the schizophrenic group of 158 families there is 1 family with 4 additional schizophrenic members, 2 families with 3 other schizophrenics, 4 families with 2 others, and 35 families with 1 other.

Taking all kinds of abnormality and all relatives, except the uniovular co-twins, there is little difference between the four groups in the total amount of abnormality observed. The psychopathic group is highest showing 27.5 per cent of relatives as abnormal, the affective group the lowest with 24.3 per cent. It is interesting that the figure is as high as 24.6 per cent for the organics, where in the surprisingly large number of six families both parents were abnormal. Although the psychopathic group is the one with the highest proportion of abnormality, it is also the group which has the largest proportion of families with no recorded cases of abnormality other than the propositus (26.9 per cent; the lowest is the affective group with 18 per cent). The abnormal members of this group are thus relatively highly concentrated in certain families. For example, there are 8 out of 52 families where both parents are abnormal.

It is possible that the percentage of families in a group where neither parent was abnormal might give an indication of the average stability of the home in the different groups. It is of interest that in the psychopathic group, where one would expect to find the most abnormal home background, only in 36.0 per cent of the families were both parents normal, while in the organic group there is a much higher figure of 57.2 per cent. The parents of the affectively ill propositi are both normal rather more frequently (50 per cent) than those of the schizophrenics (42.2 per cent) and the abnormalities from which they suffer tend to be rather milder than those of the parents of schizophrenics. In a later section (pp. 116-18) an attempt is made to analyse the chief characteristics of the abnormal relatives in the four clinical groups.

In all four diagnostic groups, however, a remarkable relation exists between abnormality in the parents and abnormality in the binovular twins. The relevant figures are set out in Table 9.6 and they have been arranged in terms of psychiatric

[6] Risk periods: schizophrenia, 15-39 years; epilepsy, 15-24; affective illness, 20-49; psychopathy/neurosis, 20-39. — *Editors.*

TABLE 9.6. RELATIONSHIP BETWEEN ABNORMALITY IN PARENTS AND ABNORMALITY
            OF THE BINOVULAR TWIN PARTNERS

Binovular twin partners	Number of parents diagnosed		
	Abnormal	Normal	Total
Schizophrenic group			
Abnormal	40	50	90
Normal	40	95	135
Affective group			
Abnormal	8	13	21
Normal	8	30	38
Organic group			
Abnormal	9	13	22
Normal	12	36	48
Psychopathic group			
Abnormal	11	5	16
Normal	25	41	66

abnormality in its widest sense. They show in all diagnostic groups that if one or both parents are abnormal the risk of abnormality for the co-twin is increased. If all diagnostic groups are lumped together, χ^2 = 10.38 for which $P < 0.01$. However, if the diagnostic groups are held separate, χ^2 is not significant in the affective and organic groups but remains significant in the schizophrenic group (χ^2 = 5.17, $P < 0.05$) and nearly so in the psychopathic group (χ^2 = 3.32, $P > 0.05$).

The simplest interpretation of these findings would be that the general constitution and non-specific genetical factors are highly important in determining the manifestation of schizophrenia or of psychopathy or neurosis, but less so the manifestation of an affective or organic illness. The environmental hypothesis, that overt abnormality in the parent has its effect on the child through the environment, cannot be excluded, but it is not plausibly reconciled with the difference between the schizophrenic and the affective groups.

In the schizophrenic group there is also a relationship between abnormality in the parent, or in other members of the family, and the mortality in the schizophrenic propositi themselves. If a parent were schizophrenic mortality was heavy and the chance of the propositus (12 cases) reaching the age of 40 was only 0.58, of reaching 55 only 0.33. If the binovular twin or if a brother or sister were schizophrenic, the propositus (28 cases) had a 0.83 chance of reaching 40 and a 0.70 chance of reaching 55. If neither parent nor sib were schizophrenic, the respective chances for the propositus were further improved to 0.93 and 0.83. This finding again suggests a relationship between bodily constitution and powers of resistance to schizophrenia.

Personality Resemblance Between Uniovular Twins [abbreviated]

Unlike binovular twins, uniovular twins are not only equipped with the same basic constitution but, by virtue of their close physical resemblance, they tend also to share a more similar early social environment. It is therefore not surprising that they frequently resemble each other almost as closely in personality as they do in appearance. In our summaries of the case histories of uniovular twins in Part II we have stressed personality differences between them. We have also demonstrated a tendency for the more submissive, the more neurotic, the more sensitive, and the less sociable twin of the pairs predisposed to schizophrenia to be the one who breaks down or becomes the more severe invalid. An attempt was made to bring out the similarities in personality and to see how far the differences of which we hear can be explained as different facets or minor variations of the same basic personality. In some instances environmental factors, such as the relations of the twins to each other, can be pointed to as influencing their divergent development.

Of the 15 male uniovular pairs for which we have relevant information, in only two, or perhaps three, were there noteworthy differences of personality.

Of the 39 female pairs there were 19 who show some difference of personality, though no pair shows a strong difference. This difference was nearly always in energy or in degree of extraversion. One may be described as more domineering, or more boisterous, more high spirited or pushing; whereas the other by contrast seems quieter, more unassuming, reserved, or sensitive. This is the nature of the difference in 14 of the 19 cases, and it can presumably be related to the twin situation. In the close attachment that often develops between the twins, it may happen that one habitually takes the lead. A similar mutual orientation occurs with ordinary friends, or with husbands and wives, and one is reminded of the "pecking order" of domestic poultry. It seems fairly safe to assume that the pattern of dominance and submission, which is set in this way in early childhood, has some effect on the way individuals react to the environment generally throughout adult life. A personality trait which much less frequently shows differences between twins is the degree of emotional lability. In this case it is not easy to see how the twin relationship could be responsible.

It is noteworthy that Galton (1883) himself observed the same tendency to disparity in energy in the first twin study of 60 years ago. He wrote:

> These differences belonged almost wholly to such groups of qualities as these: the one was the more vigorous, fearless, energetic; the other was gentle, clinging and timid; or the one was more ardent, the other more calm and placid; or again, the one was the more independent, original, and selfcontained; the other the more generous, hasty, and vivacious. In short, the difference was that of intensity or energy in one or other of its protean forms; it did not extend more deeply into the structure of the characters.

Summarizing the material as a whole we can say that uniovular twins, in the absence of any pathological change, develop into closely similar personalities. There are nearly always differences, but these are ones of degree and generally slight — though relatives tend to emphasize them in a natural effort to award each twin his distinctive personality. Such slight and quantitative differences may affect practically any feature of the personality, predominant mood state, variability of mood, firmness or vacillation, sensitivity, social adaptability, and so on. Yet these minor differences seem to be of considerable importance as, aided by chance, they may lead to very different life-careers. In one quality only, as we have said, is the tendency towards differentiation conspicuous, that is in the energy of character. The twin situation seems very frequently to be the direct cause of a development by which one twin becomes the leader, the more active and out-going, and the other the led, the more passive and withdrawn. This again may lead to a decisive difference in later life. In the schizophrenic group, for instance, it is the more active twin who was relatively more spared by an eventual schizophrenic process. Only among the psychopaths does the active twin lose the advantage, and hysterical symptoms seem more likely to occur in the more dominant partner. Dominance and submissiveness may not, perhaps, be the contrasts they appear. In ordinary clinical psychiatry we find personalities who are dominant in one environment, submissive in another, and are able to change with ease from one attitude to the other. A more important contrast lies between the dominant-submissive and the independent temperaments; and in this respect we rarely find any noteworthy difference between uniovular twins.

Twins Separated in Childhood and Later Life [abbreviated]

A comparison of twins who are brought up in different families or who later in life find their ways into different cultures is obviously of great importance to the study of problems of heredity and environment. Such studies are difficult to carry out, especially retrospectively. As cases are comparatively rare — Newman, Freeman, and Holzinger (1937), after painstaking inquiries throughout the U.S.A., could find and investigate only 19 uniovular pairs that had been brought up in different environments — it was of interest to record such information as we possess about the twins in our series who have been separated. Cases were included where the separation was of short duration only, but where it has occurred at a very early age when, according to some authorities, separation from home can sometimes cause far-reaching difficulties in later adjustment.

It can be said that only in two cases, one uniovular and one binovular , was there anything like clear evidence that the different experiences of the twins during their childhood separations contributed anything significant to their differing psychiatric fates. The findings in the cases where one twin emigrated were suggestive, but not generally applicable.

Factors Predisposing to, or Associated with, Mental Illness

Environmental Factors. In order to get a line on the influence of factors which predispose to, or are associated with, mental illness, we have classified the members of every pair of twins into those who had the more and those who had the less severe illness; we can then test whether the factor being investigated is present, or present to a greater degree, in the one or the other group. Unfortunately, information is often extremely scanty, so that the number on which we can make our test is often only a fraction of the total of all cases. The relevant figures that we have been able to obtain for the affective, psychopathic, and organic groups as well as the schizophrenic are set out in Table 9.7.

Difficult Birth. From Table 9.7 we note that being the first born of the twins, and therefore perhaps slightly more liable to injury at birth, is not significantly a disadvantage in any diagnostic group.

If, however, the birth of either twin (first or second born) was more difficult it was that twin who proved more likely to suffer, or suffered more severely, from psychiatric disorder in later life. This is equally true for uniovular and binovular twins and the deviation is in the same direction in all four diagnostic groups. Birth weight, amount of breast-feeding (about which, however, there is practically no information), and rate of infantile and childhood development seem to be almost without effect.

Physique and Health. Kallmann (1948) has reported, and laid great stress, on the finding that the twin who enjoys more satisfactory health, and who is the more athletically built, is the one who is less likely to fall ill, or, falling ill, is likely to do so later on in life, to be less seriously ill, and to recover more easily. His findings are

TABLE 9.7. FACTORS PREDISPOSING TO

	Schizophrenic						Affective					
	Uni.		Bin.		Total		Uni.		Bin.		Total	
	M*	L*	M	L	M	L	M	L	M	L	M	L
Born first	16	16	52	42	68	58	1	5	10	10	11	15
More difficult birth	7	3	10	7	17	10	–	–	4	–	4	–
Lighter at birth	3	5	10	14	13	19	1	–	2	2	3	2
Less breast feeding	2	–	2	2	4	2	–	–	–	–	–	–
Slower in early development	4	3	17	19	21	22	2	–	6	2	8	2
More neurotic child	4	4	12	6	16	10	1	–	6	2	7	2
Submissive to twin	7	2	22	8	29	10	2	1	4	1	6	2
Poorer physical health	8	3	24	22	32	25	1	1	2	3	3	4
Lighter weight	1	3	6	13	7	16	2	2	2	4	4	6
Less athletic build	–	1	7	15	7	16	–	1	1	5	1	6
Less intelligent	9	13	31	25	40	38	1	2	9	7	10	9
Remained single, twin marrying	8	2	35	5	43	7	3	1	7	–	10	1
Married later	1	2	7	11	8	13	–	2	8	5	8	7
More pregnancies	3	6	15	35	18	41	1	4	9	8	10	12
Number of pregnancies	19	24	78	113	97	137	5	11	55	55	60	66
Less stable occupationally before illness	7	4	37	4	44	8	2	–	6	–	8	–
Lower economic status before illness	2	–	9	1	11	1	–	–	3	–	3	–
More psychological stress	5	8	9	9	14	17	–	–	8	1	8	1
Generally more neurotic	13	4	32	6	45	10	–	–	6	2	6	2
Personality:												
More depressive	2	4	9	13	11	17	2	1	4	6	6	7
More labile emotionally	3	1	8	2	11	3	2	–	5	2	7	2
Less sociable	3	3	36	15	39	18	–	–	8	4	8	4
Cooler, more reserved	2	4	33	15	35	19	1	–	2	7	3	7
More paranoid, sensitive	9	2	23	11	32	13	–	1	4	1	4	2
More irritable, aggressive	3	5	18	11	21	16	–	–	6	3	6	3
More anxious	4	5	8	12	12	17	–	–	4	1	4	1
More hysterical	3	2	15	5	18	7	–	–	2	1	2	1
More hypochondriacal	–	1	5	3	5	4	–	–	4	1	4	1
More rigid	1	4	14	15	15	19	–	3	3	2	3	5
More obsessional	–	1	4	1	4	2	–	–	–	2	–	2
More eccentric	–	–	10	5	10	5	–	–	1	–	1	–
More alcohol consumed	1	–	8	4	9	4	–	–	–	1	–	1

*M = more severely ill twin, L = less severely ill (or unaffected) twin
†Excluding G.P.I. and other purely exogenous psychoses

based on large numbers and on physical examinations. The figures in our table, which are admittedly based merely on the recollections of relatives, show no sign of such a tendency, although we believe it to exist.

Neurotic Traits in Childhood. In all diagnostic groups there is a marked tendency for the more severely affected twin to have been the more neurotic child, but this tendency, however, is shown only by the binovular twins. This suggests that the difference is genetically determined and that the constitutional make up which predisposes to mental illness in the adult helps to cause neurotic symptoms in childhood. If the uniovular twins had shown the same difference as the binovular ones, it might have been easier to interpret the findings as suggesting that environmentally caused neurotic trait patterns in the child predisposed to later and graver illnesses. This is the position taken by psycho-analysis and related schools of thought, but it finds no support in our figures. Uniovular twins differ very little in

OR ASSOCIATED WITH MENTAL ILLNESS

Psychopathic						Organic†						Totals					
Uni.		Bin.		Total		Uni.		Bin.		Total		Uni.		Bin.		Total Severity		
M	L	M	L	M	L	M	L	M	L	M	L	M	L	M	L	More	Less	X^2
3	4	22	14	25	18	2	2	13	10	15	12	22	27	97	76	119	103	
2	–	10	5	12	5	–	–	4	2	4	2	9	3	28	14	37	17	7.4
2	1	6	6	8	7	–	–	1	2	1	2	6	6	19	24	25	30	
–	–	2	–	2	–	–	–	1	–	1	–	2	–	5	2	7	2	
2	1	8	3	10	4	–	–	5	–	5	–	8	4	36	24	44	28	3.3
1	2	14	3	15	5	1	–	1	2	2	2	7	6	33	13	40	19	7.5
1	4	5	7	6	11	–	–	1	1	1	1	10	7	32	17	42	24	4.9
1	2	10	6	11	8	1	–	7	2	8	2	11	6	43	33	54	39	
3	1	6	3	9	4	–	–	–	1	–	1	6	6	14	21	20	27	
–	1	6	2	6	3	1	–	–	1	1	1	1	3	14	23	15	26	
3	3	22	8	25	11	–	1	13	4	13	5	13	19	75	44	88	63	4.1
3	1	12	3	15	4	4	–	7	3	11	3	18	4	61	11	79	15	43.6
1	2	4	3	5	5	–	–	4	3	4	3	2	6	23	22	25	28	
–	5	4	10	4	15	–	4	8	8	8	12	4	19	32	61	36	80	16.7
4	11	14	36	18	47	–	9	38	41	38	50	28	55	185	245	213	300	
3	–	14	1	17	1	1	–	3	–	4	–	13	4	60	5	73	9	
–	–	4	–	4	–	–	1	–	–	–	1	2	1	16	1	18	2	12.8
2	1	1	3	3	4	1	1	3	–	4	1	8	10	21	13	29	23	
5	–	13	1	18	1	–	–	3	2	3	2	18	4	54	11	72	15	
1	1	5	2	6	3	2	–	2	3	4	3	7	6	20	24	27	30	
2	–	8	–	10	–	1	–	5	–	6	–	8	1	26	4	34	5	
1	1	8	5	9	6	–	–	2	4	2	4	4	4	54	28	58	32	7.5
1	1	5	4	6	5	–	–	2	3	2	3	4	5	42	29	46	34	
1	–	11	2	12	2	–	–	3	2	3	2	10	3	41	16	51	19	14.6
–	–	8	5	8	5	–	–	5	3	5	3	3	5	37	22	40	27	
2	1	9	3	11	4	1	–	3	3	4	3	7	6	24	19	31	25	
3	–	17	4	20	4	–	–	3	1	3	1	6	2	37	11	43	13	16.1
–	–	6	1	6	1	–	–	–	3	–	3	–	1	15	8	15	9	
–	1	2	1	2	2	1	–	2	–	3	–	2	8	21	18	23	26	
–	–	7	–	7	–	–	–	–	2	–	2	–	1	11	5	11	6	
1	–	1	–	2	–	–	–	–	1	–	1	1	–	12	6	13	6	
1	–	1	–	2	–	1	–	3	2	4	2	3	–	12	7	15	7	

the degree of neuroticism in childhood (in our series there are only 13 cases where any material difference is shown), and when there is a difference it bears no relation to differences of mental health in the adult.

It was also the more submissive of the two twins who was more severely affected in the schizophrenic and affective groups; numbers are too small in the organic groups to reach any definite conclusions, and in the neurotic and psychopathic group the tendency is rather the opposite way. In the group of endogenous psychotics, however, both the uniovular and binovular twins show the same preponderance of a severer affection in the more submissive partner. The interpretation is not easy, but it does suggest the influence of environmental, psychological causes.

Intelligence. From Table 9.7 there is no indication it is the less intelligent twin who is more likely to have a schizophrenic or affective psychosis. But it does appear that he is the one more predisposed to psychopathy and neurosis and to organic illness.

101

This is true only of the binovular twins, and would therefore appear to be connected with genetical make-up. The less intelligent twin is nearly three times as likely as his partner to be the more severely affected in later life by either psychopathic and neurotic or by organic illness, and in the binovular twins of both the psychopathic and organic groups the tendency is significant. It would seem that the gene or genes responsible for schizophrenic and affective psychoses are to this extent specific and have little effect on intelligence; whereas those genes which aid in the causation of temperamental instability and defects of personality, and of epilepsy and the dementias, might well have some effect on initial intelligence also. This supposition is supported by numerous reports by other workers which suggest that schizophrenics and affective psychotics are on the average of normal intelligence or better, whereas neurotics and epileptics tend to be of less than average intelligence.

The findings on occupational status before the outbreak of the illness can be connected with the findings on intelligence; but it is more likely that they are related to the temperamental aspects of the personality. In all diagnostic groups, including schizophrenics and affectives, the more severely affected twin had usually the lower economic position at the time of onset of the illness.

Sex Life. The figures of Table 9.7 show that the more seriously affected twin much more frequently remained single, in all diagnostic groups, and, if she did marry, though this did not occur at a significantly later age, had fewer children. This result can be regarded as in large part due to the effect of the illness itself; even affective and neurotic illnesses appear to act in some measure as a bar to marriage. It may also be true, but cannot be deduced from our figures, that the individual predestined to mental or nervous illness has a lesser urge towards marriage and is less fertile.

In the schizophrenic twins we are able to go a little further regarding their pre-morbid marriage rate. Though there was no difference between the less and the more severely affected twin in this respect in the uniovular twins, the difference in the binovular twins is well marked. At the age of the first schizophrenic illness of either twin, before the effects of the illness could have made themselves felt, 23 of the 115 eventually more severely affected twins and 41 of the eventually less severely affected, had married. The difference is significant and yields a χ^2 (Yates) of 6.26, $P < .01$. Even when twin partners are subclassified as schizophrenic, psychopathic, or normal, in each of these three subgroupings the same tendency holds, though numbers are too small for separate tests of significance.

The tendency which we observe in the social function of marriage does not extend into reproductive life. During the period between the time when both twins had married and the first schizophrenic illness of either, the eventually less seriously affected twins had a rather smaller, and not larger, number of children. It is also noteworthy that ten illegitimate children were born to the more severely affected, only one to the less severely affected.

Neurotic Traits in Adult Life. Occupational stability was less in the more severely affected twin in all diagnostic groups and in both uniovular and binovular twins, and this was a phenomenon of great regularity, holding true in 73 out of the 82 pairs in which a difference was recorded. This high proportion is presumably due to genetical and environmental effects tending in the same direction. One may assume that any environmental factor as well as any genetical factor which predisposed towards

102

illness also tended to interfere with occupational stability, and it may also be that the occupational instability was the earliest premonitory sign of an eventual illness. A poor occupational record would, furthermore, make adaptation after illness all the more difficult, and so lead to longer hospitalization and to a corresponding classification of the illness as more severe.

A result scarcely less in magnitude is disclosed when severity of illness is correlated with general neurotic traits. Again the more severely affected twin has had a more neurotic personality in 72 out of 87 cases, and again all diagnostic groups and both types of twin show the same thing.

If we take personality traits individually we can see that only certain traits seem to be associated with the gravity of the illness. Emotional lability is so most conspicuously, and this trait shows its effects in all diagnostic groups and in uniovular as well as binovular twins. Hysterical tendencies and paranoid tendencies also show a universal association of the same sort, and again the difference holds good for both uniovular and binovular twins. Lack of sociability, however, though significant in all diagnostic groups but the organic, is connected with a severer later affection only in the binovular twins. Other temperamental traits such as irritability and aggressiveness, anxiety, coolness, and reserve show correlations which, though they tend in the same direction, are not statistically significant, and some traits, such as those of a depressive kind, seem to be of no prognostic significance at all.

It cannot be claimed that much weight can be placed on this individual analysis; but taking together all our findings on the subject of the pre-morbid personality, we can say that they suggest first that the make-up of the personality affects the liability to psychotic as well as neurotic illness, and that environmental as well as genetical factors play a part in its causation.

Actual psychological precipitation, however, shows itself to be of little significance; in the uniovular pairs it has no effect on later history at all, and even in the binovular pairs it is without effect outside the affective psychoses.

Handedness. Information about handedness was obtained in only 68 out of 297 pairs (23 per cent). In one pair both members were left-handed; in 23 pairs one member was left-handed, the other right-handed; in the remaining 44 pairs both members were right-handed. Thus of 136 persons of known handedness 25 (or 19 per cent) were left-handed. This figure for twins is almost certainly higher than that found in the general population. Taking the uniovulars and binovulars separately, we find that among 18 uniovular pairs there are 5 left-handed members (14 per cent), while 49 binovular pairs contain 19 left-handed persons (19 per cent). The difference, however, is not significant. Wilson and Jones (1932) give the incidence of left-handedness in the single born as 6.5 per cent, in uniovular twins as 10.7 per cent, in binovular twins as 11.4 per cent. Rife (1950) gives higher figures: 26 per cent of left-handers in uniovular twins, 23 per cent in binovular twins.

There is no tendency for the left-handed to be more abnormal mentally than the right-handed. In fact, in 14 out of the 23 opposite-handed pairs it is the right-handed who is the more abnormal. Nor does any one of our four main diagnostic groups contain a significantly larger number of left-handed propositi than any other group.

An interesting finding relates to the uniovular schizophrenics. Of the 5 discordant pairs of known handedness 3 are opposite handed, while this is the case in only 1 of 6 concordant pairs — and in that pair uniovularity is not established with complete certainty. In other words, the only 3 certainly uniovular schizophrenic pairs where one member is left-handed and the other right-handed are all discordant. The numbers are, of course, far too small for any conclusion to be drawn. It is unfortunate that more information is not available.

THE PRESENT INVESTIGATION: CLINICAL

The Schizophrenic Twins

Concordance. There are in all 41 pairs of uniovular twins of which one member, the propositus, was schizophrenic, and in 28 of these pairs the other member was found to be likewise schizophrenic. Together these two figures give a concordance rate of 68.3 per cent. Such an estimate, however, takes no account of age, and is more inaccurate than it need be. The usual methods of allowing for age are not very satisfactory. It is customary in twin investigations to deal with the partners of the propositi as if they constituted an ordinary sample of the population. Weinberg's shorter method is used which allocates no risk of schizophrenia to persons under the age of 14, a half-risk between 14 and 40, and a full share of the risk after 40. Using this method we would reduce our total of 41 by half the number of those twins who when last observed were under 40; as 23 twins of our co-twins failed to reach this age, the concordance figure would become 28/29.5 = 94.9 per cent. Such a figure has little meaning. Alternatively we might apply the reduction for age only to the partners who never became schizophrenic. This is logically incorrect, as Schulz (1942) has shown; but in the present case it leads to a more reasonable concordance figure of 28/37.5 = 74.7 per cent.

The best estimate we can make of the concordance rate will take into account the correlation in age of onset between twins as well as the length of time they remained well before or after the illness of the propositus. In case 61, for instance the propositus fell ill at 45, and his twin was still free from schizophrenia at the age of 60. Among the concordant pairs only 4 differed in age of onset by more than 15 years so that we may calculate that the twin at the time of observation had survived (28 + 24)/56 of his chance of developing the disease.

TABLE 9.8. DIFFERENCES IN AGE OF ONSET OF SCHIZOPHRENIA IN
UNIOVULAR TWINS

Concordant		Discordant		
Difference in age of onset		Difference between age of twin when last observed and age of onset in propositus		
Years	No. observed	Case No.	Years	Weight assigned
1	9	13	+ 30	55.0/56
2	5	231	+ 22	54.5/56
3	1	61	+ 15	52.0/56
4	3	2	+ 13	50.5/56
5	1	133	+ 13	50.5/56
6	2	291	+ 12	50.0/56
8	1	164	+ 11	50.0/56
13	1	202	+ 11	50.0/56
14	1	53	+ 5	46.5/56
18	1	160	− 6	8.0/56
20	1	96	− 6	8.0/56
22	1	59	− 11	6.0/56
31	1	17	− 12	6.0/56
Total	28	13		487.0/56

Proceeding in this way, as is laid out in Table 9.8, we reach a concordance figure of $28/(28 + 487/56) = 76.3$ per cent. The procedure obviously has its own deficiencies, but further refinement would not be justified by the small total of cases.

To reach this figure of 76 per cent we have included among the concordant pairs a number in whom the diagnosis of schizophrenia in the partner is not established. The most doubtful case is 117. In this the twin's behaviour became peculiar at 43, after she had developed a goitre. Soon after this she became more seriously ill and had to go into an Observation Ward where she died. The whole of her mental abnormalities, of which we were unable to obtain an adequate account, might have been due to physical ill-health. Doubtful also, though to a lesser degree, is case 87. Here the twin at the age of 20 behaved in a strange way very suggestive of on-coming schizophrenia. However, he improved without developing acute psychotic symptoms and remained apparently normal until a sudden and inexplicable suicide a few years later. There is a gross insufficiency of information in three cases, and there are disputable qualities about two others. But it would seem captious to exclude them, as in every case schizophrenia is much more probable than normality or any other diagnosis.

To compensate for the possibility that we have over-estimated the incidence of schizophrenia in the twin partners, there is an equal possibility that we have under-estimated it. Counted to the discordant pairs is case 2, in which the twin's illness, though superficially depressive, had paranoid features, and ended in a suicide which seemed unexplained by the rather superficial depression. Furthermore in case 133 the twin brother migrated to Italy where he is said to have had nervous symptoms of unknown nature, though he never needed hospital treatment.

To refer briefly to the other discordant pairs, 4 of whom died before the propositus became schizophrenic, we note the presence of other psychiatric abnormalities. We have no reason to think that the partners in six cases are anything but normal. But the twin in case 53, as well as having congenital syphilis like the proposita, was dull and psychopathic. When she was interviewed she was sullen and suspicious and complained of a variety of neurotic symptoms. The twin brother in case 61 is a heavy beer-drinker like the propositus and has become a paranoid and shiftless psychopath. The twin sister in case 164 showed a marked but understandable anxiety reaction without schizophrenic features when her sister fell ill, and appears to have escaped anything more serious. In case 291 the twin sister resembled the proposita in many lifelong neurotic traits, for which she has had much medical advice, and is thought by her relatives to have behaved peculiarly, e.g. laughing and giggling in a strange way for no reason, and being generally unpredictable. Of case 160 little is known; the twin died about 6 years before his brother fell ill. Even when these cases are taken into account one could not regard the non-schizophrenic twin as consistently schizoid — a finding which has been reported by Kallmann (1946).

There were 10 pairs of concordant binovular twins (one with an associated mental deficiency). In addition there were 3 probable schizophrenics: a shy young man who died at home, described as unable to keep a job, "clairaudient", and as doing "silly little things"; a psychogenic paranoid state, with another schizophrenic sister; and a psychopath who became queer, dirty, "like a degenerate" and disappeared untraced. Including these probable schizophrenics, we have a concordance figure of 13 out of 115, or 11.3 per cent (14.4 per cent when corrected for age by Weinberg's shorter method).

Among the sibs there were 19 schizophrenics and 7 probable schizophrenics, giving an incidence of 4.6 per cent (5.4 per cent corrected for age). Among the parents there were 7 certain and 5 probable schizophrenics; incidence 3.9 per cent (4.1 per cent with age correction).

In other groups only occasional schizophrenics appear. One propositus with epilepsy and ? schizophrenia is counted in the organic group. A brother of a manic depressive is schizophrenic; the mother of a hysteric apparently had both epilepsy and schizophrenia; in both these cases the propositi had schizoid symptoms. The brother of an anxiety neurotic was a schizoid personality and possibly schizophrenic.

Some explanation is necessary of the high concordance figure for binovular twins compared with that for sibs. It is difficult to assess how much, if any, is due to the more similar early environment of the twins, but a great part of the difference is more probably to be accounted for by the fact that the twins of the propositi were more thoroughly investigated than the sibs. This suggestion is also supported by the fact that the incidence of schizophrenia in the sibs of the propositi is very low, judged by the values found by other workers, i.e. 8 per cent or over. However, similar findings are not noted in the organic and psychopathic groups.

A remarkable feature is shown by the schizophrenic binovular twins which is not found in other groups. Nearly all (11 out of 13) of the concordant pairs are same-sexed. Both the twins in the opposite-sexed pairs are not certain but only probable schizophrenics. Neither the sibs nor the parents who are schizophrenic show any tendency to be of the same sex as the propositus, nor, as we have said, do the abnormal binovular twins of the non-schizophrenic propositi. We can only note this fact as a curiosity and cannot offer an explanation.

Age of Onset. The differences in age of onset in the concordant uniovular twins have been recorded in Table 9.8. Taken in pairs, the ages yield a correlation co-efficient of +0.54. This figure may be compared with the correlation coefficient between the ages of onset in pairs of schizophrenic sibs, which we have calculated from our material. This is +0.39, based on 26 pairs. On other material Slater (44) found a sib-sib correlation of 0.55; Strömgren (1935) has found one of 0.19. A very striking anomaly is that the correlation given by the concordant binovular twins is +0.74. This figure is, however, based on the very small number of 13 pairs and cannot be regarded as reliable.

The ages of onset of disease in the propositi, in their twin partners, sibs and parents are given in Table 9.9. One of the interesting features of this table is the large number of persons who first became ill in later life. Even when the parents are omitted, 46 persons out of 224, 20 per cent first fell ill after the age of 40.

This table also shows the sex distribution. From the twin partners the uniovular twins may be omitted leaving 4 male and 9 female affected binovular twins. Even then it will be noted that in all groups affected females outnumber affected males by approximately 2:1.

Course and Outcome. In 18 of the concordant uniovular cases the propositus had a single illness, in 10 two or more attacks. The corresponding figures for their schizophrenic partners are 17 and 11; in 12 cases both propositus and twin had a single illness. These figures do not yield a significant χ^2. Of the 13 concordant binovular pairs 7 of the propositi and 7 of their partners had single illnesses, the remainder two attacks or more; in 4 cases both twins had one illness only. To test whether genetical factors are likely to play a part in determining the course of the illness we may add together the concordant uniovular twins, the binovular twins and the sib-pairs. Where the propositus had only one attack, 31 out of 44 schizophrenic relatives had one attack only, compared with 8 out of 23 relatives where the propositus had two attacks or more. These figures yield (with Yates' correction) a χ^2 of 6.50 which is significant at the 0.02 level, and strongly suggests that genetical factors do help to determine whether the schizophrenia takes a relapsing form or not.

We have classified the outcome of the disease according to whether it ended in a social recovery, in some form of social defect compatible with life outside hospital, or in hospitalized invalidism. Among the concordant uniovular twins, in 21 cases the propositus and in 16 cases the partner ended as hospital invalids; in the binovular twins the corresponding figures are 10 and 8. Exact correspondence in outcome was noted in 16 out of 28 (57 per cent) of the uniovular pairs, in 7 out of 13 (54 per cent) of the binovular pairs, and in 10 out of 26 (38 per cent) of the sib-sib pairs. However, if we subject the material, either taken separately or together, to statistical analysis the results are not significant and there is no suggestion that related individuals suffering from schizophrenia resemble one another in outcome. Bleuler (1941), however, found that in pairs of blood-related schizophrenics there were marked resemblances in age of onset and course, and that there was a significant though lesser degree of resemblance in end-state. Bleuler's material, which was not one of twins, was much larger than ours and contained 367 pairs of affected relatives. Slater (44) also found a marked and statistically significant resemblance between pairs of sibs in the course and outcome of schizophrenia. On the other hand Essen-Möller (1941) found no close resemblance between his uniovular twins in these respects.

Duration. There is little to be learned from a statistical examination of the duration of the illness of the twins. There are too many accidental causes of variation in this respect for a comparison to be worth while. One twin, treated in one hospital, may be released after the acute phase of the illness has blown over; the other twin, in another hospital, may have an acute illness of about the same duration, but yet, perhaps because he does not make such a good recovery, or because the hospital authorities are stricter about discharge, he may remain in hospital for many years after the end of the illness. Illnesses occurring in two twins at different ages may

TABLE 9.9. AGES OF ONSET OF SCHIZOPHRENIA AND SEX DISTRIBUTION IN
PROPOSITI AND RELATIVES

Age in years	Propositi			Twin partners			Sibs			Parents			Total		
	m.	f.	T.	m.	f.	T.	m.	f.	T.	m.	f.	T.	m.	f.	T.
0–14	—	—	—	—	1	1	—	—	—	—	—	—	—	1	1
15–19	9	18	27	1	2	3	—	2	2	—	—	—	10	22	32
20–24	16	14	30	4	11	15	3	4	7	1	1	2	24	30	54
25–29	10	23	33	2	6	8	1	6	7	—	1	1	13	36	49
30–34	4	11	15	—	2	2	1	2	3	—	—	—	5	15	20
35–39	8	10	18	1	3	4	2	—	2	—	1	1	11	14	25
40–44	3	10	13	1	2	3	—	—	—	1	—	1	5	12	17
45–49	3	11	14	—	4	4	1	—	1	2	2	4	6	17	23
50–54	—	4	4	—	—	—	—	2	2	1	2	3	1	8	9
55–59	—	2	2	1	—	1	—	1	1	—	—	—	1	3	4
60–64	—	—	—	—	—	—	—	—	—	—	—	—	—	—	—
65–69	—	—	—	—	—	—	—	1	1	—	—	—	—	1	1
Total	53	103	156	10	31	41	8	18	26	5	7	12	76	159	295

have entirely different effects on this total stay in hospital, for one is much more likely to have a prolonged stay if he has been admitted at an early age. Again, an illness may be terminated after only a brief period in hospital if one twin dies early and not the other. As a result of all these possible variations there are remarkable discrepancies, and there is no obvious sign of any correlation between uniovular twins in the duration of their incapacity. In case 129 the proposita was ill for 49 years, the first signs of her illness being at the age of 16; her twin, who fell ill at 47 was ill for only 15 years, dying at 62. In case 4 the proposita was in hospital for 46 years from 32 to 79; her twin had an illness of perhaps 6 month's duration at about the age of 26. The next longest stay is observed in case 8, where the proposita remained in hospital for 34 years; her twin's illness, which terminated in death, was for only 3 years. Durations of 28 years are noted in cases 43 and 273; in one case the illness of the twin lasted 20 years, in the other 4 months.

One might think that the matter could be pursued by examining the hospital notes more narrowly, and distinguishing between acute periods of illness and those long quiet periods when the patient is kept in hospital mainly for social reasons. This would be a forlorn task. The detail provided in hospital records is not sufficient for the purpose; and, what is just as important, in many cases there is a slow and progressive deterioration, part of which may be due to schizophrenic changes, part to what is usually called institutionalisation.

We can only conclude that we can give no evidence of a similarity between uniovular schizophrenic twins in the duration of their illness. What may be said of the uniovular twins applies equally to other relatives such as binovular twins and sibs.

Type of Onset. Disease onsets were classified into sudden, gradual with a sudden exacerbation, and gradual. The second of these groups was, however, poorly represented, not because it is actually infrequent in clinical practice but because the information available was seldom sufficient to show that gradual changes had preceded the sudden outburst which eventually led to the patient's admission to hospital. For the same reason the total number of sudden onsets may be exaggerated. Maintaining this differentiation there was conformity in mode of onset in 20 out of 27 (73 per cent) of the uniovular pairs (in one pair information insufficient), in 9 out of 13 (69 per cent) of the binovular pairs, in 16 out of 26 (62 per cent) of the sib-sib pairs, and in 7 out of 12 (58 per cent) of the parent-child pairs. Putting all relationships into a single table yields a χ^2 (Yates) of 11.72, which is significant at the 0.001 level, and so is strong evidence that the type of onset is genetically determined.

Precipitation. It is not possible to provide useful statistics on this subject, but a few clinical similarities may be noted, sometimes physical ones, sometimes psychological, often a mixture of both.

Both Pamela and Viola (273) for instance, were frail, undersized children of low intelligence, and in each case their first illness followed a physical upset: with Viola it was an inoculation while in the A.T.S., and with Pamela an appendix operation at 18. Other physical factors, such as those associated with the endocrine system, enter into a number of the cases. A common precipitating factor is childbirth. This is so in 39/47, for Rose became ill some while after an abortion, while Mollie became acutely excited and maniacal a fortnight after the birth of her baby. Freda in 11 became retarded and acutely depressed about a month after her son's birth, and, although her twin, Louisa, never had any children, it is worth noting that she accused herself of being too much of a coward to have a baby and guilt about that fear entered into her early psychotic symptoms. One twin in 115 first fell ill during her pregnancy and her

108

partner after tonsilectomy. Connie, the over-sensitive proposita of 129, was very much upset during adolescence by her mother's illness and death and she gradually became ill after this; her twin succumbed to schizophrenia during the menopause, following her father's death. Both Norah and Freda (137) had a history of overwork and had failed examinations four times before falling ill during adolescence. The illnesses of both were also associated with fluctuations in weight. In case 20 Lilian and Mary fell ill at about the same age, that is about the time of the climacteric. Mary had marked menopausal symptoms before her illness; in Lilian's case no such symptoms are recorded, but there is a tale of an unhappy love affair which may have been due to menopausal instability. In addition, both twins were going deaf.

Psychogenesis appears to have played a part in other cases. The proposita in 41 became ill while still in hospital after childbirth when her husband was killed in an accident tree-felling, while the precipitating factor in her twin's illness was a long and very unhappy love relationship. In case 14 Dora's recurrent illnesses are associated with an abortive love affair and one of her twin's illnesses with the death of her mother. The father's death was thought to have brought on Ellen's illness (168), but her twin, Constance, broke down at a much earlier age, without apparent psychogenesis, after some dental extractions. Leslie, the propositus in case 287, gradually declined into a schizophrenic state after a sun-stroke, and this illness of his appears to have precipitated his twin's breakdown. The psychogenic factor in case 117 which appears to have led to Hilda's illness was in the first place her twin's marriage and 14 years later her twin's death; the twin's own illness was attributed to a goitre.

In the remaining uniovular pairs there is no evidence of any noteworthy precipitating factor in either twin.

There are instances of concordant precipitation among the binovular pairs as well. Marcella (57/246), became ill after an occupational stress when she was governess to a small boy in Paris, while the stress in her twin's case was a marital one. The schizophrenic illnesses of two of their sibs were also precipitated by psychological strains similar to those suffered by the twins themselves. Another sib-sib concordance, and the most remarkable, is the instance of *folie à trois* in case 50. In case 37 a physical factor was present in both twins; in the one it was childbirth, in the other a poisoned finger. On the other hand, the stress undergone by both the proposita and her brother (94) was psychological. In her case it was the death of her twin, while her brother was upset by a dispute about a trust fund.

Among the binovular pairs and the sib-sib pairs, however, the frequency of some sort of precipitation in one of the pair which is not matched in the other, is much greater than in the uniovular cases.

If, therefore, we concern ourself solely with the presence or absence of precipitation there is a remarkable degree of concordance in the uniovular twins, 27 out of 28 cases. But often the precipitating factors cited are not very convincing, and they are often very different in the two twins. On the whole our evidence suggests that genetic factors play a part in determining an individual's susceptibility to physical and psychological precipitants, although one must also make considerable allowances for the consistency which springs from the mental attitude of the informants, rather than from qualities which are inherent in the cases themselves.

Clinical Symptoms. Catatonic symptoms and signs: It seems natural to subdivide catatonic signs and symptoms into positive and negative. Under the first we may include such things as catatonic excitement, overactivity, impulsiveness and aggression. The second embraces stupor, negativism, retardation and "catatonia", i.e. waxy flexibility and other abnormalities of muscle tone.

Any given subject may therefore be classified into one of four classes, as having: (a) both positive and negative catatonic signs, (b) positive only, (c) negative only, (d) neither.

Of these classes the first was most heavily represented in the propositi and also in all the relatives except the schizophrenic parents. In fact 60 per cent of the parents, 75 per cent of sibs, and 75 per cent of the binovular twins, who had schizophrenic psychoses, had catatonic signs of some kind; only one of the uniovular twins was without them. Positive catatonic signs are more frequent than negative ones, in the proportion of 5 to 4, but they tend to be associated together, so that the class of individuals with both positive and negative signs is in excess, and the class in which signs of both kinds are absent is nearly twice as well represented as random probabilities would lead one to infer. The only significance of these statistical findings is to support the commonly held psychiatric belief in a catatonic syndrome within schizophrenia.

More interesting figures become available when we compare the illnesses of related individuals. In the parent-child relationships the incidence of absolute concordance is 30 per cent; that is, in 3 of 10 pairs both members belonged to one and the same class of the categories a, b, c, or d above. In the sib-sib pairs concordance was 38 per cent, in the binovular twins 42 per cent, and in the uniovular twins 74 per cent. However, only in the last group is there a greater concordance than chance would suggest; from the relative frequencies of the four categories (a-d) in the twins taken separately we would expect 12.16 to be similar, and 12.84 to show some dissimilarity (only 25 pairs could be used for this purpose, as in the remaining 3 information was insufficient). The similarities observed were 19. The difference is significant at the 0.01 level (χ^2 = 7.49, 1 D.F.).

We may conclude that, even if other classes of relative do not show close resemblance, uniovular schizophrenic twins resemble one another significantly in the presence or absence and in the nature of catatonic signs. Resemblance between schizophrenic sibs in their liability to catatonic signs and symptoms had been previously reported by Slater (44).

Hallucinations: Information is available about 23 uniovular pairs and in 16 both were hallucinated at some time, in 3 neither at any time. This gives us a total concordance of 19 out of 23 (83 per cent). Corresponding percentages were: for binovular twins 33 per cent, for the sib-sib pairs 67 per cent, and for the parent-child pairs 58 per cent. However, although the uniovular twins resemble one another more closely than other relatives, none of the figures attain statistical significance. The great bulk of all hallucinatory experiences were in the auditory field; however, it is noteworthy that in two cases both members of the uniovular pair had visual hallucinations, and the same coincidence was observed in one of the sib-sib pairs.

There is, therefore, a suggestion that the presence or absence of hallucinations, and possibly their nature, may be affected by genetical factors, but we have insufficient information to say anything definite. Previous work (Slater, 44) also failed to show a significant resemblance between schizophrenic sibs in the tendency to hallucination.

Delusions: These are so common in schizophrenic illnesses that, like hallucinations, they do not form very satisfactory material for estimates of concordance. Of the 24 uniovular pairs in which information was sufficient, both members of the pair were deluded in 16 cases, and there was no case in which neither member of the pair was deluded. Figures of a corresponding type were obtained for other classes of relatives, and the incidence of positive concordance was so high, that of negative concordance so low, that tests of statistical significance were not applicable.

A disappointing result was also obtained when delusions were classified by form into (*a*) ideas of reference, (*b*) of passivity, (*c*) of bodily change, (*d*) of guilt, (*e*) persecutory, (*f*) grandiose, (*g*) hypochondriacal. (It proved impossible to get adequate information about the presence or absence of primary delusional experiences.) In each group numbers were small and, with one exception, showed no statistically significant concordance within pairs. However, when all pairs of relatives, both of whom had had delusions in some form, were taken together, a χ^2 test

(Yates) showed a greater resemblance within pairs in respect of passivity feelings than chance would suggest (χ^2 = 4.23, 1 D.F., $P <$ 0.05). Slater (44) found that sibs resembled one another significantly in paranoid features.

Mood changes: These, which play a prominent part in schizophrenic illnesses, may be classified as positive or negative. Under the first heading we noted in our subjects the occurrence of depressions, periods of elation, agitation or anxiety and also of any marked and rapid change in the emotional level. As negative symptoms we recorded apathy, social withdrawal, and inappropriateness or flattening of affect.

Symptoms of the positive kind are likely to occur early in the psychosis and to be associated with a florid picture. The occurrence and the nature of such an emotional change are likely to be determined also in part by the underlying personality. In 24 uniovular twin pairs for which we had sufficient information, both twins showed such a change in 15 cases, neither twin in 5, giving a total concordance of 20 out of 24 (83 per cent). The binovular twins also show 83 per cent concordance; in other relatives lower figures were reached, none of them statistically significant. Taking all relatives together, we get figures which show a significant tendency for relatives to resemble one another in this respect (χ^2 (Yates) = 4.3, 1 D.F., $P <$ 0.05). Slater (44) found that pairs of schizophrenic sibs resembled one another in their affective symptoms.

Analysing the positive affective changes separately gives confirmatory findings. Only the tendency towards rapid fluctuation of mood, which is rare, fails to give significant results. In the case of a comparatively common symptom like depression the results are rather striking, and are given in Table 9.10.

TABLE 9.10. DEPRESSIVE SYMPTOMS IN SCHIZOPHRENIC PROPOSITI AND RELATIVES

		Depressive symptoms		
	Present in both	Present in one		Absent in both
Uniovular pairs	11	7		6
Binovular pairs	8	4		0
Sib-sib pairs	7	9		10
Parent-child pairs	2	5		2
Total	28	25		18

This shows a total of 46 pairs resembling one another, while the chance expectation is only 36.2 (χ^2 = 5.41, $P <$ 0.02).

Although the figures are less striking there are also significant tendencies towards resemblance in the occurrence of elation, anxiety symptoms and agitation.

Affective changes of the negative kind tend on the whole to occur later in the illness, and are associated with deterioration. In this case, apart from the uniovular twins themselves there is no general tendency towards resemblance within pairs of relatives, and even in the uniovular pairs the tendency is not significant.

We see, therefore, that these two types of affective change behave differently statistically. While the positive signs seem to be closely connected with genetical factors, the negative changes do not. This is to be associated with the findings already reported on this material, that pairs of related schizophrenics resemble each other little in outcome.

Depersonalisation: Although depersonalisation can be regarded as an affective symptom, it is in a class of its own from the clinical, psychopathological and prognostic point of view. Information on the subject in the records of mental hospitals tends to be scanty, and if the symptom was not recorded it does not mean it was not to be found. When all pairs of relatives are taken together, in 70 pairs there is no record of the symptom in either pair, in 4 cases the symptom was recorded as present in both; in 2 cases it was present in the propositus but not in the relative and in 3 cases the reverse was the case. An exact test shows that the probability of such a distribution is approximately 1/3,000, so that the result is highly significant. The four positively concordant cases are a uniovular pair, and a binovular pair, both cases of double propositi.

Thought disorder: This was commonly present. In the uniovular pairs both showed it to some degree in 15 pairs, neither in 4 pairs, in 3 other pairs it was present in one only. This gives a total concordance of 86 per cent, which may be compared with 69 per cent in the binovular twins, 54 per cent in the sib-sib pairs, and 56 per cent in the parent-child pairs. Only in the case of the uniovular twins does a χ^2 test show statistical significance (χ^2 Yates = 5.95, 1 D.F., P < 0.02). Taking all relatives together, a two by two table shows no significant deviation.

Thought disorder, therefore, like other deteriorative symptoms, shows little sign of being genetically determined.

Organic signs: From time to time in schizophrenic illnesses one may see signs which resemble those of an organic (symptomatic) psychosis. The commonest of these are confusion, disorientation and delirious symptoms, and epileptic fits. These signs were rare, but were present in both members of two uniovular pairs and one binovular pair. Taking all relatives together, we note positive concordance in 8 pairs, negative concordance in 54 pairs, discordance in 11 pairs; χ^2 is significant at 5.92 for 1 D.F. Despite, therefore, the apparently accidental and exogenous appearance of these symptoms it may be that they, too, have some genetical basis.

Suicide and self-injury: Among the uniovular twins these symptoms are recorded in both members of seven pairs; among the binovulars in both members of one. Taking all pairs of relatives together there is significant concordance, a two by two table yielding a χ^2 of 4.92, P < 0.05. Kallmann and Anastasio (1947) have reported that they have been unable to find a single case, either in their own very large material, or in the literature, in which both members of a pair of twins committed suicide. We have no such case either; but our material would seem to show some resemblance within twins in tendencies toward self-injury in a more general sense.

Treatment. Unfortunately, it is not possible to provide information of any value about the effects of treatment, for it was mostly given very late in the illness, at a point when great benefit could hardly be hoped for. It must be remembered that the clinical material dates largely from days before modern methods of treatment had begun to be extensively applied.

In one case the proposita received at different times insulin, cardiazol and thyroid but remained a hospital invalid; her twin made a social recovery without treatment. In another pair both twins received at different times cardiazol and progesterone; one of them had insulin treatment and E.C.T. as well, the other had in addition a course of continuous narcosis. In another case, one twin had insulin treatment, the other cardiazol and E.C.T.; both remained hospital invalids. Convulsive treatment was given to one or both in 11 pairs. There is no suggestion that the treated twin did better than the other; it was in fact the twin who was more severely ill, and ill for a longer period, who was deemed to require treatment.

It is not from facts like these that we shall get an answer to questions about the effect of treatment.

Affective Illnesses in the Families of Schizophrenics. Thirty-six affective illnesses have been observed among the binovular twins, sibs and parents of the schizophrenic propositi (16 of them among the parents) and there are 4 depressive or cyclothymic personalities. These cases must be regarded with interest, even with suspicion, for their very occurrence tends to support the views of those who hold that the distinction between schizophrenic and affective psychoses is more one of convenience than of scientific validity. If there are different genetical factors for schizophrenic and affective psychoses, then we must suspect that some of these apparently affective psychoses were, genetically, schizophrenias – or, alternatively, that some of the schizophrenias were, genetically, affective psychoses. Finally, there arises the possibility that there are "schizo-affective" psychoses which may tend to be regarded either as schizophrenias or as affective psychoses, according to the balance of symptoms, but which are genetically distinct from either. These possibilities are discussed below.

When we look more closely at these 36 affective illnesses, one anomaly appears at once: no fewer than 17 are involutional or menopausal melancholias, and 3 others have been diagnosed as atypical depressions. The rest consist of 3 reactive depressions, 4 manic-depressive or cyclothymic depressions, 6 other depressive states and 3 cases of suicide in a depressive setting. Seventeen involutional cases out of 36 is high, compared with 5 out of 26 for the affectively ill relatives of the affective propositi, or 3 out of 10 for the affectively ill relatives of the organic and psychopathic propositi. Comparing the schizophrenics and the others, a two by two table gives a χ^2 of 3.92, exceeding the 0.05 level of significance. The suggestion arises that there is a genetical relationship between schizophrenia and involutional melancholia.

Atypical schizophrenic features in the affective relatives: All three atypical depressions and a few of the involutional depressions have schizophrenic-like features. The mother of the schizophrenic twins 34/124 became depressed at 38 and attempted to strangle herself. In her agitated depression she was extremely paranoid, had passivity feelings, and for a month was stuporose. She recovered, but relapsed again 20 years later with a similar illness, from which she again recovered. Both her binovular twin daughters had depressive symptoms in their schizophrenic illnesses, and Iris's illness took a remitting course. Stupor was a notable feature of the illnesses of all three.

Similarly, the sister of propositus 75 had two depressive illnesses at 32 and 57, and in the second deteriorated in habits, became noisy and violent and posed in a stereotyped way, though once more she recovered. Her brother, the propositus, had a deteriorative schizophrenic psychosis without any affective admixture.

Our one recurrently manic relative (167) is also interesting. The father of these binovular twins, one of whom had a paranoid schizophrenia without affective symptoms, and the other a menopausal depression without schizophrenic features, first fell ill at 38 with a fairly typical mania, though he was hallucinated at night; at 47 he fell ill again with a depression which changed to mania and was paranoid with passivity symptoms of a very schizophrenic quality (he felt the doctor drawing electricity from his body). In his third illness at 52 he was even more paranoid and was hallucinated in most senses. In his fifth illness at 69 there were marked catatonic features, and he repeated meaningless phrases in a stereotyped way. It is by no means impossible that all his illnesses were to be regarded as recurrent catatonic excitements, though the absence of deterioration of personality with each successive illness, and the invariable recovery are against this.

Most of the involutional melancholias occurring among the relatives of schizophrenic propositi are fairly typical and do not show any marked schizophrenic colouring; but there are some suggestive exceptions. The father in 11 fell ill at 52 with an otherwise typical melancholic psychosis, but his hypochondriacal delusions had a bizarre quality (he believed, for instance, that his nose was falling to pieces), his restless agitation took on a stereotyped monotonous character, and he remained for 14 years in the mental hospital without recovery.

The brother of proposita 216 had two depressions at 39 and 69, and apparently made a practically complete recovery from the first, though he continued to stay in the mental hospital. In his second illness he had hypochondriacal delusions and catatonic symptoms, which, however, could be attributed to organic senile changes. The proposita herself had two illnesses, at 35 and 51, and though the second was an unmistakable schizophrenia, the first was clinically a depression.

The father in 51, sib 3 in 149 and the mother in 254 also all showed anomalous and schizophrenic-like features in the course of depressions of later life.

Reviewing these cases as a group, it does seem probable that some of them were in fact schizophrenic psychoses, and might have been recognised as such if fuller clinical data had been available. The rather high incidence of affective psychosis among the relatives of schizophrenics, and particularly the high incidence of the depressive illnesses of later life, may well be due in part to schizophrenic psychoses being mis-diagnosed as affective ones.

Atypical affective features in the schizophrenic propositi: We now have to consider the opposite possibility, which is that some part of the incidence of affective psychoses in the relatives of schizophrenics is due to a mistaken diagnosis of the propositus. The schizophrenic propositi, in whose families affective illness occurred, often themselves showed a marked affective colouring to their illnesses.

The best example is the discordant uniovular pair Millicent and Elizabeth (2). Millicent fell ill at 45 with a depressive state apparently brought on by being told by her doctor that she had a growth. She remained depressed for 5 months until her suicide, but never showed any schizophrenic symptoms. Elizabeth also became mildly depressed at 20, with worries about her health, and depressed once again in the same way at 33. But on this second occasion she developed paranoid ideas of being poisoned, passivity feelings, catatonia and an unmistakably paranoid schizophrenic illness which, however, was throughout strongly coloured by a depressive mood.

Case 37 is one of two female binovular twins, Alison and Norah, both of whom became schizophrenic. The father was a reserved, sensitive and worrying psychopath; the mother became paranoid with oncoming deafness. One sister also became deaf and paranoid in middle age, and another sister had a reactive depression lasting 9 months after the death of the mother. Alison became depressed at 35 with a septic thumb, and was confused, possibly from toxaemia, but passed on into a catatonic stupor. Her long and malignant psychosis was characterised by phases both of excitement and inhibition. Norah's illness was even more depressive in colouring, so much so that her first illness at 31 was considered throughout to be melancholic. Her second illness at 34, from which she also made a good recovery, was also predominantly depressive, but on this occasion she was hallucinated. In her third illness at 37, heralded by attempted suicide, she showed for the first time a paranoid schizophrenia, receiving messages through the ether telling her that her children had been murdered, and the affective symptoms at last receded.

The family background of case 6 is interesting. The father had a psychosis at 21 of which nothing is known, but he remained well for the rest of his life. Though very reserved with outsiders, he appears to have been of a cyclothymic temperament. The same is true of his son, twin brother of the proposita, who had a mental illness of apparently affective nature at 35. The illness of the proposita, though it finally ends in a characteristically schizophrenic picture, is in many ways anomalous. Her first illness at 22 was a typical depression. Three years later she broke down again and never recovered. Schizophrenic signs are shown after the tenth month, but for 13 years a somewhat apathetic depression is in the foreground of the picture. The organic illness 16 years after her second admission, with focal cerebral signs, remains unexplained; it cannot be due to diabetes. Perhaps it was an acute catatonic excitement, in which both fleeting neurological signs and a mild pyrexia are known to occur. This is the more likely as the whole of her illness seems to proceed by a series of short, acute phases, with intervening periods of quiescence.

Other similar cases can be more briefly mentioned. Case 251 is interesting in that the propositus and his sister both had hypochondriacal reactions in adolescence. With the former it was an incipient schizophrenia, but there is no evidence that the latter was also schizophrenic. Nineteen years later, after childbirth, she had a mild depression without anomalous features. The mother of 258 had an involutional depression at 42. The daughter became worried, depressed and self-reproachful at 45, and a year later passed into a chronic catatonic state by way of increasing suspiciousness and apathy. In case 145, depression colours the illness of Edmund and the personality of Rodney, although both these binovular twins were probably schizophrenic; their mother suffered from a reactive depression. An elder sister, in case 255, committed suicide at 21 on discovering that the man by whom she was pregnant was already married. Depressive features and attempts at suicide occur in both the schizophrenic sisters in this family, and the psychopathic father was depressed later in life. Symptoms of both schizophrenic and affective type are seen in proposita 112 and in her sister. Even when she was examined at the age of 46, 29 years after the onset of her psychosis, the proposita still showed clinical resemblance to a depressive state, though the schizophrenic form of the illness could not be mistaken. Her sister's psychosis was typically depressive but for the occurrence of catatonic rigidity.

Reviewing this group of cases, we feel no temptation to think we have misdiagnosed affective psychoses in the propositi as schizophrenias. Although their psychoses are coloured more than is usual with affective features, they are in other respects quite typical, and are certainly no less malignant than the other schizophrenias we have observed. There are other possible explanations which would be more easily related to the clinical facts. It might be, for instance, that constitutional traits of personality which under some circumstances could be the basis of an affective illness, tended also to reduce powers of resistance to schizophrenia. Alternatively, the facts we have noted might be partly explained by Kallmann's hypothesis that the liability to develop a schizophrenic illness is greater if physical health is reduced and weight is lost, as might occur in the course of a bodily illness or in a psychogenic depression. In any case there is no need to wonder if an oncoming schizophrenia calls forth affective symptoms, either in the way of depression or excitement, as the capacity for affective reaction is a quality of the normal human being. A number of schizophrenic propositi, without affective illness in their families, showed marked affective features which could be regarded in this way.

"Schizo-affective psychoses": The third possibility, mentioned in the opening paragraph of this section (p. 113), should however be briefly discussed. This was that there are such things as "schizo-affective" psychoses, in which symptoms of both schizophrenic and affective type can be shown, but which depend on independent genetical factors, which are distinct from those responsible for either of the main groups. Some of the cases already mentioned could be interpreted along this line, e.g. 34/124, 216, 2, 37, 145, 255, 112. Leonhard (1934) has described several families in which anomalous endogenous psychoses were shown by several members as a distinct clinical syndrome, with indications of a dominant mode of inheritance. In the seven families we list, a parent as well as children was affected in five. Our evidence is of very little weight, but it certainly does not tend against the possible existence of schizo-affective psychoses of an autonomous kind.

The possibility is not to be ignored that an atypical psychosis may occur when the same individual carries heterogeneous tendencies to endogenous psychoses of different kinds at the same time. Smith (1925) has reported such cases, and has shown that in ascendants and collaterals psychoses of a typically schizophrenic and of a typically affective kind could be found, when the propositus had an atypical psychosis combining features of the two sorts. There are possibly such cases also in the present material. The clearest example we have of accidental coincidence of distinct hereditary tendencies is in case 149. The father had a malignant catatonic schizophrenia, beginning at 45, the mother probably had an involutional depression (though her mother, herself psychotic, had an illness beginning at 49, which is more suggestive of a schizophrenic than an affective state). Of their children, two developed involutional melancholias and two schizophrenias, and in each case the psychosis was of a fairly typical kind, without anomalous features.

There are several other families in which schizophrenias without much affective colouring and affective psychoses without schizophrenic-like symptoms coincide. In the family of proposita 131 there are a mother and a binovular twin sister who had typical depressive illnesses, while the proposita herself had a typical deteriorative schizophrenia. In the family of case 147 there is, in addition to the father who had involutional melancholia, a cyclothymic sister, energetic, easily offended, "either up in the air or down in the dumps over some trifle".

The illness of the propositus shows no genuine disturbance of mood. Although there are no affective illnesses in the family of case 94, there is a moody psychopathic father who committed suicide, and a sister with a depressive personality. Neither the proposita nor her eldest sister showed depressive symptoms in their paranoid schizophrenias. The illness of the youngest brother, however, was a mild schizophrenia with paranoid and hypochondriacal symptoms and a favourable outcome, showing also much anxiety, depression and self-reproach. The illness of father and daughter in case 28 have nothing in common. Here the father's illness might possibly be attributed to his cardiovascular degeneration and arteriosclerosis.

The only instance in which schizophrenia occurs in the families of the affectively ill propositi can be mentioned here. In case 97 the alcoholic mother committed suicide in a fit of depression; the father, sib 1 and the twin sister show cyclothymic traits. The propositus is apparently manic-depressive; but in hospital he is sometimes taken for a schizophrenic, being described as suspicious, manneristic and impulsive. Sib 5's illness also has these characteristics, but is a predominantly paranoid schizophrenia without affective symptoms.

Reviewing the whole of the evidence, it does seem that schizophrenia and affective psychoses are genetically distinct. Nevertheless we can observe syndromes which break up in their distribution over several members of an affected family. We can see, for instance, depressive features in a psychopathic setting, appearing in the course of a schizophrenic illness, and showing openly as an affective psychosis in different members. A constitutional tendency which can be of pathogenic importance in one, exercises only a pathoplastic effect in another.

To a lesser extent the same observation may be made on schizoid traits; but on the whole the occurrence of a schizophrenic psychosis seems to be less dependent on homologous personality traits than are the affective psychoses.

Abnormal Personalities in the Four Clinical Groups

The abnormal personalities found among first-degree relatives of the propositi in our four main groups can be roughly classified as (1) neurotic without gross deviation of personality, (2) alcoholic, (3) psychiatrically notable personalities (in the sense of the German term "auffällig") without social incapacity, and (4) psychopaths. Their distribution is given in Table 9.11.

TABLE 9.11. TYPES OF ABNORMAL PERSONALITY AMONG RELATIVES IN EACH CLINICAL GROUP

Relative	Propositus			
	Schizophrenic	Affective	Psychopathic	Organic
	per cent	per cent	per cent	per cent
Neurotic	13	8	13	9
Alcoholic	6	16	5	25
"Auffällig"	7	22	4	5
Psychopath	75	54	78	61
Total	101	100	100	100

It is noteworthy that the abnormal personalities in the schizophrenic families were much more markedly abnormal than those found in the affective families. They have nearly as high a proportion of psychopaths, in the total of abnormal personalities, as does the psychopathic group itself.

As abnormal and psychopathic personalities can be of very variegated hues, it is not easy to analyse differences between the clinical groups. An attempt was, however, made to do so. Individual traits of personality, shown by first degree relatives of the propositi, were classified under various headings. It was then possible, in each of the clinical groups, to say which of the individual traits were most frequently shown.

The order of occurrence was different in each of the four groups. The five most frequently shown traits for each of the groups are shown in Table 9.12.

TABLE 9.12. PERSONALITY TRAITS MOST FREQUENTLY OBSERVED AMONG ABNORMAL RELATIVES IN EACH CLINICAL GROUP

| Relative | Propositus | | | |
	Schizophrenic	Affective	Psychopathic	Organic
1.	Paranoid	Depressed	Hysterical	Alcoholic
2.	Anxious	Emotionally labile	Aggressive	Aggressive
3.	Aggressive	Alcoholic	Anxious	Anxious
4.	Anergic	Aggressive	Emotionally labile	Paranoid
5.	Hysterical	Obsessional	Alcoholic	Depressed

This table, however, hardly gives a helpful characterization. Anxiety traits, aggressiveness, etc. take rather a high place in each of the three groups and so are not very distinctive. We learn more by noting which of the traits are much more, or less, common in one group than in either of the others. Put in this way, the abnormal personalities of the schizophrenic group are more frequently paranoid, anergic, eccentric or lacking in feeling, and are less frequently diagnosed as emotionally labile or alcoholic than are psychopaths in other kinds of family. The psychopaths of the affective families are much more frequently depressive and are more frequently emotionally labile than those of other groups, but are less frequently described as either anergic, anxious or paranoid. The psychopaths from the families of psychopaths are relatively often hysterical or wastrel types, and traits of depression, reserve and obsessionality are infrequently mentioned. In the organic group depression and elation are rather unexpectedly frequent.

The greatest psychiatric interest attaches to the abnormal personalities in the schizophrenic group. The *paranoid* traits which were their most marked characteristic are described by informants in the following terms:

suspicious, sensitive, sullen, touchy, grouchy, morose, resentful, unforgiving, difficult, quarrelsome, self-conscious, jealous, litigious, critical, takes things the wrong way, has rows with all the family, doesn't get on with people, makes heartless accusations.

The eccentricities, which are almost equally characteristic, attract a different constellation of epithetical descriptions; the father and twin brother of case 271, for instance, are text-book cases. *Eccentricities* are suggested by the terms:

giggly, opinionated, pedantic, narrow-minded, meticulous, obstinate, humourless, rigid, conventional, conceited, superstitious, prudish, cranky, miserly, foxy, precise, brusque, verbose, circumstantial talker, little-minded, full of facts, learned but incompetent, old-fashioned, routine-bound, has bizarre ideas strongly held, spiritualist, believes in self-cure by hypnotism.

The quality we call *lack of feeling* comes out in such descriptions as:

impassive, cool, calculating, placid, hard and stingy, disciplinarian, unsympathetic, cold, slack, unscrupulous, withdrawn, very sane, little feeling, unkind and selfish, unconcerned about a debt.

Closely related to lack of affect is the incapacity for warmth which shows itself in qualities of *reserve*, also shown more frequently by psychopaths from the schizophrenic than from the other families:

> shy, serious, staid, haughty, snobbish, studious, unforthcoming, independent, taciturn, unsociable, quiet turns, seeks solitude, quiet old stick, exceedingly reserved, no give and take, never reveals his thoughts, absorbed in scientific pursuits, one friend only.

The *anergic* traits seen in the schizophrenic families receive such descriptions as:

> feckless, dependent, tired, slack, unreliable, subservient, a poor thing, unable to work and health gave way, separated from family and tramped, no initiative or money sense, neglected family and went downhill.

All these are descriptions by friends and relatives of actual people and from them a vague picture emerges which is very much that which clinicians describe as "schizoid". The same or similar words or phrases occur in descriptions of abnormal personalities from the other families, but much less frequently, not in such concentrated form, and they are usually submerged by descriptions of a very different tone.

SUMMARY AND CONCLUSIONS

*[An asterisk indicates that the section which the item
summarizes has been omitted in the abridged version.]*

Introductory

A brief account is given of the history of psychiatric investigations of twins, and of the purpose, the meaning and the limitations of such work. A somewhat more detailed summary is then given of those psychiatric studies which have been made on systematically collected, unselected series of twins.

The author's own investigation was begun in 1936 on a mental hospital population of approximately 20,000 and was later extended to cover the current intake of a number of mental hospitals and one university psychiatric clinic (Maudsley Hospital). Every effort was made to make the series an unselected and comprehensive one, only those cases being excluded where the twin partner failed to reach adult life. Altogether 295 propositi, born from a multiple birth, were collected. The investigation was interrupted during the war, but in 1947 was re-opened, and all previously ascertained twins were followed up. Of the propositi 266 were personally examined by the author, 5 by a psychiatric social worker only; corresponding figures for the twin partners were 156 and 46. Both among the propositi and their partners there were some who for various reasons could not be seen.

General Data

1. The incidence of twinning in the mental hospital population, estimated as 2.2 per cent, corresponds closely with the incidence of the twin-born in the general population (approximately 2.3 per cent).

2. The clinical material consisted of 67 uniovular and 224 binovular pairs, and 6 pairs of doubtful ovularity. The proportion of uniovular twins (24 per cent) is according to expectation.

3. Nearly two thirds of the propositi were female, and females were therefore in significant excess.

Finger-prints

* 4. The method of finger-print analysis used, with other criteria, for the determination of ovularity is described, and the results are presented, with a statistical analysis.
* 5. Analysis of variance, carried out by Miss Joan May, B.A. Dip. Stat., led to the following conclusions:
    (a) The resemblance within pairs is significantly greater for uniovular than for binovular twins;
    (b) The mean binovular ridge count number is significantly greater than the mean uniovular number;
    (c) The mean for right hands appears slightly higher than the mean for left hands for binovular twins only;
    (d) Mean radial counts are on the average about three times as great as mean ulnar counts, but this relationship varies markedly from finger to finger;
    (e) There are striking differences between the means for the separate fingers, considering radial and ulnar counts separately, but fingers do not differ on radial and ulnar counts combined;
    (f) There are slightly larger variations, going from one pair of twins to another, in the differences between the fingers, and in the differences between radial and ulnar counts, than there are within each pair of twins;
    (g) Uniovular twins do not resemble one another more than binovular twins in right-left differences, in radial-ulnar differences or in differences between fingers.
* 6. A discriminant function is calculated which permits of the separation of uniovular from binovular prints with a 16 per cent rate of misclassification.

Familial Aspects of Twinning

* 7. Among the relatives of the propositi there was a significant increase in the incidence of multiple births; but there was no significant difference between the incidence of same-sexed and opposite-sexed twinning in the relatives of the uniovular and the binovular pairs; and differences between the incidences in the families of male and of female relatives were not significant.
* 8. The incidence of twinning increases with birth order. The relationship does not significantly deviate from linearity and appears to be the same for uniovular as for binovular twinning.

Psychiatric Classification

9. The clinical diagnoses of the propositi were classified into four main groups:
    (a) schizophrenic psychoses, 156.
    (b) affective psychoses, 38.
    (c) organic disorders, 49.
    (d) psychopathic and neurotic states, 52.
10. There was little difference in the total amount of abnormality observed among the sibs of the four groups; but schizophrenia was commonest (5 per cent) among the sibs of schizophrenic propositi, affective mental illnesses commonest (9 per cent) among the sibs of the affective propositi, organic states commonest (5 per

119

cent) among the sibs of the organic patients and psychopathy and neurosis commonest (26 per cent) among the sibs of the neurotics and psychopaths.

11. It was found that in all diagnostic groups the risk of mental illness for the
binovular twin was increased if one or both of the parents were mentally abnormal.
In the schizophrenic group, schizophrenia in parent or twin was associated with
diminished life expectation for the patient.

Personalities of Uniovular Pairs

12. An examination of the personalities of the uniovular twins shows that as a
rule resemblance is great and differences are slight and ones of degree. Quantitative
differences may affect almost any feature of personality, but though not large may
lead to very different life histories. The one feature in which a difference was often
marked was in energy of character. The twin relationship itself, with its aspects of
dominance and submission, appeared to favour a polar development in this respect.
The more active twin tended to be relatively spared by an eventual schizophrenic
psychosis, but, in the psychopathic groups, to make as a rule the less satisfactory
adjustment.

Predisposition to Mental Illness

13. The histories of the twins who had periods of separation in early life are not
numerous and disclose no information of great value; but in some cases it appears
that the twin who had the less fortunate experience had the more abnormal after-
history.

14. The first-born of the pair of twins appeared to suffer no psychiatric disadvantage.

15. If one of a pair of twins had had a more difficult birth than his partner, he
was more likely to have the less favourable after-history.

16. Breast feeding, early physical development, physique and health showed no
such relationship.

17. Greater abnormality in later life was associated with a more restricted sexual
life early on.

18. The less intelligent of a pair of binovular twins was more liable to psychopathic states or organic illness, but not more liable to schizophrenia or affective
disorder.

19. The binovular twin who was the more neurotic in childhood had the less
favourable after-history in all clinical groups.

20. The less favourable after-history was also associated with relative occupational instability and with neurotic traits in adult life in both kinds of twins.

21. Of individual adult neurotic traits those which were associated with a graver
psychosis were emotional lability, hysterical and paranoid tendencies and, among
binovular twins, lack of sociability.

22. Psychological precipitation of the illness was not associated with its prognosis.

23. These findings suggest that the make-up of the personality affects the liability to psychotic as well as to neurotic illness, and that both environmental and
genetical factors play a part in its causation.

24. There was no detectable relation between the psychiatric history and right- and left-handedness.

Schizophrenia

25. The best estimate the data provide for the concordance rate of schizophrenia in uniovular twins is 76 per cent. Of the uniovular twins of schizophrenics who did not themselves develop schizophrenia, some only were otherwise abnormal, and there were some who appeared to be quite normal.

26. Of the binovular schizophrenic pairs 14 per cent were concordant. The incidence of schizophrenia among the sibs of schizophrenics was only 5 per cent; but the difference between the binovular twins and the sibs is probably attributable to the more thorough investigation of the former.

27. The correlation coefficient in age of onset of schizophrenia was for the uniovular pairs +0.5, for the binovular pairs +0.7, and for the sibs +0.4. The differences between these values are not statistically significant.

28. Among the relatives of the schizophrenic propositi schizophrenic females out-numbered schizophrenic males by about 2:1.

29. Taking all pairs of affected relatives together there was a significant degree of resemblance in the course of the illness, and in type of onset, but not in outcome.

30. A number of curious resemblances in mode of precipitation were noted, but no figures were obtained which could be statistically tested.

31. As regards clinical features, there were significant resemblances between blood-related pairs in catatonic features, in passivity feelings, in the extent to which positive affective symptoms were shown, in the occurrence of depersonalisation, in signs of an organic type, and in tendencies to suicide and self-injury.

32. Affective illnesses occurring among the relatives of schizophrenics most frequently took the form of an involutional depression, and in many of the affective illnesses symptoms of a schizophrenic type were seen. It is considered that the data provide support for the belief that schizophrenia appearing in later life may take the form of an involutional or atypical depression. It was also observed that, in cases where other members of the family had affective illnesses, the propositi themselves often showed affective symptoms in their schizophrenic psychoses. The possibility is considered, but rejected, that in such cases the illness of the propositus had been affective in nature but misdiagnosed.

Affective Illnesses

* 33. Four out of 8 uniovular twins of propositi with affective psychoses were affected in the same way. Concordance in clinical picture was very incomplete.
* 34. Of the binovular twins 29 per cent had affective illnesses and of the sibs 9 per cent.
* 35. If all pairs of first degree relatives with affective illnesses are taken together, there is a correlation coefficient in age of onset of +0.35.
* 36. There was little resemblance between relatives in the total number of attacks suffered, or in the length of the attacks.
* 37. Similarities of a qualitative kind were seen in the type of precipitating factor involved.

* 38. The material was insufficient to reach conclusions about resemblance in clinical features.

Organic States

* 39. Of the 14 epileptic propositi, 2 of whom were uniovular, not one had an epileptic twin.
* 40. Among the twins of the epileptics other abnormalities were found, including psychopathy, mental defect, migraine, mood disturbances, "hysteria", general paresis.
* 41. Two uniovular pairs in which the propositus suffered from an arteriopathic illness were both concordant.
* 42. Binovular partners of propositi suffering from arteriopathic and organic paranoid states were affected in the majority of instances by comparable illnesses.
* 43. The three uniovular partners of patients suffering from general paresis are non-psychotic, but one of them developed cerebrovascular disease. A case is reported in which one of a pair of binovular twins had congenital syphilis and the other schizophrenia.
* 44. The remaining cases in the organic group are too heterogeneous to allow of general conclusions; but the clinical data suggest that genetical factors may play a part both in the predisposition to organic illness and also in determining the form of the symptoms.

Psychopathy and Neurosis

* 45. Among 8 uniovular pairs in which the propositus suffered from a neurotic or psychopathic state, only 2 pairs were concordant. One of these was a pair of boys with anxiety symptoms, tics and habit spasms; the other was a pair of neurotic wastrels with life-long social and psychiatric abnormality. In neither of these pairs did psychogenic and environmental factors appear to play any significant role.
* 46. There were 3 binovular pairs in which, despite marked differences in personality, both twins developed very similar behaviour disorders in childhood. In these cases psychogenic precipitation appeared to be highly important.
* 47. In the discordant uniovular pairs environmental factors again seemed to be decisive. Thus in one pair it was the twin who made an unsatisfactory marriage who broke down; in another the twin who had to assume greater responsibilities on marriage made a better adjustment. The observation is made that the paths of uniovular twins may diverge only very slightly at first but eventually lead to entirely different circumstances, and that the consequences of one false step may lead by a vicious spiral to a progressively lower *niveau*.
* 48. On the whole, neurotic symptoms appear as exaggerations of personality traits detectable at other times. The form of the symptoms is not so closely related to the form of the stress as it is to the basic personality.
* 49. An examination of the main traits of personality shown by blood-relatives shows rather little tendency towards family resemblance. The material, however, is not well suited to an investigation of this question.
  50. Psychopathic traits, shown by the abnormal personalities among the relatives of propositi classified into the four main clinical groups, are differently dis-

tributed. Among relatives of the schizophrenic propositi, paranoid, anergic, eccentric and emotionally cold personality traits were relatively frequent, traits of emotional lability and alcoholism relatively infrequent. An excess of personality traits of the depressive and emotionally labile type were relatively common in the relatives of affective propositi; of hysterical and wastrel type among the relatives of the psychopathic and neurotic propositi; and of tendencies to elation and depression among relatives of the organic propositi.

51. A characterization of schizoid personality traits is attempted by quoting actual words and phrases used by informants.

Case Material

* 52. On grounds of clinical interest and to enable other workers to use the data, a summary follows of every case.

Epitome

Though it has certain limitations, twin research, especially when combined with family investigation and case study, is a valid method for investigating the effects of heredity and environment.

The present report was based on a systematically ascertained series of nearly 300 twins, suffering from psychiatric illnesses, and treated at hospitals in the London area. It confirms previous views on the importance of genetical factors in the psychoses. We found that 76 per cent of the uniovular twins of schizophrenics had schizophrenic illnesses, a somewhat lower concordance rate than that of 86 per cent found by Kallmann. Within concordant uniovular pairs there were often wide differences in the severity of the illness and in outcome. These facts suggest that genetical causes provide a potentiality for schizophrenia, perhaps an essential one, though environmental factors play a substantial role, which may be decisive in the individual case. Those environmental factors which affect personality and constitution appear to be the most important. Heredity is also an important factor in the causation of affective and organic psychoses.

There is a striking contrast between the psychoses on the one hand and the psychopathic and neurotic states on the other. In the latter, uniovular pairs were less frequently concordant, and some of the binovular pairs developed very similar troubles despite big differences in intelligence and personality. The dividing line between adjustment and maladjustment is not so wide as that between sanity and insanity and is more easily over-stepped, so that chance, whether favourable or unfavourable, is more important. Once maladjustment has begun, it may contribute to its own continuance. However, personality is of even greater importance in these conditions than in the psychoses.

A study of the personalities of the twins in all clinical groups shows that the basic make-up of the personality is largely determined by heredity. Degree of energy was the trait in which uniovular twins differed most, but this might be in part a product of the emotional relationship between the twins. Finally, from a comparison of uniovular and binovular twins we gain an appreciation of the genetical differences between one person and another without which a full understanding of both psychotic and neurotic behaviour is impossible and which helps us, moreover, towards that knowledge of fundamental pathology which is the basis of a rational treatment of disease.

Acknowledgments

The expenses of this investigation were met by personal and expenses grants from the Medical Research Council. The work was centered first on the Maudsley Hospital and then on the Institute of Psychiatry, both of which actively supported the project by providing the author with leisure from other duties, and with secretarial and other help of a very material kind. This was due to the interest and encouragement of the late Professor Edward Mapother and of Professor Aubrey Lewis. The author is also indebted to Professor Lewis for access to his own studies of some of the twins included here.

Much valuable assistance has been given by Miss M. A. Brown, Miss S. E. Hague, and the late Mr. C. J. Martin. The research was welcomed in the most co-operative spirit by the Physician Superintendents, medical, nursing and clerical staffs of mental hospitals and observation wards, and to them and to the Psychiatric Social Workers whose reports have been so often used, the author wishes to record his gratitude.

10

THE MONOGENIC THEORY OF SCHIZOPHRENIA

Despite the researches of thirty years, the genetic basis of schizophrenia still remains a matter of doubt. Some of the available observations suggest a recessive mode of inheritance, while others are more easily reconciled with dominance. To explain the discrepancies it has been suggested that schizophrenia is genetically heterogeneous; but even this attempt to make the best of both worlds encounters difficulties.

In his important paper on a North Swedish population, Böök (1953) proposed the hypothesis that, in this population isolate, schizophrenia was due to a recessive gene which manifested itself in all homozygotes and in about one in every five heterozygotes. This was, in fact, the hypothesis which provided the best fit for his data. It is one which involves features both of dominance and recessivity; and it is desirable to see whether hypotheses of this form might be compatible with the data obtained from other populations, whether, in fact, the monogenic theory of Böök could be applied more universally.

Böök's calculations of the frequencies of genotypes and matings are not very easy to follow; and as an alternative approach the following simple formulation is offered. We shall write A = the dominant (normal) gene, with frequency of $(1-p)$ in the population, and a = the schizophrenic gene, with frequency p. Then among the relatives of particular genotypes, other named genotypes will appear with frequencies which will be functions of p, as shown in Table 10.1.

The frequency of schizophrenia in the general population (s) is given by the formula $s = 2mp(1-p)+p^2$, where m is the frequency of manifestation of the schizophrenic gene in the heterozygote. We can take 0.008 as a fairly reliable estimate of the frequency of schizophrenia in most European countries. Using this formula, we can calculate the value of p corresponding to every value of m between its limits of 0 and 1, or, more conveniently, calculate the value of m corresponding to various values of p. It is also interesting to note at the same time the corresponding values of h, where $h = p^2/0.008$, and represents the proportion of all schizophrenics who are

Originally published in *Acta Genetica et Statistica Medica* (Basel) 8: 50–56 (1958).

homozygotes. This is a convenient measure of the degree to which the mode of inheritance approaches to recessivity, and varies between 1 and a very small value.

To every value of p, and of m, there will also correspond values for the expectation of schizophrenia among the various classes of relatives of schizophrenics, or in given types of matings. There are available the results of adequate investigations of the frequency of schizophrenia in the children of schizophrenics, in their sibs, and in the children of two schizophrenic consorts. Furthermore, Nixon and Slater (1957) have made one estimate of the frequency of schizophrenia in the children of first cousins. The theoretical expectations, calculated by the use of Table 10.1, are as follows:

Frequency of schizophrenia in the children of schizophrenics $= \frac{1}{2} (1+h) (m+p) - hmp$;
Frequency of schizophrenia in the sibs of schizophrenics $= \frac{1}{4} \{2m+h+p (2m+h+1- 2mh)+p^2 (1-2m)\}$;
Frequency of schizophrenia in the children of two schizophrenics $= \frac{1}{4} (1+h) \{2m(1-h)+1+h\}$;
Frequency of schizophrenia in the children of first cousins $= 1/16 (15s+p)$.

Values of these expectations have been calculated for eleven points of the entire range of possibilities, and are given in Table 10.2.

The relationships between p, m and h and the corresponding expectations of schizophrenia in the various classes of relative are also shown in Figure 10.1. This

TABLE 10.1. FREQUENCIES OF GENOTYPES IN SCHIZOPHRENICS' RELATIVES

Relative	of Genotype	will be	with Frequency as Coefficients of		
			p^0	p^1	p^2
Parents and children	AA	AA	+ 1	− 1	
		Aa		+ 1	
	Aa	AA	+ 1/2	− 1/2	
		Aa	+ 1/2		
		aa		+ 1/2	
	aa	Aa	+ 1	− 1	
		aa		+ 1	
Sibs	AA	AA	+ 1	− 1	+ 1/4
		Aa		+ 1	− 1/2
		aa			+ 1/4
	Aa	AA	+ 1/2	− 3/4	+ 1/4
		Aa	+ 1/2	+ 1/2	− 1/2
		aa		+ 1/4	+ 1/4
	aa	AA	+ 1/4	− 1/2	+ 1/4
		Aa	+ 1/2		− 1/2
		aa	+ 1/4	+ 1/2	+ 1/4
Children of first cousins		AA	+ 1	− 31/16	+ 15/16
		Aa		+ 30/16	− 30/16
		aa		+ 1/16	+ 15/16

makes very evident the extent to which the expectation in the sibs drops between the extremes of recessivity and dominance, instead of taking, as one might have expected, intermediate values; the minimum is seen in the neighborhood of the point where there is a 12 per cent rate of manifestation in the heterozygote. Something similar is seen in the behaviour of the figures for the children of one schizophrenic, where the minimum is found at a 6 per cent rate of manifestation; but there is very little change between the 12 per cent point and the extreme of absolute recessivity. At low gene frequencies, when m exceeds 0.2, there is practically no difference between the expectations in sibs and in children. It is also noteworthy that the expectation of schizophrenia in the children of two schizophrenics varies in a remarkable way between the extremes of dominance and recessivity, so that observational estimates are clearly capable of providing valuable information. The expec-

TABLE 10.2. THEORETICAL MANIFESTATION RATES AND EXPECTATIONS OF
SCHIZOPHRENIA IN RELATIVES AS A FUNCTION OF GENE FREQUENCY

p	m	h	Sibs	Ch of 1	Ch of 2	Ch of cousins
$(.008)^{1/2}$ = .0894	0.0000	1.0000	0.2967	0.0894	1.0000	0.0131
0.080	0.0109	0.8000	0.2431	0.0811	0.8120	0.0125
0.070	0.0238	0.6125	0.1947	0.0735	0.6575	0.0119
0.060	0.0390	0.4500	0.1552	0.0707	0.5412	0.0113
0.050	0.0580	0.3125	0.1239	0.0699	0.4568	0.0106
0.040	0.0833	0.2000	0.1053	0.0733	0.4000	0.0100
0.030	0.1219	0.1125	0.0993	0.0841	0.3696	0.0094
0.020	0.1939	0.0500	0.1166	0.1121	0.3723	0.0088
0.015	0.2631	0.0281	0.1444	0.1429	0.3957	0.0084
0.010	0.3990	0.0125	0.2071	0.2070	0.4558	0.0081
0.004	1.0000	0.0020	0.5034	0.5030	0.7510	0.0078

tation of schizophrenia in the children of cousins, on the other hand, varies very
little and shows itself to be an insensitive measure of dominance-recessivity.

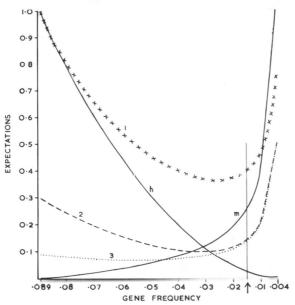

Figure 10.1—Theoretical expectations of incidence of schizophrenia in relatives of schizophrenics
(broken lines), with varying gene frequency and varying penetrance. 1 = children of two schizophrenics; 2 = sibs of schizophrenics; 3 = children of one schizophrenic; h = proportion of all
schizophrenics who are homozygous; m = manifestation rate of gene in heterozygote [modified
by author from original].

We may now compare the expectations with the frequencies that have been
actually observed. The frequency of schizophrenia in the sibs of schizophrenics has
been estimated by Kallmann (1953) as 0.142; other workers have found a slightly
lower figure. This expectation is found on the curve for sibs both at gene frequency
0.015 and again at 0.055. If the frequency were lower than 0.142, a corresponding
expectation could be found with a p value between these limits. Kallmann, again,
has found the frequency of schizophrenia in the children of schizophrenics to be
0.164; this point is found on the curve for children at gene frequency 0.013. The
estimate of Elsässer (1952) for the frequency of schizophrenia in the children of

two schizophrenic consorts is 0.392. This point is found on the corresponding curve at values of p of 0.015 and 0.038. Finally, Nixon and Slater estimated that the frequency of schizophrenia in the children of cousins was 57/40 of the frequency in the general population = 0.011, which corresponds with a gene frequency of 0.055.

When one takes into account the magnitude of the statistical errors to which all these estimates are liable, it is seen that they are all readily compatible with a gene frequency of about 0.015, and a manifestation rate in the heterozygote of about 0.26. At this point, all but 3 per cent of schizophrenics are heterozygous.

There is one important group of observations of which so far no mention has been made, i.e. the data relating to the incidence of schizophrenia in the MZ twins of schizophrenics. The concordance rate within MZ pairs has been estimated as lying between 76 per cent (Slater, 63) and 86 per cent (Kallmann, 1953). If we merely thought of the MZ co-twins of schizophrenics as a group of persons of whom 3 per cent were homozygous and 97 per cent were heterozygous, then we might conclude that the concordance rate should be 28 per cent. However, the MZ co-twins of schizophrenics are identical with their partners, not only in respect of the hypothetical specific schizophrenic gene, but also in respect of the total genetic equipment. If a much higher concordance rate than 28 per cent is actually found, this is a matter for no surprise. But the fact that the genotypic milieu should play such a part deprives the data obtained from twins of any value for the testing of the monogenic hypothesis.

If it were desired, it would be a simple though slightly laborious task to calculate expectations for other classes of relatives than those discussed above. It seems improbable, however, that information of much critical value would be thereby obtained. Furthermore, the observational data for comparison would be less reliable. In the case of one class, that of parents, the observed frequency of schizophrenia could not be safely used for such a purpose, since parents are a group of persons who have been selected for survival and for health.

Taking the material we have, it would seem that some at least of our knowledge of the incidence of schizophrenia in the relatives of schizophrenics could be adequately explained by the hypothesis of a single partially dominant gene, such as Böök proposed for the special circumstances of a North Swedish isolate; and that this hypothesis therefore merits further investigation.

SUMMARY

The consequences are examined of a hypothesis which proposes a single partially dominant gene as the genetical basis of schizophrenia. It is shown that a simple relationship connects gene frequency and rate of manifestation in the heterozygote, if the frequency of schizophrenia in the general population is held constant; a series of values for these two variables has been calculated, when the frequency of schizophrenia is taken as 0.008. The expectation of schizophrenia in certain classes of relatives of schizophrenics also varies with the gene frequency and with the manifestation rate, but in a complex way such that, between high values at the extremes of complete dominance and complete recessivity, not intermediate values but minima are found. The observed frequencies of schizophrenia in the sibs of schizophrenics, in the children of one schizophrenic parent, and in the children of two schizophrenic parents, are compatible with this theory, and would correspond with a manifestation rate in the heterozygote of about 0.26 and a gene frequency of about 0.015.

Acknowledgment.   I am much indebted to Mr. W. L. B. Nixon for valuable help.

128

11

A CASE OF TURNER MOSAIC
WITH MYOPATHY AND SCHIZOPHRENIA

This patient, a single girl aged 19 (Case No. 87810), was admitted to the National Hospital on 20.4.60. Her parents were first cousins; her three sibs are normal, but a maternal uncle's child had had a schizophrenic illness.

The patient, whose I.Q. is 92, did not do very well at school; and since then has never been fully employable, owing to her slowness. Menstrual history has been normal. Curvature of the spine was first noted at 13 but has not changed significantly since. Some weakness of the muscles appeared at the same age, and since then she has had difficulty in raising the head from a lying position.

The psychosis began in 1959, when she changed in attitude to her mother and would lock herself in her room and refuse to see anyone. In May 1959 she had her room redecorated but suddenly starting stripping off the new wallpaper and wrecked the room. In July she burnt all her best clothes and went off to Brighton. Having arrived there she found nowhere to stay, slept at the railway station and returned home next day. A few days later she cut off all her hair as close to the head as possible. On 13.8.59 she was admitted to Netherne Hospital where she was very agitated and disturbed. She was diagnosed as suffering from schizophrenia and treated with Stelazine and reserpine. Affect was recorded as incongruous; at times she was smiling to herself, at times near to tears. No delusions or hallucinations were noted; but there was thought disorder with difficulty in concentration and her talk was at times confused, with frequent interruptions. She eventually settled down, and was then transferred to the National Hospital for investigation of the weakness of the neck.

On admission, though quiet and slow, she showed no mental abnormality of a schizophrenic kind. On neurological examination there was bilateral facial weakness, severe weakness of both sternomastoids, weakness of the right scapular muscles, the

---

By E. Slater and K. Zilkha. Originally published in the *Proceedings of the Royal Society of Medicine* 54: 674–75 (1961). Photographs showing the myopathic facies and scoliosis omitted.

right deltoid and both triceps muscles. Dr. E. A. Carmichael thought the muscular weakness was due to old poliomyelitis; but this was thought unlikely by Dr. R. W. Gilliatt, owing to the symmetrical weakness of the facial muscles and wasting of the sternomastoids. EMG studies of the right deltoid, pectoralis, and rhomboid muscles on two occasions showed in all three muscles slight reduction in motor unit interference pattern on maximal voluntary effort; the motor units were brief, polyphasic, of reduced amplitude. The changes resembled those of a myopathy. A biopsy specimen from the right deltoid showed no abnormality. The EEG was normal. Otological examination showed moderate bilateral deafness, chiefly in the band 4,000-8,000 c/s. Vestibular function was normal, apart from some slight general reduction of caloric responses. Dr. C. S. Hallpike reported that the cause was obscure. The Ishihara test was normal. Blood-films showed typical 'drumsticks' in 10/500; but buccal epithelial cells were chromatin negative. Professor Penrose reported that the blood culture cells might be those of a mosaic Turner's syndrome with about one-fifth of the cells lacking one X chromosome, while the others were probably normal: "The skin culture cells did not seem to support this view, although there seemed to be quite a number of abnormal karyotypes. As this occurs in cultures not infrequently, I am inclined to discount them and to consider that she probably has the karyotype of a normal female."

The syndrome is interesting, combining unaccountable deafness, an unusual form of myopathy and a scoliosis not accounted for by muscular weakness. In view of the positive family history, the schizophrenic illness may be coincidental; as far as we know this is the first case in which schizophrenia has been reported in a case of Turner's syndrome, pure or mosaic. The fact that the patient is the child of first cousins is curious. We wonder whether parental consanguinity can be expected to show in excess in such cases.

12

THE SCHIZOPHRENIA-LIKE PSYCHOSES OF EPILEPSY

I. Psychiatric Aspects[1]

INTRODUCTION

In 1953, in an article intended for the general practitioner, Denis Hill made a brief reference to the chronic paranoid psychoses which may develop in association with temporal lobe epilepsy. He described the condition as likely to come on when the seizures were diminishing in frequency, as appearing gradually with onset in middle age, and as resembling a paranoid schizophrenic state. In 1957, D. A. Pond, from the same department of applied electrophysiology at the Maudsley Hospital, gave a more detailed account of the clinical features. He described the psychotic states as closely resembling schizophrenia, with paranoid ideas which might become systematized, ideas of influence, auditory hallucinations often of a menacing quality, and occasional frank thought disorder with neologisms, condensed words, and inconsequential sentences. There were, however, also some points of difference, of a quantitative rather than qualitative kind: a religious colouring of the paranoid ideas was common; the affect tended to remain warm and appropriate; and there was no typical deterioration to the hebephrenic state. All the patients had epilepsy arising from the temporal lobe region with complex auras; occasional major seizures occurred in sleep only. EEG foci, always present, were sometimes only to be demonstrated in sleep-sphenoidal records. The epilepsy began some years before the psychotic symptoms,

By Eliot Slater, A. W. Beard, and Eric Glithero. Originally published in the *British Journal of Psychiatry* 109: 95–150 (1963). This five-part paper has been abridged by the omission of the following: Part II (Physical Aspects), by Dr. Beard alone, except for its summary; a lengthy table, listing the main clinical features of each case, and most of the references to case numbers from that table; case summaries of centrencephalic epileptics from Appendix of Part I; one table from Part III and one from Part IV; descriptions of lobotomised patients from Part IV. The summary of the paper was reprinted in the *International Journal of Psychiatry* 1: 6–8 (1965) and discussed at length.

[1] By Eliot Slater and A. W. Beard.

usually in the late teens or the twenties; and the latter often seemed to begin as the epileptic attacks were diminishing in frequency, either spontaneously or with drug treatment.

This is the first explicit recognition of the syndrome which is discussed in detail in the paper which follows; but the occurrence of schizophrenia-like psychoses in association with epilepsy has been reported again and again over the last half-century, usually with a good deal of bewilderment on the side of the author. In his excellent review (1936), Gruhle quotes a total of 23 authors, most of them describing cases in ones and twos, going back to Giese who reported six cases in 1914. Gruhle remarks that to report further cases would only have a purpose if this were done from a new viewpoint. The particular form of association between epilepsy and schizophrenia which struck him with great force was that in which patients who had been observed for years or decades as undoubted epileptics then developed chronic paranoid psychoses. In his own material there was one case in which the psychosis antedated the epilepsy, and in seven others a schizophrenic psychosis followed the onset of epilepsy at intervals of 1, 6, 10, 18, 19, and 38 years, with one case not known.

Gruhle, who was one of the pioneers of phenomenological analysis of the symptomatology of schizophrenia and an observer of outstanding sensitivity and acumen, said that the form of delusional experience in these schizophrenic epileptics was not clinically distinguishable from the true schizophrenic delusion. Delusions were mostly of a simple persecutory kind, lacking a paraphrenic fantastic quality; they were mostly expressed in states of altered mood, but they could be elicited by questioning at all times. They bore no relation to epileptic personality change, by degree or quality. Finally he formulated his own opinion, that these cases did not constitute a combination of two diseases, but were all symptomatic schizophrenias. "Es liegt also nur ein Grundleiden vor: eine toxisch endogene Epilepsie." [There is therefore only one basic disease present: a toxic endogenous epilepsy.]

In reviewing past work, we propose to confine ourselves to the more important contributions of an observational kind. Reviews of the literature, and discussions on such points as whether or not the combination of epilepsy and schizophrenia occurs with more than random frequency, will be ignored. Papers reporting EEG abnormalities of an epileptic type occurring in schizophrenics, or noting without adequate description the occurrence of abnormal mental states in association with an EEG focus, will not be reviewed here.

Of the early reports, those by Krapf (1928) and Glaus (1931) are the most interesting. Krapf reviewed the cases described in the literature before that time in a critical or even hypercritical spirit. As an example he abstracts Giese's fourth case, in which a man who had epilepsy from the twenties first became psychotic at the age of 53; but while he admits the diagnosis of schizophrenia he throws doubt on the epilepsy. He emphasizes the similarity of the experiences of the epileptic twilight state with those of schizophrenia; here too one may see withdrawal of thought, imposition of thoughts, thoughts heard aloud, feelings of being hypnotized, etc. In other cases, he thinks, schizophrenic-like symptoms may be interpreted as reactive delusion-formation on the basis of an epileptic personality change. He himself reports six cases, of which five are very similar to the cases which are the subject of the present paper; in his fourth case, however, overt epileptic symptoms were first shown only after the onset of a schizophrenic-like personality change. In these cases he succeeds in rejecting the double diagnosis by arguments along the lines mentioned. Where such an argument is not possible he proposes the alternative of a latent predisposition to schizophrenia which is temporarily mobilized during the psychosis; in two of the cases reported, the existence of schizophrenic relatives in the families is noted.

The paper by Glaus is a better documented one, and 12 cases are described in detail. Again there was one case, and one case only, in which the schizophrenia antedated the epilepsy. In the remainder, the onset of epilepsy was in the age range 6-35, with mean of 17 years, the schizophrenia appeared between the 22nd and 42nd year, with mean of 31 years, the mean duration of epilepsy before onset of schizophrenia being 14 years, with extremes of 5 and 36 years. In these cases schizophrenia had been diagnosed by clinicians of Bleuler's clinic, some of them by Eugen Bleuler personally. Again the cases bear a strong resemblance to our own, with paranoid syndromes predominating. A marked deficiency of the report, judged by present-day standards, is the lack of information bearing on the possibility of a focal origin of the epilepsy. There are, however, indications of a focal origin in several cases, in which an aura of vertigo or of an olfactory kind, or the occurrence of automatisms are mentioned. Like Krapf, Glaus attempts to evade where he can the necessity of making a double diagnosis. Thus his first case is one in which a man, who had had grand mal attacks from the age of 12, at the age of 23 entered on a chronic paranoid psychosis in which he believed that he was the creator of the world, had been twice born, and had a ring of electricity around his head; on grounds which are obscure to us, this is interpreted as an uncomplicated epileptic psychosis without even schizophrenic colouring. Three other cases are regarded as epileptic only, though showing some schizophrenic colouring to the picture. In the remaining cases, however, the combination of epilepsy and schizophrenia, either simultaneously or successively, is accepted. In one of these cases there was a schizophrenic mother, and in another a schizophrenic father.

The classic paper by Feuchtwanger and Mayer-Gross on brain injury and schizophrenia (1938) also contains relevant material. This consists of 23 patients who before the onset of their schizophrenic illnesses had all had open head injuries, mainly penetrating shrapnel wounds, all but two sustained during the 1914-18 war. The first nine patients described all developed epilepsy within one to three years after the injury. The "schizophrenic" psychosis was predominantly paranoid in seven cases, predominantly catatonic in two. In these cases the injuries were either frontal or temporal.

Other papers may be more briefly discussed. That by Jasper et al. (1939) is principally concerned with EEG abnormalities discovered in 82 patients with typically schizophrenic psychoses. One case is described of an ingravescent paranoid state in a woman subject to myoclonic epileptic attacks. Rey et al. (1949) in a paper on 82 cases of temporal lobe disturbance mention that there was a schizophrenic impression in 14 cases, and one patient had been diagnosed as schizophrenic. Ervin et al. (1955) found that 81 percent of 42 patients with temporal spikes on the EEG were schizophrenic. However, transient psychotic episodes, which may well have been epileptic twilight states, were so diagnosed. Karagulla and Robertson (1955) have discussed in detail the schizophrenic-like symptoms which may appear in association with a temporal lobe attack, with a number of striking illustrations; but the chronic paranoid psychosis of epilepsy, with its similarity to paranoid schizophrenia, is not referred to.

This is the subject explicitly dealt with by Bartlet (1957). Examining the literature, he found no evidence to support the hypothesis that schizophrenia was more or less likely to occur in epileptics than in the general population. He examined the records of all patients with a diagnosis of psychosis following epilepsy and those with a combined diagnosis of psychosis and epilepsy attending the Bethlem and Maudsley Hospitals, 1949-53, in which epilepsy antedated the onset of psychosis and the patient continued to suffer from delusions for a year. He concluded that the eight schizophrenics so found were not a larger number than could be accounted for by chance, since they constituted 0.75 percent of the total material. The argument is fallacious, since the concepts of prevalence and incidence are confused; the 0.8 percent risk of schizophrenia which applies to the general population refers to the whole life-time, and not to a single delimited year. More interesting is the short clinical description which is provided for each of these eight cases; seven of them had clinical or EEG evidence of a temporal lobe lesion.

A somewhat fuller description of six cases, five of them paranoid and one predominantly hebephrenic, is provided by Rodin *et al.* (1957). In the hebephrenic case onset was at the age of 11; in the remainder it was in the span 16 to 42, the epilepsy having antedated the schizophrenia by many years in every case.

In his monograph on 415 cases of brain injury Hillbom (1960) reports 11 psychoses diagnosed as schizophreniform. Of these only two patients were subject to epilepsy, and in both of them there had been a penetrating wound in the right temporal or fronto-temporal region. It is interesting that, as in the material of Feuchtwanger and Mayer-Gross, there is no great difference between the schizophrenia-like psychoses of the head injury patients, whether these patients had epilepsy or did not. In his comments Hillbom says that in nine of the cases there was a chronic disturbance reminding one of schizophrenic paranoid-hallucinatory psychoses, while in two the picture was more reminiscent of the defect state left behind by such a psychosis. When there were such psychotic symptoms as primary delusions and hallucinations, which might appear even in a quite clear state of consciousness, there was always a lesional cause, most likely an irritation caused by the injury in temporal, frontal or parietal lobes, most frequently the temporal lobe.

From this review it may be seen that the appearance of psychoses resembling schizophrenia during the course of a chronic epilepsy has been a phenomenon which has repeatedly attracted psychiatric attention. Those who have observed them have described these illnesses in much the same terms; and the duration of the epilepsy before the onset of the schizophrenia-like psychosis has tended towards the same mean figure in a number of reports. It has, in fact, long been recognized that we have here an important problem for which no generally acceptable solution has yet been proposed.

EPILEPSY AND SCHIZOPHRENIA
AS A CHANCE COMBINATION

It has been argued that, as neither schizophrenia nor epilepsy are excessively rare, the appearance of both conditions in one individual should at least be sufficiently frequent to account for the cases which have been reported in the literature. This argument has never been backed by any adequate statistical reasoning. In the attempt to account for our collection of 69 epileptics who developed schizophrenic-like psychoses, we may consider the matter as follows.

For a member of the general population the expectation of schizophrenia is approximately 0.008 and the expectation of epilepsy is 0.005. The expectation of a combination of both disorders on the basis of chance coincidence is therefore 0.00004. Forty per million of the population can expect over the course of their lives, provided they live through the entire risk period, to become either schizophrenic epileptics or epileptic schizophrenics. As epilepsy has an earlier age of onset than schizophrenia, though the ranges of age of onset largely overlap, the former of these two combinations will be commoner. We may make the rough guess that there will be three epileptics who become schizophrenic for every schizophrenic who becomes epileptic. If this is accepted, the expectation for the development of first epilepsy then schizophrenia, a process we shall call ES, will be 0.00003.

The ages of our probands at the time of onset of psychosis lay between the limits of 12 and 59. We shall assume:
1. that there is zero probability of becoming ES under the age of 12;
2. that between the ages of 12 and 59 the probability of ES having occurred increases arithmetically from year to year;
3. that after the age of 60 there is no further risk of ES;
4. that, although this is very unlikely, ES individuals have the same expectation of life as other members of the population, this assumption being one that maximizes the number of ES individuals one might find in the population.

Other more complex assumptions could be made, but would make little difference to the result of the calculation that follows.

From the estimated age distribution of the total population of England and Wales for mid-year 1957 given by the Registrar General's Statistical Review, we may calculate that in the 36,733,000 individuals over the age of 12, 22,209,000 risk-lifetimes will have been survived, with the expected appearance of 666 ES individuals. Of the 45 million population of England and Wales we may suppose that two-ninths, or approximately 10 million, live in Greater London, or rather in the area served by the Maudsley and National Hospitals. In this area accordingly we estimate that 148 ES individuals will be living; and that fresh cases will be appearing at the rate of about one-fiftieth of this number per annum, i.e. three per annum. Ordinary clinical considerations suggest that of the standing ES population the great majority will be living as chronic patients in mental hospitals.

Alternatively we may look at the matter in the following way. The mean age of our probands at the time of onset of psychosis was 29 years. Twenty-nine years before the time of our enquiry, in the year 1928, 660,267 persons were born. If we suppose that this was the number of persons born yearly on the average from 1900 onwards, and that all individuals destined to become ES survived until their twenty-ninth birthday, and then became psychotic, there would be 20 fresh ES cases every year in the total population of England and Wales. Two-ninths of these would be appearing in the London area, i.e. four to five fresh cases per annum.

The National Hospital and the Maudsley Hospital are, of course, hospitals to which psychotic epileptics might well be preferentially referred. But it is inconceivable, if such an exiguous supply of cases was the only source to be drawn on, that we could so easily have ascertained as many as 69 fresh cases in two only of all the neurological and psychiatric clinics, the observation wards, the psychiatric wards of general hospitals and the mental hospitals which serve the London area.

On the basis of these considerations we concluded that patients suffering from epilepsy develop schizophrenia-like psychoses with a frequency much greater than chance expectations would permit. The suggestion which then arises, that a schizophrenia-like psychosis may be the consequence of epilepsy, was greatly fortified in our minds by clinical observations which were made quite early in the enquiry. These were special features, both of the epilepsy and of the psychosis, and of the way in which they were combined, which could not be accounted for, except on the basis of a causal relationship. Although we were looking for "schizophrenics" with a past history of epilepsy, without being too particular about time relationships, in all our cases the epilepsy was continuing at the time of the onset of the "schizophrenia." Although any type of epilepsy would have satisfied our criteria, focal epilepsy was very much commoner in our group than petit mal and centrencephalic epilepsy. While any psychosis which, in the absence of epilepsy, would have been diagnosed as schizophrenic was admitted to the series, paranoid schizophrenic pictures greatly preponderated, and even considered as such were anomalous for relatively good preservation of affective responsiveness. The extent to which these early impressions were borne out as the series grew to completion, and the other clinical findings of a specific kind which were later made, will appear from the account which follows.

COLLECTION OF DATA

The work of the present authors, though it came to be intimately connected with the work proceeding at the Maudsley Hospital, was independently inspired; cases of the type described here were being demonstrated as epileptic psychoses at least by 1952. The motivation for the investigation and the way in which it was conducted have been described elsewhere (Beard and Slater, 1962). At this point it is sufficient to say that 31 of the cases to be described were ascertained in the course of routine clinical work at the National Hospital, where both authors were working in the psychiatric department. The larger number of 38 cases were made available at the Maudsley Hospital, where Professor (then Dr.) Denis Hill and Dr. D. A. Pond gave this investigation every facility and support. A. W. B. attended at the Maudsley Hospital, and saw the patients being investigated there, and was able to select those who came within our terms of reference. In this way it was possible to reach approximately the same standard of neurological and psychiatric investigation in both series of patients.

The case material from which the selection was made was the intake of the two hospitals between the years 1948 and 1959, and the study itself extended from March 1957 to August 1959. It is certain that not all the patients who attended the two hospitals from 1948 to 1959, and who would have fulfilled our criteria, have fallen into our net. The ascertainment, in fact, was not fully systematic. In brief, all the patients whom we got to hear of were included who fulfilled the criteria: (1) that the diagnosis of epilepsy was supported by EEG or unequivocal clinical evidence; and (2a) that the diagnosis of schizophrenia had been made by psychiatrists of experience; or (2b) that, in our opinion, the diagnosis of schizophrenia would have been the diagnosis of choice in the absence of a history of epilepsy. From this it will be seen that we took only a narrow selection of epileptic psychoses, and excluded all those in which psychotic symptoms had been confined to episodes in which confusion or some alteration of consciousness could have been regarded as playing some part. We were interested only in patients whose schizophrenia-like state had persisted for weeks or months in a setting of apparently complete mental lucidity. When the collection of material was closed, we had accumulated a total of 83 cases, of which 14 had subsequently to be excluded, either because it was not certain that the patient had at some time suffered from epilepsy, or because the mental disorder, out of context with the epilepsy, might have failed to pass muster as schizophrenic in the judgment of a competent psychiatrist. When the list was closed 47 of our 69 patients, or more than two-thirds, had been given a diagnosis of schizophrenia at some other psychiatric centre.

One of the purposes of the survey was, of course, to see whether a definite clinical syndrome could be delineated. First impressions suggested the formation of four groups:

1. a group of 11 patients whose chronic psychosis had been preceded by the repeated recurrence of short-lived confusional episodes;
2. a group of 46 whose psychosis was highly typical of a paranoid schizophrenia;
3. eight patients with a picture resembling hebephrenic schizophrenia; and
4. four patients whose epilepsy was of the petit mal type.

TABLE 12.1. CLINICAL CLASSIFICATION AND PROVENANCE OF CASES

Group	Hospital		Total
	Maudsley	National	
A. Chronic psychosis with recurrent confusional episodes	8	3	11
B. Chronic paranoid states	29	17	46
C. Hebephrenic states	1	11	12
Totals	38	31	69

On further investigation, the distinctions between these groups became somewhat blurred, no one group having a monopoly of any single symptom, and the differences between the groups being quantitative rather than qualitative. In the following pages, however, we have retained a part of this classification. The first and second groups are retained as Groups A and B; but the third and fourth groups are combined in Group C which, as will later be seen, shows points of difference from the others. The clinical classification and the provenance of our cases are shown in Table 12.1.

PAST PSYCHIATRIC HISTORY:
PREVIOUS PERSONALITY

The family histories of these patients were subjected to a special investigation, which will be reported in the third paper of this series by Slater and Glithero; and the past medical history, and the history relating to the epilepsy, are reported in the second paper by A. W. Beard. The previous personalities of these patients may be discussed here.

If there were a common aetiological basis for the schizophrenia-like psychoses of epilepsy and for other types of schizophrenia, one would expect to find evidence of it in the prepsychotic personality, e.g. in "schizoid" traits. This would be true whether one supposed that the epilepsy had released a latent predisposition or that epilepsy and schizophrenia co-existed in the one patient as a result of chance. The recorded account of the patient's prepsychotic personality was therefore examined with this in mind. Examination of the pre-morbid personality, i.e. the personality before onset of epilepsy, was not possible in the large majority of cases in which epilepsy had come on before the personality had fully matured.

In Table 12.2 the relevant observations are entered, and in reading it it must be borne in mind that the majority of case records will contain no statement in respect of any single named trait. The psychiatrist describes the personality by noting salient features, and does not mention character traits in which the patient differs little from the generality of mankind.

TABLE 12.2. DISTRIBUTION OF PERSONALITY TRAITS

Personality Traits	Number of patients
Schizoid	
1. Outgoing, sociable, good mixer	20
Shy, withdrawn, unsociable, seclusive	23
2. Affectionate, kind, considerate	15
Cold, selfish	2
3. Easy to get on with	3
Touchy, sensitive, paranoid, suspicious	9
4. "Not schizoid"	1
"Schizoid"	2
Epileptic	
5. Placid, good-tempered	5
Irritable, bad-tempered	14
6. Unaggressive	1
Aggressive	4
7. (a) Stubborn, obstinate	4
(b) Impulsive, improvident	5
(c) History of delinquency	2
(d) Religious interests	8
Affective	
8. Cheerful, happy disposition	25
Moody, liable to depression	14
Anxious	15
9. Hardworking, energetic	15
Lacking energy or initiative	9
Obsessional	
10. Perfectionist, very tidy, obsessional	19

An examination of these figures shows no excess of schizoid traits of personality. Of the two patients recorded as "schizoid", one was a girl who had had epileptic attacks from the age of three months, and the other was a woman who had had fits from the age of 10 years. Paranoid traits also are associated with early onset of epilepsy, none of the nine patients recorded having an onset later than the age of 18. It is reasonable to suppose that where these traits were shown they were in part caused by an epileptic personality change.

The same is true of the epileptic personality traits; irritability, aggressiveness, stubbornness were noted in a total of 13 patients, all of them with onset of epilepsy not later than 17. They too can be regarded as the result of personality changes, and not as signifying any pre-existing constitutional deviation.

Affective traits show no deviation from expectation, but there is a high proportion of patients with obsessional traits. Pedantry, circumstantiality, rigidity and other obsessional phenomena are commonly seen in patients who have suffered some organic impairment of central nervous function, and as an epileptic personality change; and of the 19 patients showing such traits 14 had an early epilepsy with onset not later than 15.

We conclude that the premorbid personality was of a normal type, with a normal amount of variation; but that when the onset of epilepsy was early, epileptic personality changes could be found in the prepsychotic personality. There is no evidence of an unusual abundance of personality traits of a kind which might indicate a predisposition to schizophrenia.

138

THE ONSET OF MENTAL ILLNESS

As will be shown in the paper by A. W. B., the age of onset of psychosis was related to the age of onset of epilepsy and the duration of epilepsy. The mean age of onset of psychosis was at 29.81 years of age, after the epilepsy had lasted for a mean duration of 14.10 years. There was a highly significant correlation coefficient between ages of onset of epilepsy and "schizophrenia" of +0.6, indicating that the duration of the epilepsy is likely to be one of the causative factors.[2] Exceptionally, the psychotic symptoms began very soon after the first recognizable epileptic fits: in less than one year in four cases, and in less than two years in two cases.

In some of these six cases the relationship between the onset of epilepsy and of psychosis is dubious. Thus in Case 11, the patient was first admitted to hospital at the age of 32 with a history of having had both fits and ideas of reference for the past 10 years. In Case 27, the patient came under observation at the age of 53, with a history of having had a fracture of the skull in an explosion at Woolwich Arsenal at the age of 38; within a year his eventual epilepsy was showing itself in periodic nocturnal incontinence and automatisms, and his psychosis in suspicions of his wife's fidelity. In Case 41 it is impossible to date the onset of the epilepsy with certainty. At the age of 12 the patient began to have inexplicable attacks of temper which would end in a deep sleep, and also at times to fall from her pony. In one of these falls at the age of 15 she sustained a subdural haematoma; and after this came attacks of unconsciousness without convulsion, and periodic rages and moods of depression.

In Case 60, at the age of 19 the patient had a single convulsion which passed off into a prolonged confusional episode with disorientation and hallucination. She misidentified people, was emotionally labile, noisy and aggressive. The psychotic state persisting, she was eventually diagnosed as suffering from schizophrenia, and given electro-shock and insulin coma treatments.

In the remaining cases the epilepsy and the psychosis can be dated more accurately.

RELATION BETWEEN FREQUENCY
OF FITS AND PSYCHOSIS

In all cases epileptic fits persisted up to the onset of the psychosis, with the exception of Case 36, mentioned below. In the great majority it was not possible to relate the onset of the mental illness to any change in the quality or frequency of the fits. In some cases, however, some such relationship was at least suggested. In two cases, there was an increase in the frequency of the fits shortly before the appearance of psychotic symptoms; but in a larger number the reverse was true.

Thus in six cases the psychotic symptoms appeared at a time when the fit frequency was falling or was being successfully controlled by medication. In four cases the fluctuating courses of both the epilepsy and the psychosis showed a relationship, in that paranoid symptoms were more prominent when the fits were fewer. In another patient there was a suggestion of an inverse relationship between the

---

[2] As stated in 1969 by Slater and Moran (136), the calculation of a correlation coefficient was illegitimate here, since cases in which psychosis might have preceded the epilepsy were excluded from observation. Using an appropriate method of calculation, Slater and Moran showed that in each sex the psychosis occurred earlier than expected, but the departure from expectation was significant in females only. — *Editors.*

psychotic episodes and the amount of subcortical epileptic brain activity shown on the EEG. In two patients, both with a centrencephalic petit mal, there had been no epileptic fits for a year before the onset of the psychosis. In one of them improvement in the psychosis followed on the occurrence of two spontaneous grand mal attacks. In the other (36), after a year of freedom from fits, the patient became depressed, made a suicidal attempt, and on recovery from this depression began to suffer from auditory hallucinations. In two other patients the mental state improved every time a fit occurred; in the second of these the patient would begin to get olfactory hallucinations if for a time there had been no fits.

MODE OF ONSET

Data relating to mode of onset and course of the psychosis are shown in Table 12.3. The most usual onset was very insidious; and as a rule there was the gradual appearance of delusions as a first symptom. The following case is representative.

Case 19

This man had had epilepsy since the age of 10. At 38, when he was having one major attack a month, he began to complain of depression. He told the psychiatrist he didn't know whether he was coming or going. Someone had told him he was being a Billy Muggins. For six months he had had the idea he was being followed; people had followed him round who looked like foreigners. At a tea-bar the man who served him had said "thank you very much, your Majesty;" and he was only a plain mister — as far as he knew. These vague ideas in course of time became systematized into the delusion that he was a scion of a noble family, and could expect a vast sum from a will. He became auditorily hallucinated, and heard voices in his head which said "Duke of York," "Duke of Cambridge" (the names of pubs in his neighborhood), "Duke of Salisbury," and "Squire". The voices knew everything he had done, and they must have recordings of his entire life. There was a pick-up in his body, "a pin in my body to pick up the nerve vibrations," which transmitted thoughts from the brain, and also made the brain receive.

TABLE 12.3. ONSET AND COURSE OF SCHIZOPHRENIA-LIKE ILLNESS

		Group A	Group B	Group C	Total
Onset					
Acute		3	6	2	11
Episodic		7	12	1	20
Subacute		1	3	5	9
Insidious		—	25	4	29
Course					
Towards improvement		5	13	3	21
Fluctuating		2	11	2	15
Towards chronicity		3	21	7	31
Not observed		1	1	—	2
	Totals	11	46	12	69

In 18 patients the first psychotic symptoms took the form of apathy, depression, lassitude, and forgetfulness. In these cases the psychosis manifested as the culmination of epileptic personality changes. The following may be cited as an example.

Case 47

This patient had had screaming attacks as a little girl, and grand mal attacks without aura or focal signs since 13. Her attacks practically ceased at the age of 32. From this time on there was a progressive personality change. From being normally affectionate and active, she became unaffectionate, sulky and aggressive, and lost all her interests. When admitted to hospital at the age of 38, she was becoming more and more difficult, refusing her food, refusing her tablets, refusing to get out of bed or to wash herself. In hospital she showed thought blocking, incongruities of thought and affect, grimacing and fragmentary delusional ideas. The state persisted even when the possibility of drug intoxication, which had first been thought of, had been eliminated; and she was then found to be also auditorily hallucinated.

In four patients auditory hallucinations in a clear state of consciousness were the first psychotic symptom. Thus one patient (23), who had been epileptic since 17, had nervous breakdowns at 21 and 23, on the latter occasion receiving deep insulin treatment. He was first seen by us at the age of 31, and had then been almost continuously auditorily hallucinated for 10 years, hearing women's voices that constantly questioned him, leaving him only for a few hours at a time. During the past seven years they had become quieter and quieter till they were now little more than a distant mumble. Delusional ideas were restricted to a few ideas of reference. He was first regarded as a burnt-out schizophrenic, and only under investigation showed the signs which led in the end to a temporal lobectomy.

In 17 cases the chronic psychosis appeared as a sequela after a series of epileptic confusional episodes. Thus one patient was subject to epileptic attacks since the age of 17, mostly nocturnal, without convulsion, and followed by a period of confusion. At the age of 40 he had attacks on three successive days. On the two intervening days he was normal, but on the third day his behaviour changed. He got up and went to his work as a gardener as usual; but there he felt that all his friends were plotting against him. After that he began to get suspicious of his wife. He refused to drink his tea, saying she had poisoned the sugar. On attending at the hospital, he felt that the magazines in the out-patient department had been specially chosen to test patients. The delusional state persisted for more than three years, before it gradually began to fade.

An episodic mode of onset was shown by 20 patients, the following being a well-marked example.

Case 6

This man was subject to epileptic attacks from the age of 17. There were short-lived psychotic episodes of 11 days in 1950, 14 days in 1951 with a second episode lasting 26 days in the same year, 38 days in 1957, and 16 days in 1958. Most of these started with a confusional state, in which he would be shouting in the street. In 1950 he was described as excited, talking about Christ, deluded, manneristic and confused. In 1951 he was regarded as showing epileptic dementia, and was agitated, hilarious, excited, uncontrollable, grandiose. In 1957 he was suspicious and secretive, said he had been in touch with Scotland Yard about a woman across the way, and thought that people wanted to kill him. His speech was vague and incomprehensible; he smiled at times for no apparent reason. In his illness in 1958 catatonic signs were shown, sitting up in bed with arms flexed in a boxing stance, sitting up and lying down, posturing; he was auditorily and visually hallucinated, his talk jerky, rapid, incoherent.

Acute and subacute modes of onset were shown by a total of 20 patients. This most usually took the form of the more or less rapid appearances of paranoid ideas over the course of days or weeks, accompanied by corresponding anomalies of behaviour. However there were examples of other modes of onset, e.g. with sudden acute excitement or religious ecstatic psychosis, with an attempt at suicide, and on recovery from status epilepticus. An onset taking the form of an acute catatonic state was shown in the following case:

Case 26

This girl, who had had fits since infancy, at the age of 17 went into a psychotic state which developed rapidly in the course of a few days. There were first a tendency to make odd and inappropriate remarks, and bizarre behaviour such as sitting the whole of a morning with a newspaper, apparently reading it but in answer to questions being unable to say even what was in the headlines. She then kept her eyes closed, her mouth in a fixed smile; in the night she was found kneeling naked in a position of prayer, apparently having been there for some time, as she was very cold. Admitted to hospital she remained negativistic and catatonic. At times she would eat if a piece of bread was put into her hand; at other times the food had to be put into her mouth. She had to be taken to the toilet, but would walk with assistance; if pushed too hard she would become aggressive. Investigations showed a focus in the right temporal lobe, and in due course a lobectomy was carried out with removal of an atrophic lesion.

If we compare the modes of onset of psychosis in the three groups, we note that an episodic mode of onset was predominant in Group A, an insidious onset in Group B, and either a subacute or an insidious onset in Group C. Differences between the groups in these respects are statistically significant; but they may well have been determined in part by the principles on which the cases were classified, and if so would not be very meaningful.

The different types of course which the illness took are also shown in Table 12.3. The commonest development was towards chronicity, or even to deterioration (46 per cent); but in 31 per cent of cases there was a tendency to improve, even to the point of recovery from the psychosis. A fluctuating course was observed in 22 per cent of cases. In respect of these characteristics there are no significant differences between the three Groups A, B and C. Nevertheless, course and mode of onset are themselves correlated, as is shown in Table 12.4. As the illness began, so it tends to go on. The best chances of improvement or recovery are found in patients with an acute or subacute onset (observed 10, expected 5.96), patients with an episodic onset tended to a fluctuating course (observed 8, expected 4.48); and those with an insidious onset tended towards chronicity (observed 18, expected 12.96). These differences are statistically significant (χ^2 12.19, 4 d.f., .02>p>.01).

TABLE 12.4. CORRELATION OF MODE OF ONSET WITH TYPE OF COURSE OF THE SCHIZOPHRENIC-LIKE PSYCHOSIS

Mode of onset	Course			Total
	B towards improvement	F fluctuating	C towards chronicity	
Acute and subacute	10	4	5	19
Episodic	4	8	8	20
Insidious	7	3	18	28
Totals	21	15	31	67

SYMPTOMATOLOGY

The schizophrenic symptomatology shown by these patients is schematically described in Table 12.5. The more detailed description which follows relies not only on anamnestic data but also on the findings made during hospital observation.

1. Delusional symptoms

Delusion formation was shown by all our patients with the exception of two, both of them in Group C, i.e. suffering from hebephrenic-like states. The second of these suffered from auditory hallucinations, and believed in the objective reality of his experiences.

The primary delusional experience, which is supposed to be very characteristic of schizophrenia, can seldom be directly observed, but was reported by a few of our

TABLE 12.5. SCHIZOPHRENIC SYMPTOMATOLOGY, FROM SELF-DESCRIPTION OR
OBSERVED IN HOSPITAL

	Group A	Group B	Group C	Totals
Delusions in clear consciousness	11	46	10	67
Hallucinations in clear consciousness				
auditory	6	31	9	46
gustatory	—	2	1	3
olfactory	—	4	1	5
somatic	—	5	2	7
visual	3	10	3	16
total patients affected	7	35	10	52
Catatonic disorders of behaviour				
impulsive and bizarre acts	3	6	4	13
loss of mobility and volition	1	12	6	19
manneristic behaviour	3	21	10	34
negativism	1	2	2	5
total patients affected	4	26	10	40
Thought disorder, schizophrenic type	4	16	11	31
Loss of affective responsiveness	1	17	10	28

patients. Thus one man said that after three fits on successive days he had a sudden abnormal clarity of thought, "I had two thoughts side by side," and he then realised the untruth of Christianity. Another patient on a bus journey suddenly realised the conductor was whistling because he thought the patient was queer. Another had a sudden awareness of the power of the love of God, and realised he had a special mission. Another patient, during the interview, suddenly thought the examiner had "summed up" against her. Another dropped something to the floor by accident, and instantaneously found that this meant that everything would be all right. It suddenly came to another that he was God, and his fiancée the Virgin Mary.

Mystical delusional experiences are remarkably common. Apart from those already mentioned, the following may be cited. One patient said that "God, or an electrical power" was making him do things; he was Christ, the Son of God. Another said that he felt God working a miracle on him. Another felt that God and the Devil were fighting within him, and God was winning. Another claimed, "All life comes from radioactivity in space. All this goes into one vast electronic brain, which gives God the power to give you life and individuality. I am the Ark of God." Another man said that because his name was John, he was like John the Baptist and was to make known the Second Coming; the patient in the next bed was the reincarnation of the Messiah. Two of the women believed they were pregnant and would be the mother of God. A good description of visionary experience was given by a patient who said that an instant came when everything all of a sudden made sense. "The next thing I was aware of was the earth revolving on its axis. I saw the mass of the earth, under the earth, and sort of in the sky. I see the symbolization of God, and God says to me 'There is no such thing as nothing'."

Related to these are the delusions which might be based on a feeling of depersonalization. One patient felt filled with a radioactive fluid; another could feel light playing through his eyes into his skull, which was empty; another said that her womb had been destroyed; another that her veins had gone back on her, her heart had shifted; another that half his head had been eaten away; another that she was turning into a diamond; another that she was changing into a man.

Derealization experiences might be the basis of other delusional ideas. One patient doubted the paternity of his children; another thought her father was not her father, her mother not her mother, her birthday presents were not hers; another said that her father had lines on his face, her mother was wearing a mask, her clothes were not her own; another that her clothes were mildewed; another man said that he was God and was crucified, his mother was not his mother. Other patients say that everything that is cooked is dirty, the patients are not patients but medical staff, the doctor is not the doctor but the Devil, people in the street look like foreigners, everybody is dressing up as in a pantomime.

Passivity feelings are prominent, and are closely connected with systematized ideas of persecution. One patient is under the control of a machine; another feels things moved under her hand, and feels she is photographed and spied on all the time; another said the neighbours influenced the quality of her voice, she could feel the drawing of the rays, drawing her towards her kitchen; another felt an external force, possibly the Devil, was taking over her brain; another that sexual feelings were being forced on her; another that people were reading her thoughts and "digging at her privacy"; another could feel people looking at her as she undressed. Into these delusions enter a number of bizarre features: rays, thought-reading, telegraphic sense, hypnosis, being filmed, being judged, electronic wires, magnetic powers.

Some of the most characteristically schizophrenic ideas which are met with in these patients are the feelings of special significance which may attach to common-place events. Two parked cars are seen, which mean that the patient is being watched. The colour green is of evil omen, so that green foods must not be touched. Other people's actions take on a special meaning; all the patient's past life is appearing in the office letters. There is a strange significance to events; it all falls into a pattern. Things have "some kind of connection." "It is all a put up affair." "Something's going on, I don't know what." People's Christian names have a significance. Things are said which the patient has heard before. The cars hoot in code.

Special powers are claimed by many: being able to heal people by looking at them, having a telegraphic sense, being able to see through walls, being able to split the atom, being able to read the thoughts of others and foretell the future. One woman said she was magnetic, and could draw the beauty out of anything, it was the crystals in her eyes that gave her the power. This delusion appeared to be derived from the illusion one has of rays of light proceeding from a source, such as a street-lamp, seen through the window or through the eye-lashes. One patient said he could pick up people's thoughts, he had a strange power coming down from the Lord, and it opened to him certain scriptures. Another patient, who had had an AEG examination, said that a fluid had been taken from him at operation which would provide a strong power, if brought into contact with a female fluid of the same amount and standard.

Persecution of an extreme kind is a dominant feeling in the minds of many. Not only are they watched, followed, made fun of, controlled from outside, but they are also poisoned, starved, raped, enveloped in poison clouds, they are being driven mad, and are on the point of being done in.

2. Hallucinations

Only 11 of our patients had, as far as is known, no hallucinatory experiences at all; and in a further 6 cases, though hallucination was probable it was not certain. A few had experiences of an illusional type, or transitional between illusion and hallucination. Thus one patient said she had seen a white dove flying round the square, which betokened the end of the world; this may have been a seagull. Another said he saw the roof-tops painted gold under the sun. Another saw colour everywhere, red on all the shops, put there to send her mad.

What appear to be visceral hallucinations are not infrequent; vaginal sensations (two patients); a feeling inside as if the bladder was full, the organs being touched, the devil having sexual intercourse with her; stomach sensations; a sensation of the body being shrivelled and constricted; the tongue being moved; the strength draining out of the head into the abdomen. Auditory hallucinations are also sometimes associated with particular parts of the body. One patient heard his stomach and his intestines speaking to him, and also parts of his mind, such as his "common sense". Two other patients heard voices coming from the stomach or abdomen, and another said the voice came from the abdomen and from the top part of the head, and his left eye would tell him what he was reading.

Olfactory and gustatory hallucinations were experienced by six patients: tea tasting like hair shampoo; saliva poisoned, gas in the throat; bread soapy; scent being thrown on her; "a holy smell."

Visual hallucinations were most commonly experienced in what was probably a dream-like state, although one in which there was no confusion and a subsequent clear recollection was retained. These hallucinations were often extremely complex, and were usually full of meaning, often of a mystical type. Nearly always there was auditory hallucination at the same time. One patient saw God, heard voices and music, and received a message that he was going to heaven. Another had a vision of Christ on the Cross in the sky, and heard the voice of God saying "You will be healed, your tears have been seen." No fewer than eight patients had these complex mystical experiences, half of them being in Group A. Visual hallucinations, also of a complex kind, were experienced by other patients without any mystical affect. One patient saw visions of friends and acquaintances, often for as long as fifteen minutes at a time, projected, as she thought, in a three-dimensional picture in her room. She would hear the figures recounting conversations on sexual topics which she could not understand, so that they would laugh at her naivety. Other patients saw a cross in the sky and birds that flew through her, visions of faces in the sky, a star and an arm with lights coming out of the fingers, visions of male genitalia with a voice that called her a whore who was always "wanting it," horrible frightening things with glaring eyes and monkeys climbing up the walls of her room, visions of mice, crocodiles, giant legs walking with a lady in Victorian dress. The simpler hallucinations were often experienced in what appears to have been a state of complete lucidity, without any dream-like quality.

The commonest type of hallucination was in the auditory field. Such hallucination might go on continuously and without limit, provoking some emotional reaction but without any observable effect on consciousness. Thus one patient said she heard innumerable voices from everywhere, from the very walls of the house, only passing off when she fell asleep, friendly Norfolk voices, all female. Much commoner are the persecutory voices. Another female patient heard the neighbours reporting on what she was doing all day long; there was much sexual talk, and the voices would say "communist pig," "the old cat," "she is listening," and sometimes meaningless phrases. This patient was subject to multiple hallucinations. She felt pricking and pulling sensations in her eyes due to electricity, she felt a vibration in the lower limbs, needles and electricity being put into her, and saw the lights flashing as cameras went off. Other things the voices say are "We'll get him," "He's natural, I mustn't do that to him," "I suppose he will be using his bodily organ in Piccadilly tonight," "Give him double now," "she does, she doesn't," "come down to earth." Both God and the Devil are among those who speak, as also relatives, neighbours, and unknown persons. Voices that comment on the patient's actions, repeat his own thoughts and otherwise directly interfere are relatively common. Some give orders, which may or may not be obeyed. One patient repeatedly smashed the furniture at home under such commands; another was constantly urged by the voice of her mother to kill herself or kill her sister, but took no such action; another took orders from voices to do the most ordinary things, e.g. to pull the chain after going to the lavatory. Particularly interesting are the hallucinated remarks which also show thought disorder: "That's human nature, the old voicing is too much for you," "you should live up to the voices never," "truth or horribility."

3. Thought disorder

This symptom was shown by about half the patients, and then most commonly in a relative incapacity to handle abstract concepts, and tendencies to be rambling, one-idea'd, long-winded, inconsequential, repetitive, monotonous, circumstantial. These are qualities which one may find in both the organic and the schizophrenic patient, and are not considered further here; they have not been included in Table 12.5. More characteristically schizophrenic are answers beside the point, answers interrupted by thought-blocking, answers never finished or with disturbed syntax, or containing neologisms: "The spirit of God is too great in men and therefore I have epilepsy," "Regarding my permissible entry into the Maudsley, I place all confidence thus: I choose favourably," "The strange thing is you can't make up your mind what religion you are going to be; every religion you think of is different, and so is life itself," "I am not going to be transfigured, so that my face can be altered, by giving away my family history." Neologisms used by patients include "frauding," "nones," "insentiment," "antaggered," "bleedant."

The allusive answer, which seems to be hinting at abnormal experience without explicit statement, is particularly characteristic of schizophrenia; it was shown by a number of patients: "I am not where you see me, but somewhere secret"; "It's the modern world I don't understand, I don't mix with the modern people, it's the modern speech as far as I can tell"; "I'm definite it's a religion and I'm almost certain it's God because I try to act natural." Incoherence to the point where what emerges is a word-salad was shown by a handful of patients, but on occasion only. Thus one patient was speaking of being "put inside Cambridge." When asked whether he meant "Claybury" (Hospital), he replied: "It is just a different university principle. It is just a different regard in dress, isn't it? Two gentlemen, both been in the same places and they've got different ways about them, isn't it? High temperamental or egg-timing."

The subjective experience of thought disorder was reported by several patients. One said: "It's very difficult; you see, everything has a double meaning," another "my mind keeps dotting about all over the place," another complained that his thoughts stuck and he was unable to get rid of them, and several more that their thoughts could be read and thoughts were put into the mind or their thoughts interrupted. Some of these patients thought the external thoughts were coming from God.

4. Emotional disturbance

Affective disturbance of some kind was shown by all patients, if only in the form of periodic moods of depression or irritability. Moods of irritability and aggressiveness were in fact shown by 34 of the patients, and moods of depression by 33. The most typical form of the depressive mood was short-lived but frequently severe; 17 of these patients made one or more attempts at suicide. The converse mood of exaltation or ecstasy was experienced at times by 12 patients, most typically as a semi-mystical experience, such as has already been referred to. The paranoid mood, in which there is a feeling of something mysterious going on, without specific delusional idea, has also been discussed. Single patients also described sudden unmotivated feelings of intense fear and of a devastating loneliness and bewilderment.

The schizophrenic defect symptom of flatness of affect was exhibited to some degree, at least at times, by 28 of the patients. The more communicative patients described loss of interest, incapacity to find any enjoyment, the lack of warmth in their feelings for relatives. More commonly there was no such complaint, but the patient showed flat, silly, or inappropriate emotional responses, would smile without reason in a fatuous or in a secretive or superior way, or, especially in cases of Group C, show an unrelieved hebetude.

5. Disturbances of volition and catatonic phenomena

These are best considered together, since the distinction between them is in any case rather vague. Impairment of volition, shown in reduction of energy, interest, and initiative, was shown at times by 19 patients. Activity might sink to a very low level, or take on a bizarre quality. One patient would sit the whole morning with a newspaper open in front of her; she would only walk if assisted, and only eat if the food were put into her hand. This inactivity would be at times interrupted by a sudden wild dash, or a peal of laughter. Another patient began to slow up in all movements, took to walking only on the pattern of the carpet, and eventually retired to bed, where she lay answering questions only with a puzzled look or an incongruous smile. This patient also showed characteristic schizophrenic ambivalence: when the doctor on the round left her side, she called him back, but when he turned to her again was unable to say anything. Of other patients, one would sit looking at her wrists for hours, another would hold his hand in front of his mouth when speaking, or whistle instead of answering, another kept her hand pressed to her abdomen, another was constantly looking round at the door. Withdrawal from family life, going out to sit on the stairs, retiring to the bedroom to sit with drawn curtains, sitting for hours listening or staring into space were other typical manifestations.

Some degree of manneristic behaviour was shown by 34 patients: smiling, frowning, a foolish giggle, talking to oneself, screwing up of the eyes, banging of the head, clapping hands and slapping the floor with the feet, a statuesque posture, or mincing or stilted gait, holding the fingers twisted, etc. Sudden impulsive acts, aggressive or bizarre, motivated in some cases by hallucinations, e.g. a dash into the garden to fetch in a brick, suddenly putting the hand through a pane of glass, were shown by 13 patients. One patient spent the better part of 24 hours in stereotyped repetitive exercises, as he believed under the influence of an external control. Resistiveness and negativism of a schizophrenic kind were shown by five patients.

Some of the patients were able to describe the subjective experience of disturbance of the ego: "I keep finding myself with various personalities," the body feeling as if it were moved around under external control, feeling drugged, the mind revolving under the control of a machine, being told what to do.

6. Clinical summary

In summary one may say that there is not one of the cardinal symptoms of schizophrenia which has not been at some time exhibited by these patients. However, the combination of symptoms shown by individuals differs slightly from the most usual schizophrenic patterns. Although they are seen, catatonic phenomena of any gross degree are unusual, and loss of affective response does not occur so early or become so marked in the great majority of these patients as in the typical schizophrenic. By and large they are friendlier and more co-operative, and less suspicious of hospital staff, so that only very rarely do they cause a serious nursing problem. In a ward with mentally normal patients they are usually able to keep their symptoms to themselves and to spare the feelings of other patients.

SUMMARY AND CONCLUSIONS

The appearance of chronic psychotic states, clinically closely resembling schizophrenia, in epileptic patients has been recorded from time to time by many authors. The more significant of these papers are here reviewed. Most recently Pond has associated chronic paranoid psychoses resembling schizophrenia with temporal lobe epilepsy.

Patients of this type have been collected, as systematically as circumstances permitted, at the National Hospital, Queen Square, and at the Maudsley Hospital; 69 such patients were found, and have been investigated.

1. The question is examined whether the purely coincidental combination of epilepsy and schizophrenia, each of them relatively common disorders, would be sufficiently frequent to make such a collection possible. It is concluded that this is not so, and that in the bulk of cases the combination cannot be randomly determined.

2. As the appearance of a schizophrenic-like psychosis in an epileptic might be aided by a schizoid predisposition, the past personalities of these patients were examined. It was concluded that the premorbid personality was of normal type, but that when the onset of epilepsy was early, epileptic personality changes could be found in the prepsychotic personality. There was no evidence of schizoid traits in excess.

3. The mean age of onset of the psychosis was 29.8 years, after the epilepsy had lasted for a mean duration of 14.1 years. There was a significant correlation coefficient between the ages of onset of epilepsy and of schizophrenia of +0.6, indicating that the duration of the epilepsy was likely to be one of the causative factors. There was no close relationship between the frequency of fits and the onset of psychosis; but in some instances there was a suggestion of an inverse relationship, e.g. psychotic symptoms first appearing when the fit frequency was falling.

4. The modes of onset of the psychosis could be classified into acute, episodic, subacute and insidious. The last of these was the commonest (29 patients), with onset of an episodic kind the next most frequent (20 patients). The course of the psychosis was similarly classified into one with tendency to improve, a fluctuating course, and a course tending to chronicity. Of these the last was the most frequent (31 patients).

5. A phenomenological analysis of the schizophrenic symptoms shown by our patients showed delusion-formation of a typically schizophrenic kind in all but two of the patients. Typically schizophrenic hallucinatory experiences in clear consciousness occurred in 52 patients, auditory hallucinations predominating. Affective disturbances of a great variety of kinds were experienced by these patients, depressions and ecstasies being not infrequent. The most typically schizophrenic affective symptom of flatness of emotional response was observed, at least to some degree, in 28 patients. Disturbances of volition and catatonic phenomena were shown by 40 patients. The commonest form of thought disorder shown was of a type compatible with organic states, e.g. deficiency of conceptual thinking, circumstantiality, etc. Thought disorder of a specifically schizophrenic kind was shown to some degree by 31 patients. It is concluded that there is not one of the cardinal symptoms of schizophrenia which has not been exhibited at some time by these patients. It would not be possible to diagnose these patients, on psychological symptomatology alone, as suffering from anything other than a schizophrenic psychosis; the recognition of the psychosis as essentially epileptic in origin requires consideration of all the available information.

APPENDIX

The Centrencephalic Epileptics

A few words should be said about the patients with centrencephalic epilepsy. There were seven of them, and five of them are in Group C, two in Group B and none in Group A. They suffered in fact predominantly from a hebephrenic type of psychosis. The family history is negative in all but one; in Case 50, the mother was in a mental hospital for twelve months with a puerperal confusional psychosis. The personal history is negative in all cases but two; in Case 50 there was a forceps delivery, and in Case 63 there was premature birth. In these cases onset of epilepsy tended to be early, ranging from four to 17, with a mean of 11. The onset of psychosis was also relatively early, ranging from 15 to 38 with a mean of 21.

II. Physical Aspects[3]

SUMMARY

In this paper are discussed the physical aspects of a group of 69 epileptics who developed a schizophrenia-like psychosis.

1. Examination of the past medical history showed that a significant proportion of patients in group A (chronic psychosis coloured by recurrent confusional episodes) and group B (chronic paranoid psychosis) had experienced conditions liable to cause a brain lesion; this was not the case in patients of group C (hebephrenia-like state).

2. The history of the epilepsy showed that the patients of group C had an earlier age of onset (9.3 years) than those of groups A and B (20.5, 16.3). However, the duration of epilepsy before onset of psychotic symptoms was nearly the same in all three groups, ranging from 12.8 to 15.6 years, with average for the whole material of

[3] By A. W. Beard.

14.1 years. There was a correlation between the ages of onset of epilepsy and psychosis with coefficient value +0.58. The suggestion arises that duration of epilepsy plays an aetiological role in determining the psychosis.

3. The quantity of medication, the severity of the epilepsy and the degree of control of the attacks by drugs did not seem to play a part in determining the psychosis.

4. There was a tendency for the patients in group A to have all or at least some of their fits during the hours of sleep.

5. The clinical features of the epilepsy indicated in 45 out of 69 cases an origin in the temporal lobe, and in a further five cases a focal origin in a sensory or motor area.

6. Neurological examination was usually unhelpful. Altogether there were 12 cases with evidence of pyramidal disturbance.

7. Psychiatric examination showed a high incidence of personality changes indicative of organic brain lesions. The degree of personality change was proportional to the duration of the epilepsy, and the association between these two variables was statistically significant.

8. The electroencephalographic findings substantiated the clinical impression of a high incidence of temporal lobe epilepsy; and there was good agreement between the clinical and EEG diagnoses. However, the EEG using sphenoidal wires and activation revealed ten cases of temporal lobe epilepsy which were not suggested by the history. This figure is considered important, in that the temporal lobe foci so revealed are sometimes amenable to surgery, and on occasion they may indicate a tumour and facilitate its early recognition.

9. Air encephalography confirmed the impression obtained from the past medical history that many of these patients have an organic brain lesion. The commonest finding, in 37 out of 56 cases, was that of an atrophic process. In only two cases did the AEG indicate a tumour.

10. Thirteen patients were examined otologically for abnormalities affecting the central connections of the VIIIth nerve. In five of these caloric tests showed vestibular functions to be normal, and in the remaining eight cases the responses suggested that one or other of the temporal lobes was affected. Otological tests would appear to be a valuable method of examination in such cases.

11. Data obtained by psychometric tests were usually uninformative. In five cases there were findings suggestive of a slight expressive dysphasia or an auditory learning deficit.

12. Eleven patients were submitted to temporal lobectomies and one patient to a frontal lobectomy. Pathological findings were very various, including neoplasms, a dermoid cyst, circumscribed tuberose sclerosis and atrophic lesions. Some of these patients have been previously reported by Serafetinides and Falconer (1962). As a result of these operations there was usually substantial benefit to the epilepsy, some improvement of the psychosis, but a heavy incidence of organic personality changes.

III. Genetical Aspects[4]

When we face the crucial problem of the aetiological basis of the psychoses we have described, there are three main possibilities to be considered. Either they are to be regarded as symptomatic schizophrenias of purely epileptic causation; or they are

[4] By Eliot Slater and Eric Glithero.

independent schizophrenias which have appeared in these epileptic subjects coinci-
dentally as the result of pure chance; or they are forms of schizophrenic illness
which have arisen in individuals predisposed thereto by the stresses produced by the
epilepsy. An investigation of the genetical background is capable of producing evidence which would assist in answering this question. If the first hypothesis is correct, the incidence of schizophrenic psychoses in the relatives of our subjects should
be no greater than in the general population. If the second hypothesis is correct, the
incidence of schizophrenic psychoses in the relatives should be the same as in the
relatives of schizophrenics of the usual kind. If the third hypothesis is correct, we
would expect an incidence of schizophrenia in the relatives of our patients which
would lie somewhere between these two figures.

With this in mind, an investigation of the family history was undertaken along
two lines. First, all the hospital records were examined for information about illness
or abnormality among first degree relatives. Secondly, one of us (E.G.) contacted
the accessible relatives and interviewed them, either at hospital or in their own
homes. At these interviews questions were put, not only about the family history,
but also about the patient's follow-up history since last admission to hospital, a
subject which will be dealt with later. On the family history, relatives were asked for
complete data about the patient's parents and sibs, and his children if any, including
age now or at death or when last heard of, illnesses, especially epilepsy or any
mental illness, and temperament and personality. Where there was a record of
mental illness, data were obtained on the time and the hospital where it had been
treated, so that further enquiries could be made.

In this way data about the family were taken from the hospital notes in all 69
cases, from 22 patients in cases where they were capable of giving useful information, from 7 fathers, 23 mothers, 6 brothers, 15 sisters, 4 husbands, 10 wives, one
aunt, one sister-in-law, and one family doctor.

The psychiatric abnormalities discovered in this way are shown in Table 12.6.

TABLE 12.6. PSYCHIATRIC ABNORMALITIES IN PARENTS AND SIBS

Abnormality	Fathers	Mothers	Brothers	Sisters	Total
Epileptic paranoid psychosis	1	—	—	—	1
Epilepsy, non-psychotic	1	1	3	2	7
Schizophrenia	—	1	1	—	2
Puerperal confusional psychosis	—	1			1
Senile psychosis	—	1	—	—	1
Possible puerperal psychosis	—	1	—	—	1
"Psychopathic personality"	9	2	—	1	12
Alcoholism	4	1	1	—	6
Neurotic symptoms	1	3	4	2	10
Total of anomalous persons	16	11	9	5	41

The most interesting finding was that the father of one of our patients (45) had
himself had an epileptic paranoid psychosis of a type which might quite well be
regarded as schizophrenia-like.

This man was said to have had "sunstroke" at the age of three or four, having
suddenly fallen while playing with his sister and become unconscious. There is a
history of fits and fits of laughing in childhood. He was always self-willed and
obstinate, difficult to live with. He seems to have been free from fits during adolescence, and he became a skilled woodworker. The first fit in adult life was observed
by his wife at night, about nine months after marriage, when he was 27. Major

attacks were rare, but he would also have a "kind of fit" in which he would become vacant and confused for a few minutes, suck his lips constantly and noisily, and tremble. He would have numbers of these attacks at night, and sometimes during the day. In personality he was an extreme individualist, a conscientious objector, an atheist, anarchist, socialist, ardent trade unionist, public orator, and a great reader of psychology, philosophy, political theory, etc. Opinionated and bombastic, he would make a great fuss about small issues, and was excitable, irritable, fussy, and meticulous. All through his life he was extremely bitter in his opposition to authority. His habits were abstemious.

At the age of 40 he is said to have had a nervous breakdown, but he was not in hospital. From this time on he became liable to long moods of depression. At the age of 43 (in 1935) he was found to be suffering from pernicious anaemia, for which he received regular hospital out-patient treatment. The psychotic illness came on acutely at the age of 46, at a time when according to his wife he had had very great numbers of his minor attacks at night, and one night when they went on nearly all night. One day his brother was called to him in the street, where he found him kneeling in prayer with a crowd around him, sympathetic but astonished and inquisitive. He declared that some spiritual force had taken possession of his body, and a voice had said "Fear not, I am with you, go and see Herr Hitler." He thought he had a mission to lead all mankind to salvation. He believed that the end of the world had come, and that all men were not brothers. He began to shout in the street "The Jews, the Jews," and was taken to hospital.

In hospital he was found to be physically well, haemoglobin 78 percent, red cells 3.8 million, colour index 1.04; no neurological lesion detected. He remembered the circumstances of his admission, and does not appear to have been confused. He is described as pedantic and stilted. He settled down very well in hospital, and for the first few months showed no inclination to depart. His paranoid ideas slipped into the past. In reports he is described as garrulous, over-confident, etc., but without solid indication of needing hospital care. Later on, when he wished to depart, his wife made objections. Still later, on more than one occasion he made attempts to escape. Finally his son, our patient, applied to take him home; but this was thought inadvisable on account of this son's epilepsy. He was out on trial in a Mental After-Care Home for six months in 1955, but seems to have come back on his own and to be glad to get back. He died of a coronary thrombosis in 1959, aged 67. For many years his fits had been very infrequent, and there had never been a second attack of paranoid-hallucinatory psychosis.

The other epileptic histories are as follows:

Case 17
Brother disabled by infantile paralysis, also has occasional grand mal attacks.

Case 28
Father had epilepsy from mid-thirties until a few years before death at 76, grand mal attacks two or three times a week nearly always at night, so that he was able to keep his job as a policeman; never attended hospital; marked mood swings.

Case 30
Maternal half-brother had petit mal attacks from 15 to 20 (not included in statistics).

Case 33
Sister had petit mal from nine to 16, brother had petit mal from childhood till 14.

Case 41
Brother bad-tempered, violent, liable to falling attacks in which he lies for a minute and then gets up again; sister had falling attacks from 10 to 13.

Case 48
Mother had grand mal attacks from seven to fourteen.

The schizophrenic histories are:

Case 43
Mother at 54 was admitted to mental hospital, hostile, suspicious, non-co-operative; she was hallucinated and believed that the staff and patients were all laughing at her, saying she was a wicked woman; she said a microphone was installed in her house, and her thoughts were transmitted by wireless all over the place. She settled down and was discharged three years later, not yet recovered, and died of cerebral haemorrhage at 66 at home.

Case 69
Brother discharged from the Navy with diagnosis "paranoid psychosis", no further information to be obtained.

The other psychoses, or possible psychoses, are:

Case 20
It is possible that the mother had a "nervous breakdown" at the time of the patient's birth; no more precise information to be obtained.

Case 38
Mother admitted to a general hospital, for treatment to her legs, at the age of 70. She had become euphoric, confused and disoriented as to time and place. In this state she was transferred under certificate to a mental hospital, where she was diagnosed as suffering from a confusional state. After nine months she was taken off certificate and made a voluntary patient, but remained euphoric, rambling in conversation, liable to laugh inappropriately, and without insight. She was so confused that she could not be left alone, and needed constant attention. She had occasional convulsions, which had also occurred at infrequent intervals for six or seven years before her admission.

Case 50
Mother admitted to mental hospital aet. 29, 16 days after the birth of a daughter and femoral thrombosis. She was confused, restless, noisy, inattentive, resistive, hallucinated. For some months there was a variable pyrexia, swelling of the legs, purulent gingivitis. Five months after admission she was still resistive, confused, disorientated. She gradually settled, and was taken home by relatives 12 months after admission, diagnosis puerperal confusional psychosis. Since that time she has remained well, but highly-strung, quarrelsome, sometimes depressed, and liable to talk of suicide.

The "psychopathic personalities" found among the relatives were:

Case 5
Father suffered from migraine, facial pain and Parkinsonism, and is now deteriorating intellectually; he has been seen by a psychiatrist and has been diagnosed as an obsessional neurotic; he was retired on psychiatric grounds aet. 59, and lives as an invalid, a selfish man with a bitter sarcastic tongue.

Case 13
Father a rather obsessional, pedantic, moralizing, rigid personality.

Case 28
Mother very quick-tempered, spiteful, nagging.

Case 29
Both father and mother nervy, anxious, hypochondriacal, always ailing and unwell with ulcers, bronchitis, etc.

Case 32
Father lifelong alcoholic with marked paranoid tendencies, depressive, interested in Christian Science.

Case 33
Father quick-tempered, irascible.

Case 41
Father a very peculiar man who rarely left his room for many years, wouldn't let his wife in to clean it, having his food sent in on a tray; wouldn't let his wife wash his clothes, would

make threats he would leave her penniless; d. 71 without overt breakdown. Sister highly-strung, bad-tempered.

Case 55

Father a brilliant man, interested in "astronomy and other mystical subjects", wrapped up in his own world, obsessional and meticulous to a degree, committed suicide at 72, having planned it with great care, settling all his affairs to the last detail.

Case 67

Father used to have "strange temper-rages" in which he would fly off the handle for nothing, then be "as nice as pie"; he also had attacks of extreme jealousy, e.g. would not let his wife maintain contact with any of her old friends after marriage, and constantly kept an eye on her dealings with tradesmen, didn't like her even to meet her own family. He had no friends himself, but was "kind but on the odd side."

Case 69

Father a cold, unlovable, obstinate, dogmatic man.

The children of the probands were too few in number and too young to provide information of statistical value. There were 40 of them, ranging from less than one to 39 years of age, mean 18; and the only psychiatric abnormality was shown by one girl of 16, who had had out-patient treatment for an anxiety state.

The age distribution of parents and sibs is shown in Table 12.7. In order to calculate the incidence of mental abnormality, we may use Weinberg's shorter method. In this method, the total population at risk is determined by assigning a value of 0 to individuals younger than X years, a value of 1 to those older than Y years, and a value of ½ to those between these ages. The limited ages, X and Y, in epilepsy can be taken to be 5 and 19, in schizophrenia to be 15 and 39, in "psychopathic personality" to be 15 and 24.

TABLE 12.7. AGE DISTRIBUTION OF PARENTS AND SIBS AT LAST INFORMATION

Age	Fathers	Mothers	Brothers	Sisters	Total
0- 4	—	—	13	10	23
5- 9	—	—	1	2	3
10-14	—	—	1	3	4
15-19	—	—	3	7	10
20-24	—	—	5	6	11
25-29	—	—	7	7	14
30-34	—	—	15	14	29
35-39	1	1	17	17	36
40-44	1	—	10	11	22
45-49	4	4	15	8	31
50-54	11	5	11	12	39
55-59	10	16	7	9	42
60-64	7	11	7	6	31
65-69	16	9	3	3	31
70-74	7	11	—	2	20
75-79	5	5	—	—	10
80-	4	5	—	—	9
Unknown	3	2	—	—	5
Totals	69	69	115	117	370

On this basis, we have observed 333.5 risk lifetimes for epilepsy, 286 risk lifetimes for schizophrenia, and 321.5 risk lifetimes for "psychopathic personality". Having found among the relatives 8 epileptics, 2 schizophrenics and 12 "psychopathic personalities", we calculate the incidences of these disorders as respectively 2.4 per cent, 0.7 per cent and 3.7 per cent.

The incidence of schizophrenia among these relatives is approximately what would have been expected from a sample of the general population, and very different from expectations if our subjects had been schizophrenics. Estimates on the expected incidence of schizophrenia in the parents and in the sibs of schizophrenics could hardly be put lower than 4 per cent and 8 per cent, leading to an expectation of finding 5.32 schizophrenic parents and 12.24 schizophrenic sibs in our material. Our finding of 2 schizophrenics differs from the expected total of 17.56 by a margin which is significant at the 0.001 level.

CONCLUSION

We conclude accordingly that, for a parent or sib of an epileptic who develops a schizophrenia-like psychosis, the risk of schizophrenia is no greater than for a member of the general population. The risk of epilepsy may well be raised, though our value is subject to a large sampling error; we have found it to be of about the same value as has been found by previous investigators for the first-degree relatives of "symptomatic" epileptics.

These findings support the first of the three hypotheses enunciated, that the psychoses which we have investigated are to be regarded as symptomatic schizophreniform psychoses of purely epileptic causation — that they are, in fact, epileptic psychoses and not schizophrenic ones from the aetiological standpoint.

IV. Follow-up Record and Outcome[5]

Between 14.4.60 and 30.9.60 a follow-up enquiry was carried out, combined with the genetical investigation which has been reported in previous pages. The informants for the genetical enquiry were also the ones who gave information about the patient's recent history. The period covered by follow-up was therefore from one to three years after the time at which hospital investigations had been carried out; and if related to the onset of the schizophrenia-like psychosis was at a mean period of 7.8 years later (range from 2 to 25 years). In addition to this the National Hospital patients have continued to be followed up from that time to the present date, as they and their relatives are asked to attend regularly at a follow-up clinic at the hospital. What is reported here relates to the findings in the special enquiry; but the data that have come in since do not suggest any modification of the conclusions that will be based on the survey of 1960. A synoptic view of these findings is given in Table 12.8.

At the time of follow-up, five patients could not be traced or refused to be seen. In the remaining 64 cases, both patients and relatives were interviewed as far as possible, and reports on any recent hospital attendance were obtained. Four of these 64 patients had died by the time of the survey; but as up-to-date information was obtained about them, they are included in the assessment. The interviews with patient and relatives were directed, apart from the genetical enquiry, towards getting a clear picture of the patient's present psychiatric state and his level of social adjustment. Most of the relatives were co-operative and helpful witnesses, and with few exceptions gave the impression of being normal and reliable people.

[5] By Eric Glithero and Eliot Slater.

TABLE 12.8. FINDINGS OBTAINED IN FOLLOW-UP SURVEY, 1960

| | Clinical Groups | | | |
	A	B	C	Total
Domicile				
Living at home permanently	5	20	5	30
Living mainly at home	4	10	2	16
Mainly in hospital	1	7	1	9
Permanently in hospital	–	5	4	9
Of these died	(–)	(2)	(2)	(4)
Lost sight of	1	4	–	5
Outcome of Epilepsy				
(0) No fit within a year	3	6	1	10
(1) Constitutes no problem	3	28	4	35
(2) Moderately troublesome	2	5	5	12
(3) Severe problem	2	1	–	3
Lost sight of or died	1	6	2	9
Outcome of Schizophrenic-like Symptoms				
(r) Passed off or recovered	5	12	4	21
(i) Improved	4	13	3	20
(s) Remained the same	1	15	3	19
Lost sight of or died	1	6	2	9
Organic Personality Changes	4	18	7	29

Clinical groups: A, 11 patients with chronic psychoses, complicated by confusional episodes; B, 46 patients with chronic paraphrenic psychoses; C, 12 patients with hebephrenia-like psychoses.

DOMICILE AND SOCIAL ADJUSTMENT

Of the 64 patients who were successfully followed up, 30 lived at home permanently. Some of them were attending hospital out-patient departments, but many of them required no hospital attention whatever. Sixteen patients lived mainly at home, but had intermittent admissions to hospitals because of periodic exacerbation or recurrence of their psychiatric symptoms. Nine patients lived in hospital most of the time, going home regularly for week-ends, and occasionally for a week's holiday. Nine patients lived in hospital permanently, not going home even for an occasional week-end.

Unlike a truly schizophrenic illness, the psychoses from which these patients suffered tended to leave them preoccupied with old delusional ideas or with remnants of thought disorder, but not with bleached, washed out or vacuous personalities. Consequently they retained at least the façade of their previous personality, and found it easier to maintain reasonably good personal relationships than to take an initiative in social interests. Of the whole group one patient participated actively and with initiative in social affairs; 13 showed a moderate though passive interest; 25 would show a mild interest with encouragement; and 25 had no social interests at all. Needless to say the degree of social interest was very much better in those patients living entirely or mainly at home than in the others.

Personal relationships showed up rather better: nine patients had well preserved personalities and were able to show tact and consideration and warmth of feeling for others; 24 retained socially adequate personalities, able to cope with normal social relationships but lacking initiative and warmth of response; 26 were able to maintain no more than a reasonably presentable facade; five were in one way or another difficult. These characteristics are again correlated with domicile; all the nine best patients spent the whole of their time at home, while all of the five difficult ones needed hospital, at least at times.

The employment record was quite surprisingly good. Twenty-two of the patients domiciled entirely at home, and 25 of the total of 64 patients, were employed in full-time work. Of those living wholly or mainly at home, three more were in part-time employment, 14 earned money in odd jobs or occasional casual work, and only four achieved nothing at all. Of those living mainly or wholly in hospital, one patient was able to go out to part-time work, eight were usefully occupied doing odd jobs or in hospital work duties, and nine did little but take part in obligatory hospital routine, such as occupational therapy. Of the 30 patients living entirely at home, none had failed to maintain their previous level of occupation, and 18 of them had actually achieved a marked improvement in their employment status.

Who actually carries the burden, or gives the necessary support to these patients, so that they function at their present level? We find that in the patients wholly or mainly living at home, 12 were entirely self-sufficient, requiring no support at any time; 11 were largely self-sufficient and required only occasional support or solicitude from their family, e.g. at times of mental upset; and 22 needed constant though limited support from their families. The patients living mainly or wholly in hospital were of course carried mainly by the hospital, though the families also took a share of responsibility.

Ranking after the success or otherwise of medical treatment in preventing progressive impairment, it was the nature of the family relationships, and the amount of support that the relatives could provide if needed, which made the difference between capacity or otherwise to live outside hospital. And in socio-economic terms it is clear that it is these families and patients that justify the support, help and guidance of the social service departments of the hospitals to which the patients are attached.

DEATHS

The four deaths which occurred in this series merit brief description:

Case 14

This man was transferred from the National Hospital to a mental hospital in 1957, and died there a year later from his cerebral tumour. He continued to have infrequent epileptic attacks, became less aggressive and more like a vegetable, but remained paranoid.

Case 21

The patient left hospital in 1958 and died in March 1959, living at home as an invalid until admitted to the local hospital where he died. He continued to have major and minor attacks until death, of which the certified cause was "bronchial pneumonia, obesity, and epilepsy". During the last year of his life his psychotic symptoms receded completely.

Case 57

The patient was discharged to a mental hospital in February 1958, and remained there till transfer to a general hospital for investigation of oedema of the legs and albuminuria. There she went downhill and died. The autopsy was carried out on the coroner's orders, and no detailed examination of the brain was made. There was, however, "an area of softening in the left lateral ventricle and extending towards the basal ganglia". Though she was found to have died of tuberculosis, there was no indication that the left hemisphere lesion was tuberculous. In the mental hospital she was quiet, withdrawn, talked beside the point, and probably continued to be hallucinated.

Case 62

After discharge from hospital he lived at home. Mentally he was uncommunicative, withdrawn, suspicious and hostile, though not aggressive. He denied his epilepsy, and gave up taking drugs. His fits increased in number till he was having several a day; these involved movements of the head and upper limbs but no general convulsion. In June 1959 he walked out of the house without saying where he was going. He did not return home, but once or twice wrote letters, not giving addresses, but saying he was sorry for all the trouble he had been, that he felt he had to go away, and asking sensibly about the family. In August 1959 he was found dead in an empty house in Deal. An inquest was held, but the Coroner said that no cause of death could be found.

EPILEPTIC AFTER-HISTORY

A striking feature of the after-history in these cases was a tendency for the epilepsy to become less troublesome, or to be better controlled, after discharge from hospital. In no fewer than 10 cases at the time of follow-up there had been no fit observed during the past 12 months or longer. In half of these cases this satisfactory result could be attributed to a temporal lobectomy; in the other cases a remission, perhaps temporary, seemed to have occurred spontaneously. The excellent epileptic result was accompanied by a favourable development in the psychosis, though not so striking. Four of these patients showed a remission of psychotic symptoms, two of them after lobectomy; five showed an improvement; and in one patient, not lobectomized, there was no change.

The best result was seen in Case 11. The patient was described as "a completely different woman from what she used to be". She was doing a full-time job as well as looking after the home. She had had no fit, blackout or "equivalent" for six years. There was no mention of paranoid ideas, though she did not feel the people at work were as friendly as they might be; and there were occasional periods of mild depression. In Case 49 the patient was working as an accountant, and was a quiet, conscientious man, free of symptoms. Discussing his previous experiences he took a guarded attitude, and still thought they could have been religious revelations. The patient in Case 67 had had no fit for 15 months, though there had been occasional outbursts of irritability. She was no longer paranoid; but she led a flat and empty life without social contacts, and lacked all warmth of feeling. In Case 45 the patient was left with a damaged personality, ponderous, pedantic, religiose, over-precise and orderly, and very slow to get to the point. He had had no fits for five or six years; but he said he had had two visions whilst asleep about four years ago, so vivid and real it couldn't have been a dream, which had given him an understanding of why things exist. In one he had seen a genie composed of bubbles, which said to him, "You are a good boy, George. Listen to your heart." The second was of the earth revolving on an axis in the arms of God, who said, "There is no such thing as death and everything is eternal." In Case 61, though the patient had had no fits for the last year, she had become worse psychiatrically and was now able to come home from the mental hospital only on week-end leave. She was as paranoid as ever, but in addition had become disoriented in time and place and unable to recognize members of her own family.

In a further 35 cases, epileptic attacks had become infrequent or so mild as to constitute no problem, medically or socially. In 12 cases the epilepsy has remained a moderate handicap, and in three cases a severe one. The degree of the epileptic disability does not have any relationship to domicile; the proportion of the more disabled and of the less disabled who live entirely at home is approximately the same.

OUTCOME OF SCHIZOPHRENIC-LIKE SYMPTOMS

As will be seen from Table 12.8, if we omit the cases where a follow-up was not possible and the four patients who had died, we are left with 60 patients of whom slightly over one-third had attained a complete remission of specifically schizophrenic-like symptoms, while in one-third these symptoms had improved. In nearly one-third of the patients the symptoms had not got any better during the time under review. The results are best in the A group, in which half the patients had a remission and all but one improved; but in all groups the majority of the patients made some move for the better. Unfortunately we cannot rely on this improvement being permanent. Thus in two of the lobectomized patients (23, 26), there has been some recurrence of schizophrenic-like symptoms since the follow-up of 1960. However, it would seem on this evidence that over the course of time there is a distinct tendency for the schizophrenic-like symptoms, which have appeared at one stage in the development of the case, to settle down again at a later stage.

Unlike the degree of epileptic disability, which was not correlated with domicile, the schizophrenic symptomatology was found to have a bearing on the degree of liberty and responsibility enjoyed. Of the 41 patients whose schizophrenic-like symptoms passed off or improved, 24 (59 percent) lived wholly at home without needing any hospital treatment; of the 19 patients whose symptoms did not improve, only 4 (21 percent) were able to live wholly at home. A χ^2 test shows a difference significant at the 0.01 level.

In some cases paradoxical results were found. There was no patient whose schizophrenic-like symptoms totally remitted, who yet had to live entirely in hospital; but there were four who had to live mainly in hospital. The following may be taken as an example.

Case 40

This patient had been an in-patient at a mental hospital for the last three years. She was admitted there following a gross exacerbation of her religious preoccupations, which had been brought on by her placing as a domestic in a Pentecostal Nursing Home, where religious devotion was the main interest of the residents. In the hospital her mother was visiting her regularly, and she came home for two weeks' holiday three to four times a year.

For some years she had had only minor turns; she got no warning, would give a slight moan, fall to the ground on the left, get up within a few seconds, be slightly confused after it and behave in an automatic fashion for three to four minutes, after which she would be perfectly all right. These attacks might occur two in one day and then none for a week or two.

When not otherwise occupied, both in hospital and at home, she would sit around reading or looking at the Bible. She liked to discuss God and religion with anyone interested, but did not go on about it inappropriately at other times. She insisted on having religious tracts hung around their living room, and listened to all the religious broadcasts. At hospital it was her daily job to clean the day room and she went out and about with other patients. At home she was very helpful, and would do the bulk of the housework without guidance, a reliable clean worker. Both at hospital and at home she was found by everyone to be kindly and friendly, going out of her way to help people; but she had no hobbies or interests other than religion. She never made paranoid remarks, but was said to be getting a little depressed lately at the prospect of remaining in the mental hospital for the rest of her life.

The above shows that special circumstances may require continuation of hospital care when the psychosis has passed off. The example that follows illustrates the possibility of life at home being combined with continuation of psychosis.

Case 68

This patient, single, was living with his elderly mother and spinster twin sisters. He did not work after coming out of the mental hospital two years ago, until a few weeks before the visit. Then after months of refusing all chance of work, he suddenly decided to apply for a portering job; and since taking it he had much improved.

He could go many months without having a fit, but usually had a fit or a batch of two or three fits about once a month. After a fit, he would be confused for half-an-hour or so; but as far as he was concerned they were not a major problem.

His conversation, at home or at hospital, consisted almost entirely of nebulous religious rambling remarks. Except for short periods, it was impossible to hold an ordinary conversation with him, since he would simply change the subject to his own preoccupations. He continued to believe in a great variety of grandiose religiose delusions, e.g., that he has been in intimate communication with the supernatural since he was born, that he can recall his christening, that he has conversations with God, hears his voice and replies, that God plants ideas in his mind; and he was prepared to talk on these themes with a gentle, sardonic and infinitely superior smile. These delusions have shown little change for several years.

The continuation of schizophrenic-like delusions and hallucinations is not the only psychiatric hazard for these patients. Apart from the frankly organic symptoms, to be discussed shortly, several patients suffer from depressive and obsessional symptoms. Depressive moods, sometimes severe, are reported in 11 cases, and in some of these the depression is the worst symptom. Thus in Case 32, the patient who had made a very good recovery since his temporal lobectomy in 1955, was free of schizophrenic-like symptoms and epilepsy, though about twice a year he got a feeling that some event was very familiar. He was the manager of a small factory, and got on well; but at times he got depressed, and felt that he could not cope with the demands made on him, though nonetheless he did.

Minor degrees of repetitiveness and similar symptoms rather of the obsessional kind, are common in the organic sequelae; but in two cases (39, 63) obsessional routines dominated the picture. The former may be taken as an example.

Case 39

The patient was living at home with her mother and going out to work. She had two major fits last Christmas following a row at work, but none before that for a very long time. She was having occasional minor attacks without warning, in which she would go blank, slump, grind her teeth for a few seconds, and then be all right; these were occurring about once a month.

She was obsessed with a fear of cancer; she wouldn't look at an uncle, who recently had a heart attack, in case it was really cancer, and wouldn't touch a newspaper if it had the word cancer printed on it. She could not bear the thought of germs of any kind, and would scrub herself from head to foot with soaps and disinfectants if she thought she had touched any germs. When she went to the cinema she would put a big scarf tightly round her head, so that the smoke and other germs wouldn't affect her. When going to bed at night she had a number of long rituals. She would go through everything in her bag very thoroughly two or three times, then put it behind her pillow and pat it a number of times. In putting on her (four) hairnets she had another long ritual. Filling the kettle, she would fill it and empty it at least six times before being satisfied. This patient was also subject to irritability, but her paranoid symptoms had largely receded.

PSYCHO-ORGANIC SEQUELAE

Paranoid and schizophrenic-like symptoms continued to be a source of disability to 34 out of the total of 60 surviving patients; and organic symptoms and signs of personality change were present in 29. These two varieties of symptom were independent of one another, as is shown in Table 12.9. Thirteen patients are shown as being handicapped neither by paranoid-schizophrenic symptoms nor by organic symptoms; but this does not mean that they were normal. Four of these patients have a moderately severe disability from their epilepsy alone; three of them are liable to short depressive moods, which may well be based on an epileptic disorder

TABLE 12.9. SEQUELAE FOUND ON FOLLOW-UP

Organic personality changes	Paranoid and schizophrenic symptoms		
	Present	Absent	Total
Present	16	13	29
Absent	18	13	31
Total	34	26	60

of function; two patients are handicapped by obsessional rituals; one patient is a recurrent drinker, and usually goes into a paranoid-hallucinatory phase after a drinking bout. There are, in fact, only five patients who appear to have made a full social recovery. The first of these patients at the time of follow-up was living at home, doing a full office job; she was engaged and intending to get married soon. She was having about one major epileptic fit every six months, and also premenstrually two or three minor blackouts per day, preceded by a feeling of someone standing behind her, followed by an automatism of a few seconds duration. Paranoid symptoms had entirely receded; she was optimistic and happy, getting on well with everyone. The second and third cases (40, 49) have already been briefly described. In the fourth case the patient, an elderly woman, was living alone and looking after herself very well; her epileptic attacks were rare, one every few months or so. Paranoid ideas had entirely receded, and she now got on perfectly well with the neighbors who she used to believe persecuted her. In the last case, the patient was living at home and looked after her husband and son; she had had no fits in the preceding nine months at the time of the visit. Psychiatric symptoms had all passed off, and in the interview she was friendly, chatty, bright, very much to the point, and appeared to have an excellent relationship with her young boy.

The nature of the psycho-organic personality changes shown by these patients does not need to be described in detail, as the symptoms are the familiar accompaniments of long-standing epilepsy: perseverative tendencies, dullness and retardation, rambling conversation, difficulty in keeping to the point, pedantry, and circumstantiality; flatness of affect was marked in a few cases and religious preoccupations in others. The quality of irritability and aggressiveness was not uncommon, and was reported in 16 cases. A few patients were handicapped by impairment of memory. In general the organic symptoms were of the same kind as those noted at the time of ascertainment and examination, but now often more severe and socially damaging.

LOBECTOMY OPERATIONS

Eleven of these patients were submitted to a temporal lobectomy, and one patient had a right frontal lobectomy. Some of them have already been reported by Serafetinides and Falconer (1962), and the remainder have been described in the second paper of this series by Beard [summarised on p. 149]. Nevertheless it seems desirable to give a short account here of the follow-up results obtained at the time of the survey in 1960.

Four of these patients were then at home, without the need of any hospital care; and a further five patients spent substantially the whole of their time at home, with only occasional visits to hospital at times of exacerbation of illness. The remaining two patients were looked after almost entirely in hospital, with occasional visits home.

Five of these patients had had no epileptic fits for the past year or longer, and in all but one of the remainder the epilepsy was now no material handicap or problem; in only one patient was the epilepsy still a serious matter.

The schizophrenic symptoms had completely receded in only three of these patients, but in another five they had improved; in three patients they had not changed for the better. Indications of organic personality changes were present in six patients. Four patients had both schizophrenic and organic symptoms, two patients organic symptoms only, three patients schizophrenic symptoms only, two patients were free from both.

SUMMARY

A follow-up survey on these patients was carried out in mid-1960, at a mean interval of 7.8 years after the onset of the psychosis. The state of the patients had by no means stabilized then, as readmission to hospital with improvement and discharge was continuing to occur. Five of the patients could not be contacted; four patients had died, but data relating to them are included in part of this report.

1. Of the 64 patients followed up, 30 were living entirely at home, 16 mainly at home with periodic readmission to hospital, 9 mainly in hospital, and 9 entirely in hospital.

2. Social interests were mainly impaired, with 1 patient participating actively, 13 with moderate interest, the remainder needing encouragement or being without interest.

3. Personal relationships were at a better level, 9 patients having well preserved personalities, 24 being socially adequate, the remainder moderately or severely impaired.

4. Work records were surprisingly good; 25 patients were in full-time work, and 4 more were in part-time work, i.e., 45 per cent having some paid employment.

5. A short account is given of the 4 deaths.

6. The follow-up showed that the epilepsy had tended to get less troublesome with time; 10 patients (5 of them after lobectomy) had had no fits in the past year, and in a further 35 patients fits constituted no problem medically or socially.

7. Schizophrenic symptomatology was closely related to social capacity and freedom. One-third of the patients had had a remission of schizophrenic-like symptoms, and a further third had experienced improvement in this respect. A few of these patients, however, are known subsequently to have relapsed for a time. The evidence suggests that the schizophrenic-like symptoms, which have manifested at one stage in the life-history of the epilepsy, tend to settle down at a later stage.

8. Psycho-organic sequelae in the form of personality changes such as perseverativeness, dullness, retardation, circumstantiality, impairment of memory, etc., were present in 29 cases. Paranoid and schizophrenic-like symptoms constituted a source of disability in 34 cases. These two forms of after-effect appeared to be independent of one another.

9. A brief account is given of the follow-up histories obtained on the 11 patients who had had a temporal lobectomy and the one patient who had had a frontal lobectomy. It does not appear that the lobectomized patients had done any better than other patients not operated on, except in their reduced liability to fits.

10. The total impression gained from the follow-up study is that these patients have an illness which runs a stormy course towards an end-state of general impairment. This impairment is of an organic type, affecting both intellectual functions and affective aspects of the personality, and is of a kind commonly seen in late stages of chronic epilepsy.

V. Discussion and Conclusions[6]

The task now arises to indicate the significance which should be given to the findings described in earlier pages. There are three possible theories by which the combination of a schizophrenia-like psychosis with a pre-existing epilepsy might be accounted for. First the combination might be co-incidental, due purely to chance,

[6] By Eliot Slater and A. W. Beard.

in which case there would be no medical problem of any consequence. Secondly the occurrence of epileptic fits might tend to precipitate the psychosis in individuals genetically predisposed, who otherwise would have had better chances of escaping such a development. Thirdly the psychosis might be the direct consequence of the epilepsy, and therefore to be regarded as an epileptic and not a schizophrenic disorder in the aetiological sense. Fourthly it would be possible to suppose that in any given collection of cases representatives of more than one of these causal chains could be found. These theories may be discussed in turn.

EPILEPSY AND SCHIZOPHRENIA
AS A CHANCE COMBINATION

The proposition is advanced that the theory of chance combination is so improbable that it must be abandoned. This is on the following grounds:

On a basis of chance combination one would expect the appearance of three to five fresh cases of epileptics becoming schizophrenic per annum in a population of ten million. If the incidence of such cases had been no greater than that, it is hardly thinkable that the authors would have been able to collect 69 cases in the course of a few years.

The theory of chance combination leads one to expect to find in our material the indications of a predisposition to schizophrenia in the same proportion of cases and to the same degree as if our patients had been schizophrenics of the ordinary kind. One of the fields in which these indications would have been found would be the family history. Specifically, the hypothesis leads to an expectation of finding a total of about 17 secondary cases of schizophrenia among parents and sibs. What was actually found was 2 such cases, the figure to be expected if the patients had been a sample of the general population, or epileptics of the ordinary kind. On the other hand, the incidence of epilepsy in the parents and sibs of our patients was approximately the number which might be expected from a group of "symptomatic" epileptics.

Indications of a predisposition to schizophrenia should also have been found in the pre-psychotic personalities of our patients. We found no excess of "schizoid" traits of personality before the onset of the psychosis. No good account was usually available of what the personality had been like before the onset of epilepsy. After that time and before the onset of psychosis, the abnormal traits which were found in excess were those known to arise in epileptics as a long-term effect.

Finally, the theory of chance combination leads one to expect in a material of schizophrenic epileptics a fairly normal representation both of epileptic and schizophrenic disorders. This expectation is not borne out. Though both hebephrenic and catatonic states are seen in these patients, the clinical picture in the great majority of cases tends to conform to a fairly typical paraphrenic form. The epilepsy is also of a special type: the great majority of patients have been found to have a focal epilepsy, and three-quarters of all the patients had a temporal lobe focus.

EPILEPSY AS A PRECIPITATING FACTOR
FOR SCHIZOPHRENIA

We now turn to the second hypothesis, that we are observing genuinely schizophrenic psychoses, which have been facilitated by the pre-existing epilepsy.

On this basis we can predict a rather more frequent appearance of the combination of the two conditions than on the hypothesis of purely chance combination. Thus on one theoretical model (Slater, 82) it is estimated that about one in four of the individuals with adequate genetical equipment for schizophrenia actually develop the illness. Pre-existing epilepsy might increase the figure of one in four to one in one; and in that case we could expect in a population of ten million the annual appearance not of 3 to 5 schizophrenic epileptics but of 12 to 20. This still seems a very small incidence rate when put in conjunction with our 69 cases gathered over a few years in only two of the many hospitals which serve this region.

The hypothesis that a pre-existing epilepsy predisposes to the development of schizophrenia leads also to the expectation that one will find some indication of a relative abundance of schizoid traits in the pre-psychotic personalities of schizophrenic epileptics and some increase in the incidence of schizophrenia among their relatives. The finding that there is no shift at all towards a raised incidence of schizoid traits of personality, and no increase at all in the incidence of schizophrenia among first-degree relatives counts heavily against this hypothesis.

The hypothesis that a pre-existing epilepsy predisposes to the development of schizophrenia seems to be compatible with an unrepresentative and rather special group both of epileptic and schizophrenic disorders. Thus, on this hypothesis, it might be that a temporal lobe epilepsy was the one which specially favoured the development of schizophrenia, and that it was particularly a paraphrenic type of schizophrenia which was predisposed to. There is, however, nothing in the theory which would lead to such special features being hypothesized *a priori*; and when they are found, subsidiary hypotheses become necessary to explain them.

If the psychoses from which our patients suffered are to be regarded as schizophrenic in an aetiological and not merely descriptive sense, then they must be expected to conform to schizophrenic norms in their main features. While it is true that these patients have shown at times all of the cardinal features of schizophrenia, and indeed over two-thirds of them coming into the hands of independent psychiatrists had been diagnosed as suffering from schizophrenia, the psychoses observed deviate from schizophrenic norms in some interesting respects. During the psychosis itself, as has been emphasized by Pond, affective responsiveness tends to be preserved to an extent which is unusual in schizophrenia. The second principal difference from schizophrenia is in the later stages of development of the psychosis, which tends in the fullness of time to pass off, leaving a personality sometimes substantially undamaged, more often damaged by the personality changes we associate with organic disease of the brain and with long-standing epilepsy rather than with the post-schizophrenic state.

THE SCHIZOPHRENIA-LIKE ILLNESS
PURELY EPILEPTIC IN ORIGIN

If, then, we exclude both the hypothesis of chance coincidence and the hypothesis of a genuine schizophrenia merely predisposed to by epilepsy, we are reduced to the third of our hypotheses, i.e. that the schizophrenia-like psychosis is not, aetiologically regarded, schizophrenic at all, but an epileptic psychosis. This hypothesis also has to be examined on its merits, and the question must be asked whether there is evidence to be brought either for or against it.

All the evidence we have considered so far, i.e. the data bearing on the frequency of schizophrenia-like illnesses in epileptics, on the pre-psychotic personality of these patients, on the incidence of both schizophrenia and epilepsy in their first-degree relatives, on the predominance of paraphrenia-like psychotic pictures and of epilepsy of the temporal lobe focal variety, and even on the long-term follow-up results, all this evidence is compatible with the view that the psychoses observed are aetiologically different from ordinary forms of schizophrenia and constitute a special kind of epileptic psychosis. Some of these findings could have been predicted on the basis of that theory, e.g. that schizoid traits would not be found to any great extent in the pre-psychotic personality, and that schizophrenia would be no more frequent in first-degree relatives than in the general population; so that these particular findings can be regarded as supporting the theory. Other points, e.g. that temporal lobe foci should be so frequently found, could not easily have been predicted in advance, but once found seem to fall into a consistent picture of aetiological relationships. Their significance will be considered in due course.

An aetiological relationship could exist between the epilepsy and the psychosis in either of two ways. First, the epilepsy itself, i.e. the occurrence of epileptic fits, could be the adequate cause of the psychosis; secondly the basic disorder of function, which manifests itself in epileptic fits, could be the cause of the psychosis. In the first case we should expect the occurrence of a schizophrenia-like psychosis to be associated with special features of the epilepsy, with its long duration, its unusual severity or frequency of fits, with fits of a special clinical type, or occurring at special times such as during the night. Some of these expectations are fulfilled; others are not. These psychoses seem to arise in epileptics conforming to usual patterns in respect of frequency of fits, severity of epilepsy, amount of anticonvulsant drugs consumed, etc. But there is a relatively high correlation coefficient between the age of onset of epilepsy and age of onset of psychosis, with a mean interval of 14 years between the one and the other. Though there was no general tendency in this group of patients for the occurrence of nocturnal fits, such fits were found specially associated with a psychosis complicated by recurrent confusional episodes. The fits from which these patients suffered were also of a rather special type since, as temporal lobe fits, they involved a good deal of abnormal psychic experience. Twilight states with visionary experiences, for instance, were certainly much commoner in this group than in the general run of epileptics. On this basis, therefore, there is evidence to suggest that an aetiological relationship may exist between the epileptic fits as such and the psychosis.

If the psychosis and the epilepsy are related aetiologically in a less direct way, by the psychosis being a late product of a disorder of function of which the epilepsy is an earlier manifestation, then our expectations will be rather different. It is no longer surprising that there should be no relation between the psychosis and severity of epilepsy. The correlation between age of onset of epilepsy and age of onset of psychosis becomes an observation that could not have been predicted. Having been observed, it would suggest that underlying the epilepsy there was a process of some kind, with autonomous developmental tendencies, liable to produce fits at one stage and psychosis at a later one. But if the psychosis is caused by some factor underlying the epilepsy, then one would expect to find evidence of what that factor was. Here again we are rewarded. In the bulk of these patients there is evidence, convergent from a number of quarters, of a lesional basis for the epilepsy.

One such source of evidence was the past medical history of these patients, which showed a history of moderate or severe head injury in 11 cases. Commenting on this, Hill (1962), while accepting the lesional basis of the epilepsy, expressed doubts whether the history of head injury was significant. He remarked that head injury is a rare cause of temporal lobe epilepsy in the young, and that the lesions in our cases lie in the medial structures of the temporal lobe, which is not a site for injuries produced by head injury. This view may very well be correct.[7] Nevertheless, the history of definite head injuries in as many as 11 cases seems too important to be wholly disregarded. Closed head injuries are exceedingly common, and they are known to cause epilepsy in about 5 per cent of cases. In a large and recent study, Hillbom (1960) reported that 20 per cent of 2,047 patients with closed head injuries developed certain epilepsies, and a further 11 per cent developed uncertain epilepsies and attacks of undetermined nature. Hillbom made a representative selection of 415 patients for special study. Of these 56 had suffered only concussions and contusions, and of them 18, or over 30 per cent, became epileptic, though none of them with temporal lobe attacks. If we bear such facts in mind in conjunction with the belief of many authorities that the occurrence of epileptic attacks over years may cause a temporal lobe lesion and temporal lobe attacks, then the frequent history of head injury in our cases may not be finally dismissed as irrelevant.

The frequent occurrence of head injury in the past was only one of the anomalous features of the medical history; this also included histories of birth trauma, middle ear and mastoid disease, encephalitis, etc. The lesional basis of the epilepsy was also supported by all the evidence of focal origins, the existence of minimal neurological changes in one-fifth of the patients, the evidence of organic personality changes, the findings of air encephalography indicating atrophic processes in 37 out of the 54 patients tested, the pathological findings in those patients submitted to a lobectomy, and the follow-up results showing a tendency for the psychosis to settle down into an organic deficit syndrome.

Taking all the evidence we have been able to collect, we find that a great part of it is in conformity with an aetiological relationship between the epilepsy, or a pathological process causing epilepsy, and the psychosis; and that there is no evidence against this hypothesis. The evidence is however ambiguous in value and insufficient to let us decide on the nature of the relationship, whether the epileptic fits themselves tend to cause the psychosis, or whether the cause of the epilepsy tends to cause the psychosis. The latter seems on the whole to be the more probable view, but there could be some validity in both.

POSSIBILITIES OF HETEROGENEITY

There is finally the fourth hypothesis of heterogeneity. On this basis we would suppose that some of these psychoses were purely chance combinations of epilepsy and schizophrenia, some would be genuinely schizophrenic psychoses predisposed to by the epilepsy, some would be epileptic psychoses. This hypothesis is really a complex of hypotheses and so is undeserving of attention unless solid evidence can be brought for it. Is there any suggestion of heterogeneity in the material we have described?

The answer to this question is very largely in the negative. There are of course heterogeneities, but little suggestion that they are significant ones. Thus we find among the established pathological lesions both neoplastic and atrophic lesions; but these cases do not distinguish themselves from one another or from the rest of the

---

[7] There are differences of opinion. For instance Landolt (1960) regards the temporal lobes as particularly liable to damage, directly or by contrecoup, in closed head injuries and concussion. All parts, including the anterior poles, may be so affected. Relevant literature is quoted.

material in any other way. The best we can do in the way of demonstrating hetero-geneity is to draw attention to the differences between the three clinical groups A, B and C. It will be remembered that the A group was characterized by frequent occurrence of confusional episodes before the onset of the schizophrenia-like psychosis proper; the B group consisted of patients with predominantly paranoid and paraphrenia-like syndromes; the C group consisted of patients all of whom had hebephrenia-like illnesses. This method of classification naturally brought with it symptomatic differences. Thus the mode of onset was mainly episodic in group A and insidious in the other groups; and the incidence of such symptoms as schizo-phrenic thought disorder and flattening of affect was disproportionately heavy in the C group. Other differences between the groups, not directly caused by the mode of selection, were not very striking. Only one of the patients in group C had a history suggestive of brain trauma, and in this respect the difference between C and the other groups was highly significant. The age of onset of epilepsy was also significantly earlier in group C than in the other groups, at 9 years on average as against 20 and 16. Finally, nocturnal epilepsy was particularly common in group A.

In his discussion of our material, Hill observed that the cases now included in group C might well be different aetiologically and symptomatologically from the rest, and he suspected that the fortuitous combination of schizophrenia and epilepsy would be found, if at all, in this group. Unfortunately, the group is not large enough to provide evidence whether this is so or not. Thus an examination of the family histories, as suggested by Hill, does not show any difference between the relatives of patients in this group and the relatives of the patients in the other groups, either in incidence of schizophrenia or epilepsy; numbers are too small for an adequate mate-rial to be available. All we can say is that, while it is far from unlikely that there are one or two genuine schizophrenics in our total material, it is very improbable that there are more than a handful. It would seem to be a practical impossibility to distinguish them individually from the others.

THE PATHOGENESIS OF THE SCHIZOPHRENIA-LIKE PSYCHOSIS

We now have to consider whether we can formulate any meaningful and testable conception of the pathogenesis of these states on an epileptic basis, and whether we can suggest any reason for their close similarity to schizophrenic states caused other-wise. These are two distinct questions, both of great importance.

Let us take the first of these problems. There are three outstanding clinical findings, which may be arranged in an order of reliability and significance. First is the focal origin, usually in the temporal lobes. This origin was demonstrated elec-trically in about three-quarters of the cases; but in the cases in which it was not demonstrated it seems very likely that temporal lobe functions, or limbic lobe functions, were disturbed. This may quite possibly have been the case with origins of fits shown in frontal or central subcortical regions. Thus in two cases, in which the EEG diagnosis was not one of temporal lobe epilepsy, tests of vestibular function showed an abnormality. The limbic lobe system is closely connected with the emo-tional life of the individual, and when it is disturbed he is liable in a state of clear consciousness to experience affects not connected with external reality, of a com-pelling and disquieting kind: *déjà vu*, depersonalization, fear, etc. There is also a liability to abnormal perceptual experiences, derealization, hallucination, etc., also occurring without detectable clouding of consciousness. Symonds (1962) rightly emphasized that there is hardly one of the most characteristic symptoms of schizo-

167

phrenia, of a positive kind, which may not be experienced as an aural phenomenon in temporal lobe epilepsy. Such aural symptoms occurred in a large majority of our patients, and in a number of them were explained by the patient in a delusional way; the aural symptom in fact had entered into the content of the delusional psychosis. Furthermore, a whole group of our patients, group A, had recurrent confusional episodes, and some patients in groups B and C had occasional episodes of this kind. Many of these episodes could properly be called twilight states, since consciousness is dreamlike rather than obscured, and it is possible for the dream material to be retained into recollection the next day with great completeness. Those patients who had religious or mystical experiences of this kind were convinced of their reality and validity, and only regained partial insight years later. Thus one patient (49), who had had no fit and no mystical experience for four years, still felt that his religious revelations had been veridical and regretted that he had had no more. Another, who had heard God say "There is no such thing as Nothing" (a rebuttal of existentialist philosophy!), felt that since then he had been given an understanding of why things exist.

There is accordingly much to be said for the point of view advanced by Pond (1962), that there is a causal relationship of a psychological kind between fits and psychosis. Pond suggests that "years of attacks of clouded consciousness might lead to a confusion of reality and autistic thinking and experience". The paranoid hallucinatory psychoses which are not uncommon in alcoholics and narcoleptics could be accounted for in this way. These conditions, he says, seem to have in common only disturbances of consciousness which are partial and not of the total kind seen in petit mal.

In its essence, this theory regards the epileptic schizophrenia-like psychosis as depending in the first place on abnormal emotional experiences physically caused, which are then integrated into the totality of psychic life as a psychodynamic process. For the development of a complex and lasting paranoid psychosis out of primitive single abnormal experiences a number of other conditions would probably be necessary. Thus the experience itself should have a strong reality value, so that at the time it occurs the patient does not easily recognize it as hallucinatory, but puts it down to a real event. It should have a strong affect accompanying it, so that it impresses the mind, and once remembered is not easily forgotten. It should occur in such a state of consciousness that it is not subsequently obliterated by an amnesic gap. It should not be easily dismissed by the patient as of trivial importance, nor seen through on reflection by subsequent use of powers of insight. It must be admitted that the aural symptoms of a temporal lobe epilepsy do tend to fulfil each and all of these conditions, whereas, for instance, the visual hallucinations accompanying a lesion of the visuosensory area do not.

On the other hand, while this theory provides a plausible explanation of the paranoid symptomatology, it seems powerless to explain such other symptoms as volitional disturbances, thought disorder and hebephrenic symptoms. Moreover it was not all of our patients who had aural symptoms or twilight states of a kind which might in time convert the mind to a totally distorted picture of the real world. A more comprehensive mode of explanation is offered by Symonds (1962). Discussing our material, this author wrote:

> "If then neither the fits nor the temporal lobe damage can be held directly responsible for the psychosis, what is the link? It may be the epileptogenic disorder of function. . . . Epileptic seizures and epileptiform discharge in the EEG are epiphenomena. They may be regarded as

occasional expressions of a fundamental and continuous disorder of neuronal function. The essence of this disorder is loss of the normal balance between excitation and inhibition at synaptic junctions. From moment to moment there may be excess either of excitation or inhibition — or even of both at the same time in different parts of the same neuronal system. . . . The EEG, though it only skims the surface, often records activity of one kind or another in the absence of seizures. The observation that epileptiform EEGs may be observed in 25 per cent of schizophrenics is not without interest in this connection. What I have called the epileptogenic disorder of function may be assumed to be present continuously but with peaks at which seizures are likely to occur. This background disorder may cause symptoms other than seizures. The presence and nature of such interictal symptoms as do occur are related to the epileptogenic focus. From this focus the synaptic disorder tends to spread along lines that are functionally determined. Thus particular systems of neurons become involved so that the disorder of function may be highly selective. [The schizophrenic-like aural symptoms of temporal lobe epilepsy suggest that] the temporal lobe includes within its boundaries circuits concerned with the physiological basis of the psychological disorder which we call schizophrenia . . it is not loss of neurons in the temporal lobe that is responsible for the psychosis, but the disorderly activity of those that remain, and this disorderly activity is of the kind that is also likely to cause seizures."

So much may be said in connection with the predominantly temporal lobe origin of the fits in our patients. The second striking finding which emerges from the clinical analysis is the correlation between age of onset of epilepsy and age of onset of psychosis. This evidence that the duration of the epilepsy in itself plays a caus ative part in bringing on the psychosis is reconcilable with Pond's psychodynamic concept, but does not seem to be suggested by Symond's physiogenic hypothesis. Once there is an epileptogenic disorder of function involving temporal lobe circuits, with abnormalities occurring interictally as well as ictally, one might expect psychotic symptoms to appear at any time. It is true that in a few of our patients the psychosis did come on very quickly after the first epileptic fits. However, the evidence seems too strong to resist the conclusion that the chronic paranoid psychosis is a phenomenon which is specially likely to occur at a particular stage during the lifetime of the epilepsy, a stage in fact at which organic damage has been done.

This brings in the third of our clinical findings of central importance, the evidence of actual destruction of nerve tissue, as shown by the AEGs and by pathological examination in cases in which a lobectomy has been carried out. The AEG was done in 56 cases; in 17 the pictures were passed as normal; in 37 cases there was evidence of brain atrophy, and in 2 cases evidence of events of another kind. This evidence of a destructive lesion is paralleled and supported by clinical evidence of a dementing process. Even at the time when these patients first came under investigation four-fifths of them showed the psychiatric indications of organic personality change. As the disease continued these indications continued to multiply; and at the time of the follow-up, just about half the patients contacted were socially handicapped by organic deficits.

It would seem to the authors that, if the illuminating hypothesis proposed by Symonds is accepted, it would need some modification. He comments that temporal lobe damage by itself is unlikely to cause a schizophrenia-like psychosis. It may be then that in the atrophic processes that we have found, it is not the cells that have died that are causing trouble but those that are dying. This suggestion falls in both with a late onset of psychosis, and with the tendency of the psychosis in the fullness of time to pass off into an organic deficit.

Our final conclusion then must be a somewhat inconclusive one. Both the modes of explanation suggested by Pond and by Symonds have evidence in their favour and seem likely to account for at least a part of the observations. Our own tendency is to think the physiogenic causation of the psychosis the more important factor, and to regard it as predisposed to by a certain stage in what is in the long run a dementing process.

SIGNIFICANCE OF THE ILLNESS AS A SYMPTOMATIC SCHIZOPHRENIA

While the occurrence and the nature of these psychoses certainly raise issues important for the study of epilepsy, their import appears even greater when the pathogenesis of schizophrenia comes to be considered. The evidence shows that these psychoses are schizophrenic in form but not in aetiology. They are not endogenous but symptomatic. Their pathological basis is not entirely unknown but partly known. They occur in individuals lacking any special predisposition to endogenous schizophrenia, and the manifestation observed can be regarded as a phenocopy of a genetically determined condition.

Psychoses resembling schizophrenia have, of course, been repeatedly observed in the presence of gross pathological processes affecting the brain, such as neoplasm and syphilis, but also in isolated cases for which so far no rhyme or reason has been found.[8] They have also been seen with chemical alterations such as amphetamine intoxication, and in this connection in a systematic way, as has been reported by Connell (1958). In this case, too, it was predominantly a paranoid form of schizophrenia which was mimicked by the organic psychosis. Features in which the amphetamine psychosis tended to differ from endogenous schizophrenia were the rapidity of onset, the dream-like quality of the experiences, the tendency towards visual hallucination, the brisk emotional reaction with emphasis on fear, and the rapid recovery on withdrawal of the drug. The resemblances to the epileptic psychosis we have discussed will not be missed. In this case it was hardly possible to argue, as had been argued with the psychoses accompanying gross brain lesions, that the illness was not only schizophrenia-like but actually schizophrenic, accompanying the other pathological events as a pure coincidence. But one might still argue, in the case of the amphetamine psychosis, that the peculiarities of an easily reversible toxic state lasting only a few days or weeks provided no useful model for the enduring changes that occur in schizophrenia. When we come to consider the schizophrenia-like psychoses of epilepsy, even this last argument cannot be applied. We are at last forced to consider what lessons we can learn from the symptomatic schizophrenias which will help towards a better understanding of the central group of schizophrenic cases, which we may call nuclear, endogenous or idiopathic.

One might take the view that with schizophrenia we are now approaching the stage of understanding which was reached half a century ago with epilepsy. It was customary then to classify the epilepsies into idiopathic and symptomatic types, and in the latter case to specify the underlying condition of which the epilepsy was symptomatic. This rather primitive stage in sub-classification may now have become possible in the syndrome we call schizophrenia. Very likely the bulk of the cases so

---

[8] Of particular interest in connection with our case material are the schizophrenia-like manifestations of Huntington's chorea. According to Panse (1942) "schizophrenia" is by far the commonest mis-diagnosis, and the schizophrenic picture may be maintained for years. In the monograph he devotes 30 pages to the description and discussion of these cases. The schizophrenia-like state is most commonly of the chronic paranoid-hallucinatory type, but catatonic and hebephrenic pictures are also seen.

diagnosed will prove to be "idiopathic", with genetical factors responsible for the specificities. But round this nucleus we would aim to define with increasing precision groups of cases in which the schizophrenia-like psychosis was traceable to known processes. A study of the mechanisms by which physical lesions and functional disturbances caused such symptomatic psychoses to appear, would then become a tool in the investigation of the main problem.

A little earlier we asked the question whether any reason could be suggested for the close similarity between the epileptic psychoses we have described and schizophrenic psychoses otherwise caused. The reason which immediately suggests itself is that the nuclear schizophrenias are themselves organic psychoses, affecting the same functional systems of the brain, or ones closely integrated with them. It would not be the place here to go into the evidence on this problem, which is constantly being added to. Nevertheless brief reference may be made to the work of Huber (1961), showing in a well-controlled material of 212 cases of chronic schizophrenia, atrophic brain changes leading to enlargement of the ventricles, especially the third ventricle. Huber found a close parallelism between the degree of the pathological change shown radiographically and the nature and severity of the psychopathological findings.

As a working programme we have to use the principle that like effects are commonly due to similar causes. It is as a mock-up of the genuine schizophrenic that the schizophrenic-like epileptic is worth special study.

Acknowledgments

The authors owe a debt of gratitude not easily expressed to Professor Denis Hill and Dr. Desmond Pond of the Department of Clinical Neurophysiology at the Maudsley Hospital and to Mr. Murray Falconer of the Guy's-Maudsley Neurosurgical Unit. Professor Hill not only made available for study more than half the patients in the series, but also discussed problems of particular patients and of the series as a whole. Medical notes and records of all kinds have been made available by these three colleagues, who have not stinted of their help at all stages.

We are also most grateful to all the Physicians of the National Hospital who have so kindly referred cases of interest, to Mr. Wylie McKissock, and to the colleagues in the Departments of Electrophysiology, Radiology and Otoneurology, Dr. William Cobb, Dr. Hugh Davies, Dr. James Bull, Dr. Hallpike and Mr. Cawthorne, on whose work we so largely rely.

We also wish to thank Miss H. Shand for the endless work of typing and retyping.

Finally, we have to thank the Mental Health Research Fund who supported this work by the award to A.W.B. of a Senior Fellowship over the whole period of the survey, and thereby made the investigation possible.

13

PSYCHOGENIC SCHIZOPHRENIA?

In 1916 August Wimmer, then the Professor of Psychiatry in the University of Copenhagen, published a monograph on the psychogenic psychoses. These he defined as a group of psychoses, independent of other accepted groups, caused by psychic trauma in individuals with a psychopathic predisposition. The psychic traumata were responsible for the appearance of the illness, its clinical "movements," its content, and very often its termination; the prognosis was regarded as favourable, never resulting in deterioration of the personality. Wimmer's monograph did not include any follow-up study. It was as a result of a suggestion by Erik Strömgren that Dr. Faergeman undertook a follow-up study of 170 patients diagnosed as suffering from psychogenic psychoses by Wimmer and his staff during the years 1924-26. He succeeded in tracing practically all of them, though this was after an interval of 15-20 years, and in personally examining 98; 53 of the patients had died. Only 10 cases had to be excluded, in the end, because it was thought the amount of follow-up information was insufficient.

The great value of Dr. Faergeman's monograph consists in the long-term follow-up information which it provides. The reviewer did not find either the introductory chapters or the discussion which follows the analysis of the results helpful in settling any of the difficult questions which are raised for consideration. Dr. Faergeman is not only an obviously exceedingly competent clinical psychiatrist; he is also a practising psychoanalyst. The trouble is that the two disciplines mix no better than spring-water and train-oil. The illuminations provided by a discussion along psychoanalytic lines are of value only within the psychoanalytic universe of discourse, and leave the non-analyst just where he was. The factual evidence supplied is, however,

Originally published as a review of *Psychogenic Psychoses: a Description and Follow-up of Psychoses Following Psychological Stress* by P. M. Faergeman (London: Butterworth, 1963) and *Die Schizophrenieähnlichen Emotionspsychosen* by F. Labhardt (Berlin: Springer-Verlag, 1963), in the *British Journal of Psychiatry* 110: 114–18 (1964).

of the greatest importance. Case summaries of all 170 patients, together with the follow-up data, are there for the reader to study.

The first point that emerges is the clinical heterogeneity of these psychoses. Dr. Faergeman classifies the clinical pictures into three main classes: (1) emotional syndromes, with sub-types of depression and exaltation; (2) disturbances of consciousness, with four sub-types, dissociations, deliria, hallucinoses and stupors; (3) paranoid syndromes, with two sub-types, with and without hallucination. As a result of the follow-up information, the cases were also classified into three groups, the verified psychogenic psychoses and probable psychogenic psychoses, the non-psychogenic psychoses, and the uncertain cases. Of the 160 cases with adequate follow-up information, just less than half, 79, could be regarded as definitely or probably correctly diagnosed; one-third of the patients, 56, were regarded as non-psychogenic; in approximately one-sixth of the cases the diagnosis remained uncertain. The biggest stumbling block to correct diagnosis by Wimmer and his colleagues was schizophrenia; in 43 of the 56 mis-diagnosed cases the illness proved in course of time to be schizophrenic. Faergeman diagnoses manic-depressive illness in 8 cases, and an epileptic or ixophrenic psychosis in 3; two patients had passed through Wimmer's clinic with undiagnosed general paresis.

Errors of diagnosis were much commoner with some clinical pictures than others. Rather more than half of the depressive psychoses were verified, less than half of the elations. Dissociations of consciousness were confirmed as psychogenic in 26 out of 29 cases; but with the deliria, hallucinoses and stupors, the diagnosis of a psychogenic state could be verified in only 22 out of 59. Worst of all were the paranoid syndromes, with less than a quarter (8 out of 34) of the cases correctly diagnosed.

The second point which emerges is, therefore, that the diagnosis of psychogenic psychosis proved a snare and delusion in slightly more than half the cases. On occasion, this must have led to clinical neglect; one of the two patients suffering from general paresis, for instance, was allowed to go home to his relatives untreated. However, the success rate for the psychogenic diagnosis, the reviewer believes, is even so presented in an unduly rosy light. When one reads through these clinical summaries, it is surprising how often the case could be regarded in an entirely different light. Dr. Faergeman does not seem to have paid adequate attention to the possibility of an acute organic illness, or to the critical significance of organic factors in facilitating extreme emotional reactions. The reviewer would regard such factors as having played an important aetiological role in 16 cases (Nos. 6, 21, 23, 50, 55, 69, 70, 73, 75, 82, 85, 86, 89, 128, 130, 131). In a further 5 cases (26, 43, 88, 90, 91) an endogenous psychosis is not to be excluded. And it is noteworthy that in 9 cases (5, 8, 16, 42, 54, 83, 84, 149, 151) there is no reported evidence of psychogenic trauma. Such considerations suggest that the more that was known about these cases the more complex they would be found to be. Writing them off as psychogenic does not do justice to the multidimensionality of the factors that have gone to their causation.

The third point of importance which emerges is that these psychoses, even in the Wimmer clinic where the diagnosis was a favoured one, are rare ones. Dr. Faergeman calculates that "verified and hospitalized psychogenic psychoses have amounted to 2.0 per cent of the total number of first admissions (1.4 per cent men, 2.6 per cent women)." The question arises, then, whether the diagnosis is admissible at all. It would seem that it applies to only a sprinkling of cases, that in making it one is as likely as not to be missing a schizophrenic or other major psychotic state, that it corresponds to no unitary clinical picture. Was Wimmer, one may wonder, doing more than apply the label "psychogenic" where the fancy took him, to an almost randomly selected series of patients?

This is to look at the matter from a severely practical point of view, that of the clinician who is faced with a difficult case. The theoretical standpoint is a different one. From this point of view we must ask what are the verified cases, and are they shown to constitute a single homogeneous group when judged by any criteria? Here again it would seem that the answer is in the negative. A considerable number of the reactive depressions and a large majority of the fugue states, amnesias, and other dissociations would be accepted by psychiatrists of any school as "psychogenic." But in these two classes of patients, personality background, treatment, and outlook are so different that it seems unwise to put them into the same diagnostic grouping. The really controversial questions are whether psychogenesis, alone or on the basis of a predisposed personality, can cause on the one hand a delirious state such as is normally seen with a toxic-infective condition, or on the other hand cause a paranoid-hallucinatory state such as is normally seen with schizophrenia. The interesting conclusion emerges that probably events of both such kinds can occur. The best example of a psychogenic delirium is in case 78, with 79–81 as also moderately convincing. The best examples of psychogenic schizophrenia-like psychoses are given, not by Dr. Faergeman, but by Dr. Labhardt; but Dr. Faergeman has some case material of interest. Among the hallucinoses, cases 117–119 present a striking picture, but one that must have had an unmistakable hysterical stamp to the onlooker; in the paranoid illnesses cases 137–140 come in question, but seem to be manifestations of markedly paranoid personalities, without that step-like change which many clinicians demand for the concept of "psychosis."

The laurels which crown Dr. Faergeman's work are earned by the long-term and extremely successful follow-up. When we come to Dr. Labhardt's case material we find other features to excite our interest. The author investigated 61 patients who had been diagnosed as suffering from schizophrenia-like psychogenic psychoses in the psychiatric clinic of the University of Basle (Professor Staehelin) between 1938 and 1958. Staehelin has defined the *Emotionspsychose* as a psychotic reaction, determined by affective breakdown, with schizophrenic symptomatology, rapid course, and exceptionally accessible to treatment. Of the 61 cases investigated, only 8 proved in course of time to have been suffering from a truly schizophrenic illness all along; but it is not certain that a higher rate of misdiagnosis might not have been established if conditions had been favourable for follow-up. In 24 of the 53 nonschizophrenic cases the after-history is unknown; and only 7 of the patients were followed up for as long as three or more years.

If there is a deficiency on this side, the reader is rewarded with full and vivid accounts of acute psychotic states of the greatest interest, which in the main justify their title of schizophrenia-like; the personalities of these patients and the traumatic events which precipitated the psychoses are also described in a satisfying way. The reviewer's greatest regret is that it was not thought necessary to give an account of every one of the 61 cases investigated; more space given to the patients, even at the expense of some of the more laborious parts of the discussion, would have repaid itself. In those cases which are described, the account is sufficiently full to be convincing more often than not. However, some cases (e.g., 17, 22, 23) do not seem particularly schizophrenia-like; and in others the psychogenic factor appears to have been overstressed. The reviewer, for instance, does not think it warranted to include among psychogenic psychoses case 21, that of a woman dying of carcinomatosis.

A number of points of general interest emerge. First is the relative rarity of the syndrome which, however, as Dr. Labhardt believes, is increasing in frequency. From 1940–50 there was an average of about one case a year in the admissions to Professor Staehelin's clinic; from 1950–56 about 3 a year, and in the three years 1956–58 about 7 a year. Professor Staehelin thinks that this is due to the increasing stressfulness of our age; it seems more likely that it is due to a greater readiness to make the diagnosis in his clinic. One of the points one misses in this account is a discussion of errors of diagnosis to which psychiatrists are liable, in both directions.

The sex ratio of the patients shows a moderate excess of women (male 20; female 33). The age distribution is interesting in showing the heaviest incidence between 20 and 29, and 70 per cent of all cases between 20 and 39. Only two of the patients were less than 20 years old, contrasting with the schizophrenic expectation which, for Switzerland according to M. Bleuler, would have meant about 10 of the 53 patients being in this age group. Unfortunately a genetical investigation was not carried out; but from the data given about family histories it is clear that a schizophrenic family background was infrequent, certainly much less frequent than in schizophrenia, though probably more frequent than in the general population. The most typical bodily build was leptosome, the most typical pre-psychotic personality was sensitive, anxious, overconscientious.

The traumata under which these patients broke down were various in nature, but drastic and immediate at the reality level. Even a stable personality, in situations of such strain, might be expected to become disturbed. The accounts of psychogenesis supplied are very convincing, though it is not apparent, as is claimed by the author, that the nature of the stress is mirrored in the content of the psychosis. Labhardt classifies these traumatic situations, which usually came to a crisis before the onset of the psychosis, under a number of heads: marital tensions, erotic and sexual traumata, religious conflicts, fear of failure, uprooting and isolation, guilt feelings, existential threats, treatment by psychoanalysis. Dr. Labhardt also discusses at length the physical factors which so commonly entered the picture. In 9 cases there were serious illnesses, nephritis, lung embolism, carcinomatosis, tonsillitis, puerperal mastitis, influenza, etc.; and in a further 4 cases the psychosis came on after surgical operation; in yet a further 5 cases physical factors entered in less easily identifiable form. Perhaps even more striking than these unmistakably abnormal conditions was the regularity of some state of emotional exhaustion, possibly including nutritional or electrolyte disturbance, preceding the collapse. It is observations of these kinds that lead Dr. Labhardt, and Professor Staehelin with him, to think of disturbance of diencephalic and mesencephalic functions as playing a part in the pathogenesis. This suggestion fits in well with what we know of schizophrenia-like psychotic states arising in connection with organic causes.

Dr. Labhardt makes out a strong case for regarding these cases as constituting a homogeneous group for the delineation of a syndrome. The onset was invariably acute, in close temporal connection with a major psychic trauma, though there might have been a prodromal state of mounting difficulties and tensions. The symptomatology was schizophrenia-like during the acute stage, though not quite typically so. There was invariably good preservation of affect, and not only a retained capacity for affective rapport with the doctor but generally a rapidly formed emotional dependence on him. The "schizophrenic atmosphere" was totally lacking. The picture was dominated by anxiety, auditory hallucinations and delusional ideas; each of these three main symptoms was present in more than half the cases. More specifically schizophrenic were the symptoms, also shown by a majority, of formal thought disorder and catatonic symptoms. The symptoms were of an extremely florid kind — ideas of impending death or world cataclysm were observed in about one third of the patients. In many ways the condition seems to resemble very closely a delirious reaction, lacking the impairment of consciousness without which most psychiatrists will not allow the diagnosis of an organic-toxic-confusional state. It is noteworthy that 14 of these 53 patients showed some clouding of consciousness at some stage.

The course of the illness is remarkable for its extreme brevity, and in this respect is unlike that of a schizophrenic psychosis. The psychotic state cleared up in 59 per cent of cases in less than two weeks, and in two to four weeks in a further 32 per cent. In less than 10 per cent was there a longer duration than four weeks, but unfortunately we are not told what was the extreme range. All these patients were treated very actively; but, though the response to treatment was highly satisfactory, it is still thought that the psychosis has a spontaneous tendency to clear rapidly. On the physical side, which is rated as very important, the treatment consisted in effective doses of tranquillizers, especially chlorpromazine, combined with a course of modified insulin treatment. No less important is the psychotherapy, to which these patients are extremely accessible. Relapse in subsequent years, so far as observed, is not the rule, but was seen in 13 of the 29 patients for whom follow-up data were available. Subsequent relapse was likely to take the form of a psychogenic illness, though, it seems, not always one of the schizophreniform kind.

A crucial point of enquiry is the possibility of distinguishing these cases from hyperacute schizophrenias. Dr. Labhardt draws up a long list of differential criteria of a quantitative kind. As already noted, with this syndrome, in distinction to genuine schizophrenia, there is much less in the way of schizophrenic illnesses in the family history. Body build is less frequently asthenic-leptosome, though still tending in that direction. Personality is never outspokenly schizoid, and tends mainly to the sensitive-anxious type. The course is of short duration, and response to treatment much more immediate than with schizophrenia. A schizophrenia-like affective psychosis is, presumably, not diagnosed in the Basle clinic without precipitating psychogenic cause of a striking kind. Such psychic traumata are also found in the cases of true schizophrenics, with probable precipitating effect in about 20 per cent of cases (as appears from Dr. Labhardt's control material): the nature of the psychogenic factors found does not differ in the two syndromes. The final conclusion emerges that, at least at some times, the differential diagnosis may be impossible; as a rule it can only be made on the basis of family history, personality type and pre-psychotic personal history.

There are other syndromes from which the differential diagnosis may be difficult. Labhardt discusses in this connection the paranoid and catatoniform reactions, neuroses and hysterical reactions, acute organic-toxic psychoses, involutional psychoses, puerperal psychoses, acute epileptic psychoses. From the theoretical point of view, the differentiation from organic states is the most interesting. Organic aetiological factors were prominent in a number of cases, as has already been noted; perhaps very thorough routine investigation of all cases might have come up with still more information of this kind.

The mysterious nature of the pathogenic mechanisms involved in these cases remains unsolved. The contribution made by psychogenesis seems to be non-specific in nature. This is not the view taken by Labhardt. In his general summary, he characterizes the psychic trauma as an obligatory one which touches the inner life of the personality, potentially threatening its existence, giving cause to ambivalence, and thereby inducing an internal tension between affects. The only feature mentioned which would be of practical service in distinguishing between one psychic trauma and another, is that of ambivalence. But how often is such an ambivalence actually demonstrated in Labhardt's cases?

Taking them in the order in which they are quoted, we have the following: Case 1, financial and family worries (illness of wife); Case 2, a young peasant called up for military service, far from home; Case 3, a 30-year-old woman feels neglected by her husband and becomes frigid, leading to increase of strain; Case 4, a woman, treated with extreme coldness and rejection by her husband, works to the point of exhaustion; Case 5, a tyrannical husband becomes paranoid when his wife takes a job, but it is he rather than his wife who suddenly becomes psychotic. It is unnecessary to pursue the case analysis. The attitudes of these patients may or may not have been ambivalent, and ambivalence is practically impossible to prove either one way or the other. It does not seem likely that there are any important differences between the psychic traumata which precipitate a schizophrenia-like affective psychosis and those which precipitate acute panic reactions, hysterical conversion states and reactive depressions; and Labhardt records no difference from those associated with schizophrenia.

It seems to the reviewer more likely that the specific qualities of these psychoses, as described by Labhardt, which distinguish them from acute neurotic reactions, are derived from physical factors, probably of a chemical kind. The author himself is sympathetic to this view. He notes that mental strains can lead to exhaustion states, which facilitate the psychosis; and he points out that vegetative symptoms and not infrequent clouding of consciousness suggest an irritative state of meso-diencephalic structures. Pathogenetically, he regards the psychosis as an end-product of a vicious circle in which affective and physical (vegetative) stimulation have mutually interacted to produce a state of excitation of the vegetative centres of the midbrain and diencephalon.

14

DISTINGUISHING THE EFFECTS
OF HEREDITY AND ENVIRONMENT

Many readers must have put down Hans Kind's (1966) review of the literature and judicial appreciation of the present state of our knowledge with a feeling of some disappointment. His most general conclusion is that a purely psychogenic theory of schizophrenia is as untenable as a purely genetical one, and that we should abandon this "one-sided and barren either-or." However, even this modest conclusion would not be universally accepted. To be sure, there is no one at all working on the genetical aspects of schizophrenia who would not agree to it. We all believe that genetical factors play only a part in causation, and that environmental and even psychogenic factors must be allowed for as well. We all earnestly hope that our colleagues, who are working on the environmental side, will soon come up with solid evidence we can get our teeth into. But there is a considerable body of psychiatrists who are unwilling to admit that genetical factors play any part at all in causation, and who therefore will take a great deal of convincing that Hans Kind's conclusion is correct.

While I personally accept this view, I do not think that it follows that we should in future abandon investigations conducted along specifically genetical or environmental lines; that we should focus our view on the field of interaction between heredity and environment; and that we should "in future turn to a deeper and many-sided study of single cases, whole families, or groups of patients of like kind." Biological research, e.g., in agriculture, abounds in techniques by which the effects of heredity and environment may be distinguished and measured against one another. In studying mankind we cannot set up neatly balanced experiments of our own, but there is nothing to prevent us from examining exhaustively the experiments which nature conducts on our behalf.

Originally published as a discussion of "The Psychogenesis of Schizophrenia: a Review of the Literature" by Hans Kind in the *International Journal of Psychiatry* 3: 416–17 (1967). Dr. Kind's paper originally appeared in the *British Journal of Psychiatry* 112: 333–49 (1966).

An example of such a natural experiment is Heston's (1966) report on the children of schizophrenic mothers, separated from their mothers within three days of birth and thereafter having no contact with them or with maternal relatives. By dint of very careful follow-up work, 47 such children, together with 50 control subjects from the same foundling homes, were followed into adult life. Five of the children of schizophrenic mothers became schizophrenic, none of the children in the control group. The author concludes that "the results of this study support a genetic etiology of schizophrenia"; but of course he says nothing about their rebutting an environmental etiology, which they do not do.

It seems to me that Kind is himself to some extent the victim of the very confusion in thinking which his conclusions are aimed to counter. In order to give adequate emphasis to the positive conclusions of psychogenic research, he seems to think it necessary to play down the positive conclusions drawn from genetical research. Thus the high concordance rates with respect to schizophrenia found in monozygotic twins by earlier workers are thought to be negated by the findings of Tienari who reported zero concordance. But one Finn does not make a winter. Since Tienari's work was published we have had the later reports of Kringlen (1966) and of Gottesman and Shields (1966b), in which precautionary measures were taken to avoid the biases which might have affected the results of Kallmann and of Slater, but which in large part confirm them. It is impossible to collect any clinical sample without some possible selective bias, and there are reasons for thinking that Tienari's results may have been so affected, e.g., by the circumstance that he collected living pairs only. If one examines, not Tienari's diagnoses made for statistical purposes, but the case histories he provides, one finds that his results also fall into a general picture which holds good for all twin series. This picture provides very stong support for the hypothesis of a genetical contribution to etiology, but it also leaves abundant room for environmental determinants.

Kind says that all attempts so far to equate the genetical predisposition with a particular mode of inheritance must be regarded as having failed; and on that account a specific genetic factor appears unlikely. This misstates the premise and leads accordingly to a false conclusion. The data at present available can readily be reconciled with more than one genetical hypothesis. It is extremely probable that one or another of them will in time be proved true, but at present we lack the evidence on which we can distinguish which one this will be. We can say that many theories are in the running; two are in the lead; none has yet passed the winning post, but none can yet be written off as having failed, or as worse placed than being an unlikely winner.

This situation is paralleled on the environmental side. We are beginning to get a picture in which we see that certain environmental causes (e.g., amphetamine intoxication, temporal lobe epilepsy, pre-senile regressive brain changes) appear to facilitate the appearance of schizophrenic syndromes. The specificity of some of these factors is already beginning to suggest speculations about the pathogenic mechanisms. On the psychogenic side we hope that research workers will turn up other specificities which will help to narrow the field of enquiry.

IV

NEUROSIS AND PSYCHOPATHY

EDITORS' COMMENTS: Of the seven papers appearing in this Part, four date from the war-time years when Slater was clinical director of Sutton Emergency Hospital, now Belmont Hospital. The influx of casualties from Dunkirk led to his work with Sargant on the acute war neuroses and on physical methods of treatment (17, 19, 20, 21, 29), one of which heads this section as Paper 15. Dr. Sargant has been Physician in Charge, Department of Psychological Medicine, St. Thomas's Hospital, London, for many years now.

Much of the work reported from Sutton was based on the analysis of information systematically collected on admission by clerk, social worker, or physician. In his "Demographic Study of a Psychopathic Population" (25) Slater reported data on birth order, sex distribution, and the phenomenon of twinning in the families of 1,000 neurotic patients. Of greater psychiatric interest are the papers on "The Neurotic Constitution" (Paper 16), based on 2,000 soldiers, in which background factors such as family history and previous personality on the one hand and degree of military stress on the other hand were related to diagnosis, symptomatology, and outcome. In this and the following paper in which he collaborated with his psychologist brother (now senior lecturer in the Department of Biometrics, Institute of Psychiatry), Slater put forward and elaborated what would now be termed a diathesis-stress theory of neurosis. To our knowledge this was the first time in which a polygenic theory was put forward in any detail to explain the constitutional background to neurotic breakdown. Like others before him, Slater also had observations to make on "Neurosis and Sexuality" (Paper 18).

Opportunity arose for the comparison of neurotic and non-psychiatric patients admitted to the hospital (43). The most intensive study on these lines was the book *Patterns of Marriage* (57) in which the co-author and field-worker was Mrs. Moya Woodside. Here the backgrounds of 100 neurotic soldiers and their wives were compared with those of 100 control couples. A chapter from the book appears as Paper 30 in Part VI, Society and the Individual.

If "A Heuristic Theory of Neurosis" (Paper 17) emphasized in an original manner the role of heredity in neurosis and psychopathy, Slater's earlier twin work (63), summarized in Paper 9, highlighted the environmental side of the coin. It showed how large differences in behavior, sometimes set in motion by apparently small causes, can occur in genetically identical twins and conversely how, given a poor environment, genetically dissimilar twins can both become delinquent. However, the monozygotic pairs on which the conclusions were based were few in number. Since the war a much larger series of neurotic and personality disordered twins has been accumulated in the Psychiatric Genetics Unit at the Maudsley Hospital, and it is on the investigation of these twins that Papers 19 and 21 are based. Here attention has been focused on the nosological or taxonomic aspect of the twin method. Although attention is given to factors associated with discordance in MZ pairs and although MZ and DZ concordance rates are compared in order to assess the likely importance of genetic factors in neurosis in general, these are not the main points of interest. It is the validity of the classification of illness that has been studied by the twin method as much as the aetiology of each given diagnosis, and the degree of specificity of genetic factors involved as much as the heritability of neurosis as a whole. In the Maudsley twin study a hospital diagnosis of hysteria (usually in the sense of conversion symptoms) did not have any of the characteristics of a valid disease entity. Later, a follow-up of patients diagnosed as hysteria at the National Hospital for Nervous Diseases (109, 112) led to the same conclusion. The first of these papers, the first Shorvon Memorial Lecture, was given in honour of Slater's late colleague at the National Hospital, Queen Square. It is ironical that the lecture was given on the day on which Slater terminated his appointment at this neurological hospital where he had been head of the Department of Psychological Medicine since 1946. The lecture contained an interesting historical account of the concept of hysteria. We have, however, for reasons of space, chosen to reproduce as Paper 20 the shorter account of this investigation, in which Eric Glithero collaborated.

If hysteria as commonly diagnosed appeared to be a symptom rather than a disease and as such to have no genetic significance, the situation as regards anxiety turned out to be different (Paper 21). In a later paper (135) it was further argued that anxiety is a quantitative trait normally distributed throughout the population and determined in considerable part by the genetic constitution. Anxious tendencies result in illness only if they are extreme or if adaptation to the environment becomes impossible on account of the degree of stress or because it is further hampered by other personality traits. Paper 21 about diagnostic similarity in twins was originally published in French and it appears here in its English version for the first time. The much greater qualitative resemblance in MZ as opposed to DZ twins supports the multi-dimensional aspects of the genetic background to personality which was put forward in "A Heuristic Theory." The diagnoses, made in ignorance of zygosity, show how psychiatric classification, at least in Slater's hands, is not a meaningless label.

15

AMNESIC SYNDROMES IN WAR

Loss of memory is much commoner in soldiers in wartime than in civilian practice in peace. From the previous records of some of our patients, it seems that the condition is often overlooked in civil life; in the Army a stricter routine and discipline make this impossible. Attention in the past has been mainly directed to states of fugue, and civilian practice suggests that behind these there often lies a criminal act or a situation from which an immediate, even though an illusory, escape is desired. Cases occurring in war, however, indicate that other causes, such as terror, bomb blast, and exhaustion, may produce not only fugues both at the time and subsequently, but also large gaps retrospectively in the patient's memory of the past.

In the first thousand military cases admitted to the Neurological Unit of Sutton Emergency Hospital we found no fewer than 144 in which loss of memory was a prominent symptom. These comprise the complete series of states of fugue and retrospective losses of memory of a functional type: cases of interference with memory due to disease of the brain, and of transient loss of consciousness after head injury are not included. Severe psychological stress was an important factor in these syndromes, as will be seen from Table 15.1.

TABLE 15.1 FREQUENCY OF CASES SHOWING AN AMNESIC SYNDROME IN A THOUSAND SERIAL ADMISSIONS

	Cases admitted No.	Amnesia present No.	Frequency %
Severe stress	251	87	35
Moderate stress	155	20	13
Trifling stress	594	37	6
Total	1,000	144	14

"Severe stress" means prolonged marching and fighting under heavy enemy action (e.g., in the evacuation from Dunkirk, through which the great majority of these cases passed); "moderate stress" includes experiences like periodical dive-bombing at home bases and aerodromes; "trifling stress" means the normal life of a training camp or depot, involving no greater strain than an unfamiliar life and separation from home.

By William Sargant and Eliot Slater. Originally published in the *Proceedings of the Royal Society of Medicine* 34: 757–64 (1941).

Classified diagnostically, amnesic syndromes were found rarely in epilepsy and schizophrenia, more commonly in head injury, but predominantly in psychoneurotic states. This may be partly caused by the selective admission of psychoneurotics to our hospital. We have found only two cases of epilepsy, both showing a functional type of syndrome and not the classical post-epileptic automatism.

Fugues are a classical though uncommon manifestation of schizophrenia. Typically they represent a disturbance of consciousness in which catatonic phenomena or paranoid and hallucinatory experiences dominate the patient. But in the three schizophrenics in our material the fugue took a form superficially hysterical in appearance, and in one of them the patient had suffered from fugues since childhood. One of the others has points of interest.

Case 1. (2001S): A man of 24, of psychopathic family, said he had suffered from headaches for many years and had been unhappy in the Army. After a period of leave he returned to his unit; he was worried about his wife's ill-health and a day or two later took, without permission, an Army motorcycle to go home and visit her. On the way he had an accident in which he was not injured but £20 worth of damage was done to the cycle. He got back to his unit, but knew he was in for trouble. He began to feel dizzy, fell down, was taken to hospital mute, and when he came round two days later was unable to remember the events of the immediate past. Attempts were made without success to clear up the amnesic patch, both by hypnotism directly and under the influence of sodium amytal. But under the drug florid schizophrenic symptoms were for the first time revealed. Ever since he had joined the Army he had felt that it was a matter of general knowledge that his father had been in prison for raping a daughter and that he, the patient, was the object of public contempt on this account. He described auditory hallucinations and interference with his thinking by which his mind was made to go blank at times.

Head injury was a causative factor in ten of our cases. In half its effect was indirect; permanent impairment of the personality by cerebral trauma, with a resulting increased tendency to hysterical types of reaction, provided a basis for the operation of psychogenic stimuli months or years later. In the remainder the effect was more direct, the unconsciousness produced by concussion passing without intermission into the dissociation of a fugue. Besides the traumatic there is a constitutional factor: there was a history of neurosis or psychosis in the first-degree relatives of six of the ten patients, and in four the personality of the patient was psychopathic, even before any head injury had occurred. It was interesting to find that of the 129 psychoneurotic patients, 30, or nearly a quarter, date their amnesic disturbance from concussion or being blown over and dazed by a bomb. This is a high proportion. In many of these cases, though subsequent treatment cleared up the major part of the amnesic period, there remained a small gap, presumably due to organic disturbance.

CONSTITUTIONAL BASIS

From Table 15.2 it will be seen that indications of constitutional inferiority were more frequent in the 32 men who broke down in the absence of any military stress than in the remainder. Nearly all (28) had fugues; three others did not actually wander off, but passed into a confused state necessitating admission to hospital, where they were found to have lost most of their memory of their past life; and one man under examination for a minor military crime lost his memory for the events on which he was being examined. In all, 6 of these 32 men showed symptoms of hysterical pseudo-dementia on admission to Sutton. Evidence of constitutional factors was strong, a positive family history and previous nervous breakdown being very common. In the families of three men a father, a mother, and a sib were said to be subject to the same sort of amnesic attacks as the patient; in another a sib suffered from epilepsy. Six men had had fugues in earlier life, before entering the Army, two for the first time before puberty. Two others had suffered in earlier life from dizzy attacks and faints. In ten cases in all, fugues had occurred not once but several times. There were similar but less frequent findings in the men who went through stress (Groups IIa and IIb); four of these patients had had previous fugues, and eight others had had other types of disturbance of consciousness, such as sleep-walking, hysterical fits and faints. These findings suggest the possibility of a constitutional behaviour pattern.

TABLE 15.2 INDICATIONS OF CONSTITUTIONAL INFERIORITY IN AMNESIC SYNDROMES

Frequency of	Group I (32 cases) %	Group IIa (39 cases) %	Group IIb (58 cases) %
1. Family history of psychopathy	53	50	41
2. Neurotic traits in childhood	56	65	39
3. Poor occupational record	22	16	15
4. Inhibited sexual life	63	40	31
5. Poor intelligence	47	13	22
6. Previous neurotic breakdown	42	21	14
7. Abnormal personality make-up	50	41	35
8. All findings 1–7 negative	9	21	19
9. Hysterical traits in personality	44	22	13
10. Obsessional traits in personality	7	14	18
11. Malingering factor observed	23	10	5
12. Required invaliding after treatment	72	54	53

Group I = Cases occurring in the absence of military stress
Group II = Cases occurring under military stress
    IIa = Cases of fugue
    IIb = Cases of retrospective amnesia

Returning to the group of men who broke down under trifling stress, one might legitimately cast some doubt on the complete sincerity and trustworthiness of all of them; but in nine of the 32 deliberate lying was observed, or there arose otherwise a strong suspicion of malingering. This, however, generally occurred in an affective setting, in which hysterical features were as a rule combined with anxiety, depression or hypochondriasis. The following case illustrates most of the features shown by Group I.

Case 2. (414S): Aged 21. This man's father was discharged from the Army in 1918 with "neurasthenia." The patient could remember him wandering off on four occasions and being away for a period lasting from a day to five weeks. He never knew where he had been, and on getting home it might be another fortnight before he would or could speak. He was a moderate drinker, but of irritable sulky temper. The mother also was neurotic. The patient was nervous as a child, timid, frightened of policemen and soldiers, and in later life was unaggressive and would not strike another man back. Before the war he had thoughts of becoming a conscientious objector, and would lie awake at night in a pool of sweat thinking about it. He did not like the Army at all. For a week before his fugue he hardly slept, suffered from headaches and knew something was going to happen. On the Saturday morning he felt worse. He remembers going to the board to read Orders; he went away, felt faint, and knew nothing more until, feeling as if he were coming out of a faint, he found himself five days later outside a cinema in Barking, 74 miles away. Apart from needing a shave, he was clean and well-cared for. His mother let the hospital know that he had paid a flying visit on the evening of the Saturday of his disappearance, just dashing in and out again. In hospital he was unremarkable but was the life and soul of amateur theatricals among the soldiers, which he organized. He steadfastly refused to allow any attempt to be made to recover the memory of the five days of the fugue. He was invalided. There is, of course, a strong suspicion of malingering in this case, and it is quite likely that the exhibition of fugues by both father and son is not so much inheritance as imitation.

In the remaining 97 psychoneurotics (Groups IIa and IIb) who broke down under strain, the amnesic symptoms took two forms, a prolonged disturbance of consciousness, nearly always in the form of a fugue, and a retrospective forgetfulness for distressing events of the past occurring when the period of stress was over. A colleague, Dr. Denis Hill, has pointed out in private discussion an important difference between these two types of symptom. The *fugue*, he considers, is an escape from the events of the present, a gross form of behaviour disorder, very often malingered, and shown, apart from the psychotic, as a rule only by severely psychopathic personalities. The *amnesic gap* in the memory of the past is, he thinks, a simple protective mechanism by which the continued recollection and presence in consciousness of painful events is avoided, a mechanism shown in minor degree by the normal person in everyday life. There is much to be said for this view, but the two types of manifestation cannot be so simply and certainly separated. Some of these men broke down under stress and passed into a fugue which provided them with some form of escape. Others first broke down after return to safety and passed into a fugue that served no detectable purpose. In some of the cases of retrospective amnesia breakdown had occurred at the time of stress, in others only later; in some of these the amnesia for the period of stress was diffuse and patchy, in others it was so complete and circumscribed as to resemble a fugue of the past. We have seen both fugues and retrospective amnesias in the same individual, and we have not found that the fugue is exclusively associated with grosser degrees of departure from normal behaviour. Nevertheless the figures of Table 15.2, showing a slight but fairly consistently higher incidence of abnormal findings in the fugue cases (Group IIa) than in the cases of retrospective amnesia (Group IIb), indicate that the fugue is to be classed as the more abnormal manifestation. The high incidence of signs of constitutional abnormality in all groups in Table 15.2 will be noted. This is evidence against the view that the acute nervous breakdown of war is a phenomenon to which even the most normal personalities are liable. It is true that in a fifth of the acute cases of Group II no history indicating pre-existing instability was elicited. This does not mean it did not exist. A weakness of these figures is that in only occasional cases was an independent history available.

An analysis of personality traits was undertaken, but apart from two findings showed little of interest. The distribution of hysterical and of obsessional traits of personality differed sharply from expectation, the former showing a positive and the latter a negative correlation with abnormality of behaviour (see Table 15.2). There was, however, a much more important finding which could not be conveyed in crude percentages. In examining our records we were struck by the frequency of a certain type of personality among the more normal of the men who broke down under stress (Group II). This type is best described by quotation from the records: "go-getter, energetic and active"; "sociable, fond of singing"; "high-spirited, interested in sports"; "knock-about, likes parties and jokes"; "many friends, simple type"; "high-spirited, self-confident, whisky drinker"; "rolling stone, fond of company, drinks a good deal"; "devil-may-care, likes making and taking jokes"; "generally gay, low-brow interests, exaggerated idea of own abilities." Nearly half of the patients of Group II were of this type, and they made up a very high proportion of those whose personalities were regarded as within normal limits. Summarizing, one may say that they are an outgoing type, popular with their mates, perhaps overkeen on popularity, not fond of their own company, quickly responsive emotionally but with affects tending to be shallow and lacking in persistence, not gifted with insight. The personalities classed as abnormal in Group II did not conform to the same type, showing the development, relatively to other traits, of paranoid tendencies, unsociability and poverty of energy output.

CLINICAL FEATURES

The clinical picture presented by the men who broke down under severe stress (77 of the 97 patients of Group II) frequently showed a very acute neurotic disturbance combined with a state of exhaustion resembling physical illness. This was particularly true of the earliest patients admitted after the Dunkirk evacuation. Many looked pale and drawn; others wore a blank or confused expression, and occasionally some degree of disorientation and objective confusion were seen. Headache was a prominent symptom. Symptoms of acute anxiety were not infrequently combined with others of a contradictory type, such as apathy, *belle indifférence* or even a mild euphoria. Hysterical conversion symptoms were occasionally seen, such as loss of voice, paralysis or gross tremors, even of the pill-rolling type. Physical exhaustion, as shown by a weight far below normal for the individual in question, was often present; and it is probable that this physical factor is responsible for much of the deviation from familiar neurotic pictures. The history that the patient gave was often confused, hazy, and full of amnesic gaps; on other occasions it was fairly coherent, and the suppressions of memory were only found by investigations with hypnosis or barbiturate narcosis. The following patient of Dr. Debenham's is illustrative.

Case 3. (1379S): A man of 24 was admitted from Millbank Hospital, having broken down at the end of a period of leave after return from Dunkirk. He described himself later as a sociable man, fond of parties and keen on his work, but easily upset by a mistake and liable to get out of spirits. On admission he was inarticulate and it was impossible to get a connected statement from him. His head and upper trunk were constantly shaking, and he held his head bent forwards, looking out of the corners of his eyes. He muttered or mumbled to himself, or moved his lips as if in speech, but was only able to answer questions slowly and softly and with a stammer and many repetitions of words and phrases. He picked restlessly at his hands and clothes and looked round anxiously at the slightest noise. He said that a bomb had fallen near him in Belgium, and he had subsequently been much upset by the scenes of dead and dying; when speaking of the bomb tears came into his eyes. There was a suggestion of something histrionic in his behaviour. Under intravenous barbiturate he lost his inhibition, tremors and tics, and was able to give a full account of his experiences with a good deal of emotional abreaction. No one experience had upset him more than another, but he had felt deserted and helpless, harrowed by the sight of slaughtered civilians and of his own comrades being killed and, as he thought, "losing their reason." On the beach at Dunkirk he had kept a bullet in his rifle for use on himself, to save himself from being "cut up" by the Germans. After this session he was much improved; but though the retardation and apparent confusion largely disappeared for good, the tremor of the head later returned to some degree. He eventually required invaliding.

As July and August came, the post-Dunkirk cases ceased to bear this hyperacute aspect. Symptoms of physical exhaustion were more seldom seen, though the patients were still often underweight. Anxiety symptoms remained much to the fore, but the patients' complaints came to bear a more hysterical quality. These later cases have been more difficult to treat and have not done so well from the Army point of view. We sent back to duty more than half of the patients admitted in May and June, but little more than 40% of those admitted later. The following case of Dr. Craske's, admitted towards the end of July, is an example of fugues appearing comparatively late in the course of an acute neurosis.

Case 4. (1521S): A man of 24 was admitted complaining of pains in the head, giddiness, tingling feelings in the legs and hands. His mother was said to be prone to worry and depression and a brother had been nervous since the last war. After school he became an engineer, until called up from the Territorials. He married because he "had to," but the child was stillborn, and he felt cheated and has resented the loss of his freedom ever since. He described himself as a cheerful, easy-going man, a popular N.C.O., though occasionally subject to mild moods of depression. He enjoyed Army life in France, was not upset when hostilities began and at first was little affected by bombing. After a bit, however, he began to suffer from nightmares, disturbed the others by shouting in his sleep, had headaches and felt anxious and irritable. The unit was moved rapidly from place to place and they got little food or sleep. Finally the whole section of 250 men fell into an ambush and were killed or taken prisoner. He was wounded in the shoulder, and was put into an ambulance and taken to a German base hospital. He was sure that some time the Germans would kill him, and when a large number of prisoners were being moved further back, he managed to dive through a hedge and escape. He got to a farm, where he was given food and civilian clothes, and mingled with refugees. He had a number of narrow escapes from Germans and from suspicious French whom he asked for food or water; but at last he got to French occupied territory and was taken to Dunkirk hospital, where he was with a great number of other soldiers and civilians. During the evacuation from Dunkirk he was still in civilian clothes, and was repeatedly stopped and questioned; this even occurred at Margate, where he became acutely upset. He was taken to Westminster Hospital, and his wound was treated. He could do nothing but think about his experiences and cry, and could not speak to his wife when she came to see him. After leave he returned to his unit, but could not do his duties satisfactorily, and became depressed to the point of thinking of suicide.

On arrival at Sutton, he was still depressed, preoccupied with his experiences and dreaming of them at night. He said he hated the war, the Army, the sight of other soldiers. He felt completely changed, as he had always been so friendly, and now everything he did was wrong. He complained of headaches and tinglings, and was sweaty and shaky. He told his story coherently, and there were no discrepancies or signs of an amnesic gap. In the first fortnight he made no improvement, and was then put on continuous narcosis, during which he became confused and hallucinated and talked constantly, reliving his experiences. At the end of the course of narcosis he was improved, but began to have frequent attacks of dissociation, lasting about fifteen minutes, during which he was back in France, usually seeing the Germans coming through the trees at the ambush. In the semi-hypnotic state induced by amytal further details of his history were obtained. He now related how he had been put in charge by the lad's parents of a boy in his company, and had in fact kept him under his wing. The boy was very nervous and finally in a wild panic had rushed off directly into enemy machine-gun fire, and must either have been killed or taken prisoner. A letter had now arrived at the hospital from the parents of this boy, asking for news. The patient was induced to answer the letter, and was much better, particularly when he heard a little later that his friend was now known to be a prisoner of war. But the hysterical attacks still continued, and further exploration revealed facts of a different kind. He now said that even before the offensive he had felt depressed and had had "wicked" thoughts about his wife. When he got depressed in France he got drunk, and had then several times gone with other women, feeling mean and guilty afterwards. The last time his wife visited him he had told her he did not want to see her, and he now felt he must have broken her heart. More than once after this there was improvement followed by relapse, exploration on each occasion releasing painful memories with temporary improvement. In his relapses the patient several times had fugues, one of which led to his waking up in the middle of the night in a neighbouring town; he thought he was back in France, accosted a policeman in a panic, and was taken to the station. Permanent improvement was only obtained when with much difficulty the full data of an incident in which he had deserted a wounded comrade were obtained. After this the periods of dissociation were at an end. He then had a course of modified insulin treatment with much benefit. He had a month's leave at home, and returned fit, with no recurrence of the fugues; but it was thought best to invalid him from the Army. He was clearly a severe constitutional hysteric, despite his satisfactory adaptation to ordinary peace-time life.

Several points of interest are exhibited by this case. The clinical picture shows not only hysterical symptoms, but also a fairly deep degree of depression; in the past there are corresponding foci of guilt and self-reproach, inadequately dealt with by complete suppression. The amnesic gaps were not apparent on first examination, but came out only in the course of intensive treatment; nevertheless no lasting improvement was possible until the last of the suppressed material had been brought out. Treatment had to be devoted to the physical aspect as well as to the psychological, continuous narcosis and insulin treatment playing their parts, first in dealing with the depression and agitation, finally in stabilizing recovery when attained. In this case the amnesic phenomena, which appeared first only under severe stress, were finally manifesting themselves as fugues in the most facile way, as the behaviour pattern became established.

The association of amnesia with guilt was rare, but a prominent feature in some of our cases. Only seven men, six of them fugue cases, showed this association in the 77 who passed through severe stress. The events for which forgetfulness was so desired were for the most part the horrors and strains of that catastrophic retreat. However 43 of these men broke down at the time of stress, thereby becoming a burden on their fellows, which might have well been a subject for uncomfortable and undesired self-examination.

TABLE 15.3 SYMPTOMS EXHIBITED BY CASES OF AMNESIA AND FUGUE PRECIPITATED BY SEVERE MILITARY STRESS

	Amnesic group (46 cases) No.	Fugue group (31 cases) No.
Obsessional symptoms	1	—
Anxiety symptoms	38	29
Hysterical symptoms (apart from amnesia)	41	29
Depression	21	14
Hypochondriasis	20	16
Paranoid symptoms	9	2
Malingering	2	2

A classification of the symptoms shown by the men who came through severe stress is attempted in Table 15.3. Anxiety and hysterical manifestations were the most prominent symptoms, though conversion symptoms were uncommon. Symptoms resembling those of schizophrenic states were very rare, hallucinations and catatonic-like behaviour being seen in one case each. Malingering also was rare.

TREATMENT

The treatment of these states is, of course, the treatment of the patient as a whole. But we have found it best not to ignore the amnesic symptoms, to explore the gaps in memory, and to be on the look-out for them, even when they are not immediately obvious, or are denied. These patients can certainly get well without interference; but men admitted to us months after return from Dunkirk have seemed to benefit from the restoration of lost memories, from which they had suffered throughout the intervening period. The better the personality, the more is the lack of knowledge of what happened in an amnesic period a source of worry to the patient. The method of exploration is a matter of personal choice; but we have found in our unit that the administration of an intravenous barbiturate is of particular value in these acute patients, who are often rather insusceptible to direct hypnosis. Under the drug it is easier to establish a semi-hypnotic contact, a point of value to the doctor who is uncertain of his hypnotic powers. The information gained will often be a mixture of truth and fantasy, and will have to be sifted. In any case the process is only one of the steps in treatment, the next being an emotional synthesis, the restoration of normal physical good health, and the readaptation of the patient. When symptomatic recovery is attained, reconditioning should begin. For the best results the patient should be convinced by actual trial that he can face the duties he carried out before breakdown. Unfortunately this is not possible in the hospital framework, so that chances of relapse are difficult to estimate. It is here that rehabilitation centres would have one of their main functions.

The progress of these neurotic states would in the uncomplicated case normally be back towards the patient's natural base-line, whether that is one of good or ill health. Unfortunately in this interim stage in the war the complicating factors are many. The patients of Group I are largely a constitutionally inferior material, and only a partially satisfactory adaptation could be expected. But it was disappointing to find so many of the more normal personalities of Group II incapable of being brought to the point of facing renewed military duties, even in the less risky circumstances of service at home. It was here that the lack of rehabilitation camps under combined psychiatric supervision and military discipline made itself felt. Even of those whom we did send back to duty about half have had subsequently to be invalided at some other centre. So far as we have knowledge of the invalided patients, they are nearly all at civilian work, but many still suffer from anxiety symptoms in air-raids. The difficulty is that we have not as yet been able to tackle the pathogenic situation, that of the war, which awaits not psychotherapy but curative surgery.

SUMMARY

In a complete series of a thousand military neurotic casualties there was found the high number of 144 who presented an amnesic syndrome. The frequency was much the highest in those cases who had undergone severe stress, such as the Flanders retreat. Epileptics, schizophrenics, and cases of head injury were seen, but the great majority were psychoneurotic. In about a quarter of these cases trivial concussion or dazing seemed to have played a precipitating role in producing states of hysterical dissociation. Those who broke down in the absence of stress were for the most part severe psychopaths, and included many cases of malingering in an affective setting. In 83 per cent of all the psychoneurotic cases there were indications of constitutional instability. Some evidence was obtained that there may be a specific constitutional tendency to fugues and other forms of disorders of consciousness. In cases occurring under stress the amnesic syndrome showed two main manifestations, fugue and retrospective gaps in the memory of past stress. Evidence tended to show that patients developing fugues had more psychopathic traits than those who showed only a retrospective amnesia. Patients breaking down under stress were, with striking frequency, men of a simple, superficially well-adapted, extraverted type of personality. The amnesic symptoms were shown in a setting in which affective features were prominent; these were, in descending order of frequency, anxiety, hypochondriasis, depression and paranoid symptoms. The treatment and prognosis of these cases are discussed.

16

THE NEUROTIC CONSTITUTION:
A STATISTICAL STUDY OF TWO THOUSAND NEUROTIC SOLDIERS

INTRODUCTION

The emergencies of war demanded the enlistment of an army of maximum size. The National Service Boards had to work with great rapidity, and with medical standards that were not so much lowered as dropped. The doctors composing these boards seem to have had but a sketchy knowledge of psychiatry, and no knowledge of the extent to which psychiatric disabilities can unfit a man for military duties. Large numbers of men proved useless within a few months or even weeks of enlistment, and arrangements had to be made to return them to civilian life as expeditiously as possible. Most of this work has been done by Army psychiatrists; but where there was a possibility that treatment might make a man fit for further service, or where his condition had so deteriorated that he was not fit for ordinary civilian work, admission to hospital has been arranged.

The clinical picture presented by these patients has been of a monotonous character. They were admitted to the Neurosis Centre on a psychiatrist's recommendation, and neurotic symptomatology was therefore to the fore. The obviously psychotic, mentally defective, or physically ill went elsewhere; and though examples of these conditions have been seen, as is recorded, they usually showed an admixture of neurotic symptoms. In general the "neurosis" exhibited was not so much an illness as a simple failure to adapt to army routine and discipline, in part an incapacity to adapt, and a response to this incapacity. Whether ill or not, the commonest symptoms were those of anxiety, hysteria, depression, hypochondriasis, etc., and tended to be shown by members of all diagnostic groups. The causes of breakdown were of the same uniform character: separation from home and family, home worries, a life of relative hardship, army discipline, the pressure of tasks physically, intellectually, or temperamentally beyond them. Only in a minority of patients were

---

Originally published in the *Journal of Neurology and Psychiatry* 6: 1–16 (1943).

the more violent stresses of war the main precipitating factor. There have been a few who went through the Norwegian campaign, or served in the Middle East, or had to defend intensively attacked aerodromes or other places of military importance. But the evacuation from Dunkirk did provide a number of acutely ill patients; and here the operative stress seems to have been a combination of both physical and psychogenic factors: inadequate training, exposure to terrifying weapons of war (e.g., the dive-bomber, of which there had been no experience), the discouragement of defeat, prolonged marching with inadequate food, rest, and sleep, etc. These patients offered a great contrast to the others, but they still presented the same constellation of anxiety, depression, and hysteria, though in much severer degree. We have seen no single case of acute schizophrenia, as reported by Hubert (1941), or of mania or psychotic depression released by such stresses, though there was a sufficiency of acutely agitated anxiety states, exhaustion syndromes, and hysterical twilight states.

The monotonous character of precipitating cause and the clinical picture was mirrored by a monotonous uniformity of the underlying personality. There were few who did not show to some degree a psychic asthenia, a feebleness of will and purpose, coupled with tendencies to worry, pessimism and moodiness, or hysterical traits. This was indeed the fundamental disability, and indications had been shown in childhood and adult life. When one considers the large number of men who have had to be invalided for such conditions as these, one is impressed with the size of the problem. The analysis which follows attempts to give a general survey of the clinical material with which we have had to deal in one E.M.S. Neurosis Centre, and to elucidate the aetiological basis of this socially important group of patients.

THE STATISTICAL METHOD

In medicine, as elsewhere in science, statistical methods are only employed when exacter methods are not practicable. Under certain circumstances they are capable of yielding results of precision and reliability, but these are always the expression of a probability. Statistical methods can be employed in fields where the known stands in very unequal relation to the unknown, but they can be so used as to disguise ignorance and to cover the effects of factors which cannot easily be taken into account. The principal advantage of a statistical approach is that it permits the introduction of numerical methods in dealing with observations which are themselves purely qualitative. This advantage alone assures it an important future in psychiatry, where quantitative measurement of such things as degree of depression remains a dream of the future. For statistical methods to give reliable results there must be a certain uniformity in the material investigated, and there must be no biased sampling, no sources of systematic distortion of the results, whose presence is at once adventitious and unsuspected. In this material these criteria are only partly fulfilled. The patients are not a fair selection of the total psychiatric material of the Army, not to speak of the Armed Forces in general. There is on the one hand a negative selection of epileptics, defectives, and the grosser psychopaths, who could be dealt with out of hand by the Army psychiatrists, of the delinquent who tended to seep into other channels, and of the psychotic and more severely psychopathic who were mostly admitted to Army mental hospitals. On the other hand only very small numbers of men were admitted from distant theatres of war. These factors affect different parts of our material to differing degrees. The schizophrenics are clearly a most unrepresentative selection, being only admitted by virtue of an error of diagnosis on the part of the Army psychiatrist, and therefore including only the quieter, more insidious, and least typical forms of that illness. The same is to a lesser extent true of the epileptics, defectives, manic-depressives, and the psychopaths. In regard to the neuroses, our admissions represent probably a selection in favour of gravity, as the minor degrees of neurotic illness were frequently dealt with by regimental medical officers and Army psychiatrists in an out-patient capacity. Nevertheless our material, though not representative of all the psychiatric problems which face the Army organization, does give a fair picture of quite a large part.

It is frequently objected to psychiatric research that both diagnosis and the observations on which it is founded are matters of opinion and of degree, from which it is argued that the findings which are dealt with by statistical analysis must be largely subjective, and correspondingly worthless. The material here analysed is based on the day to day work of more than a dozen different psychiatrists, most of them of many years experience. Factors, then, which have a purely subjective value should be so randomly distributed as to have little influence on the results. It will in any case hardly be contended that such terms as schizophrenia and such observations as positive family history correspond to no biological reality; and in so far as they do, differences between the various diagnostic and other groups will reflect to some extent the underlying fact. Statistics operate by an analysis of frequencies observed in qualitatively defined classes. The very finding of systematic differences between one class and another is evidence in favour of the real significance of the distinctions so drawn.

Collection of Data

The patients studied below were admitted to Sutton Emergency Hospital neuropsychiatric wards between November, 1939, and June, 1941. They were nearly all soldiers, but included a few sailors and airmen, but no civilians or members of civilian defence services. They were all men and below commissioned rank. In the course of ordinary history taking the psychiatrist filled in a summary form, in which specific yes/no answers were demanded to a considerable number of questions, with space for amplification where deemed necessary (e.g. on personality, symptoms, etc.). What these questions were will appear from the following tables. Not every psychiatrist was equally punctilious in filling the form, and definite information was not always available to every question. The consequence was that on a certain number of forms there were some queries or blanks where questions had been left unanswered. It is further clear that the detail in which questions were answered depended to some extent on the interest of the individual doctor, and the frequency of a positive family history, the number and even type of personality traits noted down, among other observations, varied from clinician to clinician. Eventually the summary forms of the first two thousand serial admissions were taken, about a hundred excluded as containing too many blanks to be useful, and a further hundred or so forms from the next admissions added to make up the number to exactly two thousand. Where yes/no answers had not been possible, the relevant material was codified for counting. The Scientific Computing Service Limited[1] prepared summary tables using the Hollerith Punched Card System. The information given on each form was coded and punched on a card, and special machines (tabulators) then

[1] With the aid of an expenses grant from the Maudsley Research Fellowship.

sorted the 2,000 cards into the various classes (of diagnosis, etc.), counted and printed the frequencies in each class. Finally the tables were submitted to statistical analysis.

In this paper the results will be discussed of analysis by diagnosis, by degree of stress undergone, and by outcome. It is possible that at a later time it may be worth recording the results of other counts that were made, e.g. by age, religious confession, sexual life. In the tables that follow, to avoid an excessive cumbersomeness, the presentation of absolute figures has been avoided and only percentages are given. But the totals on which the percentages are based are available in every case and from these absolute figures could — if desired — be derived. Furthermore, although the standard errors of these percentages have been calculated, they have not been included in the tables; percentages which differ from that of the general average by more than twice the standard error of the difference have been taken as statistically significant and are marked with an asterisk in the diagnostic tables. In a certain number of patients a double diagnosis had to be made (e.g., mental defect + anxiety state, psychopathic personality + hysteria, head injury + depression), which has resulted in two thousand soldiers providing 2,037 diagnoses. In the diagnostic tables we have therefore the equivalent of 2,037 patients, and percentages have been calculated on this total. In later tables only those particulars are entered which provided statistically significant deviations from the norm.

Diagnostic Classification

Diagnoses were classified into the following groups:

1. *Organic States*, inclusive of general paralysis, arteriosclerosis, neurological disorders, post-meningitic syndromes, and cases of cardio-vascular, respiratory and alimentary disorders incorrectly admitted as suffering from neurosis without physical basis. To have dealt with these groups severally would have made numbers too small for statistical handling.

2. *Head Injury*. Under this head come patients in whom there was thought to be a cerebral contusion or other lesion, old or recent, responsible for some at least of the symptoms. Grounds for this view were sometimes backed by an electroencephalogram, by the opinion of a consulting neurologist, or by indications of a typical change in personality dating from the time of the injury, but were sometimes rather nebulous; nevertheless patients in whom there was no evidence at all of neurological damage or anything more than concussion were excluded.

3. *Epilepsy*. Diagnosis was made on observation of a fit, of a typical history of fits or of periodic psychomotor attacks, or of petit mal waves in the EEG.

4. *Schizophrenia*.

5. *Endogenous Depression*. In this group were also included two cases of hypomania. The distinction between this group and that of the reactive depressions was based on such clinical findings as relative unimportance of precipitating factor, retardation, refractoriness of the depression to influence by suggestion, etc. The patients in this group could be regarded as manic-depressives or as suffering from involutional depression, with comparatively mild illnesses.

6. *Mental Defect*. Nearly all the patients so diagnosed were not so defective as to be certifiable, but they were all so dull and backward that it was considered that their defect was the main cause of failure in the Services and of admission to hospital.

7. *Psychopathic Personality*. This miscellaneous group included all patients in whom there was held to be a constitutional abnormality of personality of fairly severe degree, mainly responsible for any neurotic symptoms of failure of adaptation. The abnormality might be of any type, and included, for instance, cyclothymics, long-standing hysterics, the severely and chronically anxious, as well as those usually included under this head.

8. *Anxiety Neurosis*.

9. *Hysteria*.

10. *Reactive Depression*.

There were in addition three other small groups, too small to be dealt with severally: 20 obsessional neurotics, 16 enuretics without obvious other abnormality, 9 malingerers. The obsessional neurotics were a distinct group, though some patients of the same kind were admitted with a fairly severe degree of depression and have fallen into groups 5 or 10. Enuresis was a fairly common symptom but was usually accompanied by mental defect or the signs of a chronic neurosis, justifying inclusion in one of the other groups; but it may appear alone in the likeness of an "organic neurosis," perhaps with a specific heredity, perhaps accompanied by spina bifida occulta. The malingerers were men who deliberately pretended to an illness they did not have. Cases on the borderline between hysteria and malingering were not included, nor those who exaggerated symptoms to some extent certainly present (a very common finding). Though nothing certain can be said of them owing to the smallness of their number, they seemed to be more normal constitutionally than the neurotics and psychopaths. All these three groups, though not dealt with separately, have been included in the totals and general averages.

AGE, RELIGION, OCCUPATION, RANK, UNIT

The different diagnostic groups showed no significant differences one from another in respect of age. The average age of the whole group, which varied from 16 to 59, was 28.3 years. Patients with organic states (31.4), manic-depressives (30.2), and reactive depressives (30.5) were older than the average; epileptics (26.2), schizophrenics (26.9), and enuretics (23.4) were younger.

No significant differences were noted between the various groups in respect of religious confession, except that psychopaths belonged to the Church of England with a frequency significantly less than the average. Of all the patients taken together, 1.6 per cent were Jews, 12.6 per cent were Roman Catholics, 13.2 per cent Non-Conformists, and 72.5 per cent belonged to the Church of England.

Occupations have been classified into only four groups. The fourth of these included men belonging to the professions (37), clerical workers (162), persons having their own shops and businesses (109), and other types of work or unstated (63). These subdivisions were too small to handle separately and were therefore combined into a group which is characterized by a more sedentary type of activity than those of the other three. From Table 16.1 it may be seen that the defectives came, as might have been expected, preponderantly from the unskilled labourers. It is surprising to find that manic-depressives also come with significantly high frequency from the same group, in direct contrast to the reactive depressives who do so with a frequency significantly less than the average. Schizophrenics come from sedentary occupations with a frequency almost double the average, which accords well with what one knows of the "schizoid" personality. Psychopaths are but rarely skilled workmen, perhaps because a psychopathic personality would be a hindrance in completing an apprenticeship.

The frequency of N.C.O.s is highest in the obsessionals (35 per cent), in the manic-depressives and reactive depressives, in that order, although the numbers in the first two of these groups are too small to be significant. These are findings that might have been expected. Clinical experience suggests that manic-depressives are often superior men, and statistics gathered in Germany by Luxenburger (1933) have shown an association with better types of occupation, in contrast to our material. Epileptics, schizophrenics, and defectives have seldom won themselves promotion, again an expected finding.

TABLE 16.1. OCCUPATIONAL LEVEL AND DIAGNOSIS

Diagnosis	Number observed	Occupation				
		Unskilled %	Semi-skilled %	Skilled %	Other %	N.C.O.s %
1. Organic states	51	27.5	50.5	5.9	15.7	21.6
2. Head injury	109	24.8*	46.8	16.5	11.9	23.9
3. Epilepsy	70	40.0	38.6	8.6	12.9	8.6*
4. Schizophrenia	50	32.0	26.0	8.0	34.0*	6.0*
5. Endogenous depression	51	49.0*	17.7*	3.9*	29.4	29.4
6. Mental defect	137	59.1*	27.8*	5.8*	7.3*	4.4*
7. Psychopathic personality	265	37.7	34.0	6.5*	22.6	20.0
8. Anxiety neurosis	647	31.9	41.7	11.3	15.1	18.2
9. Hysteria	384	30.6	38.8	9.9	21.1	17.4
10. Reactive depression	228	26.4*	40.4	11.8	20.6	26.8*
Total	2,037	33.2	38.4	10.1	18.2	18.4

* = significantly different from total percentage

The data with regard to unit have been omitted from the table, as not sufficiently interesting. Of the total material 40.2 per cent of the patients came from non-combatant units, obsessionals with the lowest frequency (25 per cent), cases of physical disorder and head injury with the highest (47.1 per cent and 45.9 per cent).

PHYSICAL AND SEXUAL CONSTITUTION

The differential diagnosis of asthenic, athletic and pyknic habitus was made on impressions only. Elaborate and exact methods of physical measurement have led to confusion in the past, and hardly seemed worth the trouble of making. On the other hand well-marked representatives of all types are easy to recognise at a glance and though there are many men of whom it is difficult to say that they belong to one group rather than another, it was thought worth while to make the distinction where possible. No great value is claimed for these figures. In only about half the patients was any entry made in the record of the bodily habitus, which has necessitated doubling the figures by adding a further series from later admissions to get significant results. One notes the high preponderance of the asthenic habitus, the endogenous depressives singling themselves out from the rest by having a marked preponderance of persons of pyknic habitus.

Investigation of the sexual lives of our patients indicated that this was at least as important from the point of view of constitution as of psychogenesis. The number of men in whom sexual relations began at a late age, occurred with unusual rarity and were associated with little interest or satisfaction, was so high as to attract attention and to lead to the inclusion of a specific question in the summary form. "Inhibited" is really the wrong word, and "impoverished" or "inadequate" would be a better one, because the infrequency of sexual activity was far more often caused by lack of libido than by self-restraint. In general it may be said that complete abstinence was not regarded as "inhibition" until full adult life, say 25 years of age, was reached. The majority of our patients were married, and in these a coitus frequency of less than once a fortnight would generally be regarded as evidence of inhibition. In the analysis of the total material by sexual life several interesting correlations were found, for instance of inhibition with the asthenic and pyknic physiques, and with a poor outcome; but it is hoped to combine these with a genetic and biochemical investigation which is being undertaken at the present time, and will be made the subject of a later communication. From Table 16.2 it may be seen that an inhibited sex life is especially frequent among mental defectives and psychopaths, especially infrequent in cases of head injury. It is clearly a quality of deep biological significance, and it may be that it is genetically associated with the factors that make for inferiority of intelligence and temperament.

TABLE 16.2. BODY BUILD AND SEXUAL INHIBITION IN DIAGNOSTIC GROUPS

Diagnosis	Bodily habitus				Sexual life	
	Number recorded	Asthenic %	Athletic %	Pyknic %	Number recorded	Inhibited %
1. Organic states	74	39.2	33.8	27.0	36	50.0
2. Head injury	87	36.8	34.5	28.7	60	23.3*
3. Epilepsy	60	38.3	35.0	26.7	50	44.0
4. Schizophrenia	56	39.3	37.5	23.2	35	54.3
5. Endogenous depression	52	25.0	23.1	51.9*	28	53.6
6. Mental defect	131	51.1	35.9	13.0*	85	57.6*
7. Psychopathic personality	311	46.3	33.8	19.9	193	51.8*
8. Anxiety neurosis	710	47.7	30.4	21.8	469	38.6
9. Hysteria	392	38.3*	34.4	27.3	280	42.1
10. Reactive depression	232	44.4	29.3	26.3	176	40.9
Total	2,105	43.8	32.3	23.9	1,412	43.1

* = significantly different from total percentage

MENTAL CONSTITUTION, AFFECTIVE

As seen in Table 16.3, in 55.7 per cent of our patients there was a positive family history, i.e., one or more of the first-degree relatives, parent, sib or child, had suffered from definite neurotic illness or psychosis or epilepsy or from some form of psychopathy (such as drunkenness, shiftlessness or violent and brutal habits) which had entailed undesirable social consequences. As information was obtained almost exclusively from the patient himself, no claim can be made that the figures are of any absolute value; they would indeed appear to be minimum ones. It is of interest that a family history of fits is given not only by a third of the epileptics but by 10 per cent of the defectives, and that comparatively high frequencies of a family history of psychoses are found in the schizophrenics and endogenous depressives. Generally, a positive family history is found with significant rarity in the physical states, with significant frequency in the psychopaths. The remarkably high figure provided by the latter supplies a strong suggestion that genetic factors productive of mental abnormality can reinforce one another and act cumulatively.

TABLE 16.3 FAMILY HISTORY AND PRE-MORBID PERSONALITY IN
DIAGNOSTIC GROUPS

	Positive family history				Previous personal history		
Diagnosis	General %	Epilepsy %	Psychosis %	Neurosis %	Childhood neurosis and minor neurotic traits %	Previous nervous breakdown %	Abnormal personality %
1. Organic states	37.3*	2.0	6.8	13.7*	35.3*	13.7	31.4
2. Head injury	32.1*	3.7	1.8	6.4*	27.5*	9.2*	22.0*
3. Epilepsy	55.7	28.6*	2.9	24.3	47.2	12.9*	35.7
4. Schizophrenia	52.0	4.0	8.0	24.0	60.0	34.0	62.0*
5. Endogenous depression	62.8	2.0	9.8	13.7*	45.1	68.6*	41.2
6. Mental defect	56.2	10.1	5.8	26.3	55.5	16.1*	49.6
7. Psychopathic personality	72.5*	8.7	6.4	45.7*	76.6*	28.7	—
8. Anxiety neurosis	56.7	5.9	3.2	26.4	62.4	23.2	39.9
9. Hysteria	50.8	4.9	4.1	24.7	55.4	22.9	43.2
10. Reactive depression	55.7	3.1*	4.8	21.1	57.5	22.4	45.2
Total	55.7	6.4	4.4	26.3	58.8	23.1	41.4

* = significantly different from total percentage

Some degree of childhood neurosis is shown by 58.8 per cent of the total material, the frequency of definite neurosis being significantly high for the psychopaths, significantly low for the two organic groups and for the manic-depressives. This is one of the many ways in which the endogenous depressions distinguish themselves from neurotic states. It is to be remembered that the frequency of some degree of nervousness in childhood is probably quite high in the average population, even in children who grow up to be quite normal adults; but from the facts provided here it seems clear that neurotic symptoms in childhood, especially if they reach at all a severe degree, are of considerable significance for later life.

Almost a quarter of our patients had had a previous nervous breakdown, and of the endogenous depressives over two-thirds. It is probable that in these latter this finding was used as a diagnostic criterion.

The frequency of an abnormal personality is also shown to be high, over 40 per cent in the whole group, and in no category less than 20 per cent. Persons so marked were held to show a degree of abnormality of personality, in structure and development, which could not be regarded as within the normal limits of variation of the population. A fairly well adjusted man, with some but no very serious neurotic or psychopathic traits, would not come within this definition. It will be seen that the organic syndromes score comparatively low figures, while the schizophrenics distinguish themselves by showing a high frequency of abnormality of the pre-morbid personality. The total frequency of abnormal personality in the whole group, including the psychopaths, is 48.3 per cent.

The individual personality traits are tabulated in Table 16.4, which is one of exceptional interest. It will be seen that throughout, with one nonsignificant exception, the organic syndromes do not reach the level of frequency of the general average, and for the most part are significantly below it. Epileptics score low values for all traits, except paranoid and impulsive tendencies; in the latter they have a high figure, and one which only just fails of significance. Schizophrenics are markedly lacking in hysterical traits, markedly rich in paranoid and unsociable tendencies, which would seem, from this admittedly unrepresentative material, to be the main features of the "schizoid" personality. The endogenous depressives score figures consistently lower than the average, and often significantly lower, in all qualities but obsessional tendencies and instability of mood. The latter is an expected finding, the former much less so, although some relation between manic-depressive syndromes and obsessional neurosis and the obsessional character has long been suspected. In this respect the reactive depressives resemble the endogenous depressives, as also in the low frequency of hysterical and impulsive and aggressive tendencies. But in general they deviate much less sharply from the average, and show a much higher incidence of anxiousness of disposition, in which the endogenous depressives rank significantly low. The mental defectives score figures which are for the most part rather lower than the average, significantly so in obsessional tendencies, instability of mood, and unsociability; it is a little surprising that they do not show up more for anergic tendencies and lack of initiative, which would seem therefore to be almost purely a temperamental quality. It has often been asserted and denied that obsessional neurosis is rare in mental defectives; there is some evidence here that there is a negative association between mental defect and the obsessional character. Anxiety neurotics in general approximate to the average of the whole group, but show as was to be expected a higher incidence of anxiousness of personality, and also a low incidence of hysterical tendencies and aggressiveness. The hysterics conform fairly well to the general average, but rank low in the frequency of obsessional traits, lability of mood and unsociability; as was to be expected they show a high incidence of hysterical traits of character. The psychopaths score very high figures throughout the table, with the single exception of obsessional traits. It is interesting that, taking the material as a whole, the most common abnormal traits of personality were undue lability of mood, lack of interest in and talent for mixing socially with the rest of mankind, an anergia and spinelessness of character, and tendencies to anxiety; the least frequent traits were hypochondriasis and paranoid traits.

TABLE 16.4. DIAGNOSIS AND PERSONALITY TRAITS

	Personality traits									
Diagnosis	Obsessional %	Anxious %	Hysterical %	Unstable Mood %	Hypochondriasis %	Paranoid -sensitive %	Impulsive -aggressive %	Unsociable %	Anergic %	Number of abnormal traits per patient
1. Organic states	13.7	3.9*	11.8	23.5	2.0*	7.8	17.6	17.6*	7.8*	1.1
2. Head injury	9.2*	9.2*	7.3*	15.6*	1.8*	9.2	26.6	19.3*	16.5	1.1
3. Epilepsy	15.7	10.0*	7.1*	31.4	1.4*	20.0	31.4	28.6	20.0	1.7
4. Schizophrenia	26.0	16.0	4.0*	38.0	10.0	32.0*	30.0	46.0*	22.0	2.2
5. Endogenous depression	37.3*	11.8*	5.9*	60.8*	3.9	7.8	11.8	25.5	7.8*	1.7
6. Mental defect	5.8*	30.7	9.5	23.3*	6.6	9.5	16.8	23.4*	25.6	1.5
7. Psychopathic personality	23.0	30.2*	20.0*	47.2*	12.8*	24.5*	36.2*	44.9*	36.2*	2.8
8. Anxiety neurosis	20.6	29.1*	9.6*	32.1	6.5	10.5	14.5*	32.0	24.3	1.8
9. Hysteria	14.6*	19.3	26.9*	26.0*	7.8	10.7	20.8	25.5*	22.4	1.7
10. Reactive depression	30.3*	22.4	7.5*	44.3*	9.2	11.0	14.5*	32.5	20.6	1.9
Total	20.0	23.5	13.6	33.4	7.4	13.0	20.2	31.0	23.8	1.9

* = significantly different from total percentage

199

MENTAL CONSTITUTION, INTELLECTUAL

The school record shows, expectedly, conspicuous failure on the part of the defectives; cases of head injury, endogenous and reactive depression are associated with records better than the average. In Table 16.5 a poor school record was taken as failure to reach the top standard of an elementary school by the age of 14, a good record as education at a Central or Secondary School, or better. The intelligence ratings were based for the greater part on a simple clinical impression and such intellectual tests of a brief character as are commonly applied in the course of a routine examination. Group intelligence tests were performed on a fair minority of the patients, but they themselves were not entirely reliable. Some patients, particularly those of a hysterical disposition, who were out to show themselves as unfit as possible, did conspicuously badly on the intelligence test; a repeated test would frequently produce a ten point rise or more in the I.Q. It will be seen that the intelligence ratings mirror fairly closely the school record. The epileptics and the hysterics tend to be of lower intelligence than the average; the organic patients, depressives of both kinds, and the schizophrenics tend to do better than the rest of the material. The low rating obtained by the hysterics is of interest. As has already been stated, the figures are of rather doubtful validity but they cannot be entirely disregarded. The psychopaths, who, as will be shown, were as anxious as the hysterics to earn their discharge from the army by fair means or foul, do not show the same association with a low intelligence rating. Furthermore, as will appear later, mental defectives tend particularly to a hysterical type of neurotic symptomatology. There is a definite suggestion, then, of a real association of hysteria with subnormal intelligence. The most important finding given by the table is, however, that provided by the general averages. It will be seen that about a third of these patients were of poor intelligence and that the frequencies of the various groups differ sharply from the "normal" type of curve provided by the general population,[2] and in this population of neurotics the curve is markedly skewed, persons of low intelligence being represented in far greater numbers than those of superior intelligence.

TABLE 16.5. MENTAL ABILITY AND DIAGNOSIS

Diagnosis	School record		Intelligence			
	Poor %	Good %	Recorded No.	Poor %	Average %	Good %
1. Organic states	29.4	17.6	38	21.1	60.5	18.4
2. Head injury	20.1*	13.8	76	25.0	69.7	5.3
3. Epilepsy	37.1	10.0	57	47.4*	42.1*	10.5
4. Schizophrenia	22.0	18.0	40	20.0	65.0	15.0
5. Endogenous depression	19.6*	13.7	33	18.2	69.7	12.1
6. Mental defect	85.4*	0.0*	—	—	—	—
7. Psychopathic personality	30.2	15.5	212	33.5	55.2	11.3
8. Anxiety neurosis	28.1	15.5	546	29.9	60.6	9.5
9. Hysteria	29.7	11.9	322	39.8*	52.5	7.8
10. Reactive depression	21.0*	17.1	181	23.8*	64.1	12.2
Total	31.2	14.2	1538	31.2	58.5	10.3

* = significantly different from total percentage

[2] And by Army entrants tested with the same methods by the Directorate of Selection of Personnel. For a detailed examination of our material on this point, see Halstead (1943).

The only groups to conform fairly closely to the normal distribution are the organic states, the schizophrenics and the endogenous depressives. It seems probable that subnormality of intelligence and of temperamental stability reinforce one another in producing failure of adaptation, and that in any collection selected on this criterion one will see the intermingling of both factors. The more stable defectives and the more intelligent neurotics will as a rule more easily escape the net spread for either.

PRECONDITIONING

The frequency of a bad home environment, of a bad relationship with the father, of previous army service, and of previous war service were analysed, but are not included in a table. These were the only factors whose effect in the environmental predisposition towards neurosis could be attacked, and the result was inconclusive. We found a bad home, in the sense of excessive poverty, drunkenness or family disagreement in 20.9 per cent of patients, a bad relation with the father in 15.6 per cent. Both findings were significantly more frequent in the psychopaths (30.6, 26.8 per cent), significantly less so in the two organic groups (group 1: 5.9, 5.9 per cent; group 2: 13.8, 8.3 per cent). But although a bad home environment may certainly predispose to neurosis, the finding is entirely ambiguous, as it is probably also an expression of neurosis or psychopathy in the parents, and thereby a function of bad heredity. The two effects, environmental and hereditary, cannot be disentangled, as they are necessarily bound up together. The number of men who served in the last war, 12.4 per cent, is surprisingly high. They were nearly all volunteers, and all middle-aged men, most of whom broke down under the severe weather conditions of the first winter in France, and a reactive depressive illness was significantly more common among them.

PRECIPITATION

The innumerable external factors which may actually precipitate a breakdown do not readily lend themselves to analysis, but more easily so in the present than in a normal peace-time material. They were most commonly the stresses of war, comparatively hard life and discipline in the army, separation from family and home, home worries of various kinds (e.g., the illness of relatives, financial stress, destruction of the home by bombing, worries about a possibly unfaithful wife, etc.), and physical ill-health, as seen in Table 16.6. Some factor of one of the above kinds had fairly clearly played a part in nearly half the patients. In the remainder, breakdown had occurred under military conditions which were far from onerous, and these subjects must be regarded as being of a very low level of constitutional adaptability. The lowest figure is scored by schizophrenia, which would therefore in this material appear to be almost wholly endogenous. Epileptics, those suffering from organic states other than head injury, mental defectives, and psychopaths all became unfit with comparatively little in the way of additional environmental stress. In contrast to the other reactive states, the anxiety neuroses show themselves as associated with special frequency with some definite precipitation. They manifest the same phenomenon in their association with military stress, being the only diagnostic group to show a positive correlation there. Although anxiety neuroses constituted only 32 per cent of the total material, they were diagnosed in 46 per cent of the patients who went through some degree of military stress. This particular precipitating factor will be discussed in greater detail later on. The incidence of head injury provides interesting figures. Head injury, perhaps only a moderate degree of concussion, had occurred at some time in 13 per cent of all patients, excluding those specifically diagnosed as traumatic syndromes. The incidence is low in the endogenous depressives and schizophrenics, but significantly high in the epileptics. Other physical disabilities (orthopaedic abnormalities, such illnesses as chronic bronchitis, etc.) were present in a further 14 per cent, and one notes that a relatively high proportion of the reactive depressives were handicapped by physical factors, and that many of the hysterics hung their symptoms on to some genuine physical disability. The psychogenic factors associated with adverse home situations show no predilection for one diagnostic group as compared with others, except that they were especially frequent in the psychopaths; this is presumably to be taken as an expression of the psychopath's tendency to make unhappiness for himself wherever he goes, rather than as evidence of any causative relation in the other direction.

TABLE 16.6. EXTERNAL PRECIPITATING FACTORS

Diagnosis	Precipi-tation %	Head injury %	Physical factors %	Unsat. home %	Military stress		
					Severe %	Moderate %	Trifling %
1. Organic states	31.4*	13.7	—	13.7	5.9*	21.6	72.5*
2. Head injury	—	—	—	11.9	27.5	20.2	52.3
3. Epilepsy	20.0*	27.1*	15.7	11.4	7.1*	8.6*	84.3*
4. Schizophrenia	10.0*	6.0*	6.0*	22.0	8.0*	12.0	80.0*
5. Endogenous depression	35.3	5.9*	9.8	15.7	7.9*	7.9*	84.3*
6. Mental defect	31.4*	18.2	17.5	13.1	16.1	10.9*	73.0*
7. Psychopathic personality	33.2*	12.8	9.8	28.7*	13.6*	18.8	67.6*
8. Anxiety neurosis	61.4*	11.4	14.7	12.2	32.3*	28.7*	38.9*
9. Hysteria	48.4	19.0*	19.3*	11.7	20.3	18.2	61.5
10. Reactive depression	47.8	11.0	21.9*	14.9	19.3	21.5	59.2
Total	47.6	13.0	14.3	14.7	21.5	21.0	57.5

* = significantly different from total percentage

SYMPTOMATOLOGY

Roughly half our patients had been ill for periods of less than six months, a quarter for six months to two years, and a quarter for over two years. By this is meant not the duration of the condition, but of obvious disability or active symptoms caused by it. It will be seen that clear signs of epilepsy, mental defect, and psychopathic personality had been present in a high proportion of those diagnostic groups considerably before the time the men concerned were enlisted. Very large numbers of these men, who were as a rule useless as soldiers from the beginning, might have been kept out of the army had they been given even the most cursory psychiatric examination, with a corresponding gain in efficiency in their units and in the medical services. Of all the diagnostic groups, the anxiety states distinguish themselves by being most frequently of recent origin.

Turning to the symptoms themselves in Table 16.7 we note that by far the commonest symptoms are depression, anxiety, and hypochondriasis in that order. These symptoms are shown with considerable frequency by every diagnostic group and therefore seem to have a rather non-specific character, although they are relatively less frequent in the organic and endogenous states. Hysterical symptoms, next in order of frequency, show a sharper differentiation and are very rarely found in schizophrenic and manic-depressive syndromes. All these symptoms, with the exception of hypochondriasis, are shown by the psychopaths with a frequency considerably greater than the average. Paranoid symptoms are less frequently shown, most abundantly by the schizophrenics and psychopaths. The great rarity of obsessional symptoms will be noted. The only groups to show them with any frequency are the schizophrenics, the psychopaths, and the reactive depressives. In this point there is a sharp cleavage between the reactive and endogenous depressions. The association between obsessional personality traits and the occurrence of a depressive illness has already been shown in this material; and it may be that some of these reactive depressives with obsessional symptoms might have been as suitably diagnosed as cases of obsessional neurosis. Symptoms of a non-neurotic, i.e., psychotic or organic, nature are but rarely seen in the neurotic states, with the exception of the psychopaths. They are symptoms which one knows from clinical experience have a highly specific nature and great diagnostic value. Finally, the quality designated by the term "scrimshanking", i.e., the wilful exaggeration of symptoms and illness to secure some aim, such as invaliding from the army, is recorded as grossly obvious only in little more than 5 per cent of the patients, but with more than double that frequency in the hysterics and psychopaths. The interesting amnesic and dysmnesic symptoms have been dealt with in a previous communication (Sargant and Slater, 1941) [Paper 15].

TABLE 16.7. DURATION OF DISABILITY AND SYMPTOM SPECIFICITY

Diagnosis	Duration in months				Symptomatology (%)									
	under 1	1–6	6–24	over 24	Obsessional	Anxiety	Hysterical	Amnesia	Fits and faints	Mood change	Hypochondriacal	Paranoid	Organic and non-neurotic	Scrimshanking
1. Organic states	15.7	29.4	25.5	29.4	0.0*	21.6*	13.7*	7.8*	9.8	25.1*	17.6*	11.8	—	0.0*
2. Head injury	13.8	36.7	26.6	22.9	0.9*	38.5	26.6	—	13.8	33.9	56.9*	17.4	55.1*	1.8
3. Epilepsy	4.3*	18.6*	15.7*	61.7*	1.4	22.8*	21.4	18.6	—	27.1*	20.0*	14.3	32.9*	1.4
4. Schizophrenia	6.0*	34.0	34.0	26.0	8.0	20.0*	2.0*	14.0	4.0	38.0	24.0*	36.0*	—	0.0*
5. Endogenous depression	17.6	43.1	17.6	21.6	0.0*	35.3	2.0*	7.8*	2.0*	—	31.4	21.6	51.0*	0.0*
6. Mental defect	10.9	27.7*	27.7	33.6*	3.7	44.7	38.7*	11.7*	16.1*	38.7	38.0	11.7	16.1*	2.2*
7. Psychopathic personality	10.0	34.3	22.3	32.9*	7.2*	54.7*	46.8*	16.2	8.7	56.6*	40.0	30.6*	10.6	13.2*
8. Anxiety neurosis	15.9	42.3*	26.0	15.7*	1.7*	—	27.2	13.0*	4.8*	53.0*	40.3	11.4*	1.2*	2.5*
9. Hysteria	18.2	37.2	25.0	19.5	2.1	45.1	—	34.4*	13.1*	35.2*	49.0*	15.4	0.5*	13.3*
10. Reactive depression	15.8	42.1	25.4	16.7*	6.6*	42.6	19.7*	12.7*	2.6	—	43.4	14.9	5.3	2.6*
Total	14.4	37.2	25.0	23.4	3.2	43.7	27.9	19.1	7.4	45.0	40.9	16.4	9.8	5.7

* = significantly different from total percentage.

Statistical figures reflect the uniformity, but not the fluidity of the symptomatology in the neuroses. Apart from its dependence on the underlying personality, there was nothing fixed and stable in the clinical picture. A man admitted in a state in which anxiety symptoms were to the fore, might pass in the course of a week or two into one of listlessness, apathy and mild depression, or into one of dissociation with conversion symptoms or gross hysterical display. In general as the days passed and the patient settled into hospital, saved for the time being from the situation of stress, affective features tended to recede into the background and in their place hysterical aspects of the personality showed up for the first time; in the endeavour to remain in his asylum, the patient hollowly repeated complaints which had long lost their basis in feeling and reality, endeavoured to claim the sympathy of the doctor or became resentful and disgruntled and threw the blame for his failure on the shoulders of others. Experience constantly fortified the impression that symptoms in themselves are of secondary importance. They may indicate a line of approach and determine the immediate treatment but are of significance for progno-sis and ultimate disposal only in so far as they act as indicators of something more fundamental. An exception is to some extent provided by the depressives. In patients suffering from depression it might be only after some weeks that the nature of their illness became apparent, when attempts at therapeutic influence had failed to change their state. This was particularly likely to be observed where there was an endogenous factor in the illness which was not at first apparent. Most of these men took longer to get better than the average, and official restrictions on the possibility of convulsive treatment were a handicap.

TREATMENT

Analysis of the figures by the method of treatment employed has been done but the results are not of sufficient interest to publish. Nearly 60 per cent of the patients received no specific treatment other than that provided by the usual hospital routine, physical training, occupational therapy, etc., and perhaps a few short thera-peutic interviews. Psychotherapy of a rather more intensive degree was given in nearly a fifth of the patients (18.7 per cent), with especial frequency in the hysterics (36.2 per cent); only half as many (18.2 per cent) of the anxiety neurotics were so favoured. About 5 per cent of the anxiety neurotics received continuous narcosis, which was otherwise little employed, for the most part with the quick inrush of acutely ill patients after Dunkirk. But some form of specially directed sedation was of much more general use. Eighteen per cent of the schizophrenics were found fit for insulin coma treatment, a high figure considering the rather insidious nature of the illness in our patients. A modified form of insulin therapy (Sargant and Craske, 1941) was found useful as a form of physical rehabilitation in a wider variety of patients, particularly those who had undergone considerable loss of weight. Previous papers by Cameron (1940), Sargant and Slater (1940) and Debenham et al. (1941) have discussed the methods of treatment most generally used in dealing with these patients; but by and large they constituted a therapeutically unfavourable material. The possibilities of treatment were limited on the one hand by the frequency of a rather low intelligence and firmly anchored constitutional instability, on the other hand by working conditions. There was great pressure on beds and a rapid turnover. The time which the physician could spend with any one patient was very limited. The patients had every incentive not to improve, because thereby they might ensure escape from return to duty; and the concentration of large bodies of men of low morale in one hospital aided the spread of this attitude.

RESULTS

In only one tenth of the patients could complete recovery be obtained, but great improvement resulted in a further quarter. Complete recovery was most frequently seen in the endogenous depressives and in the hysterics, although it must be ad-mitted that in both groups it was symptomatic, and the fundamental constitution was left unaltered. Great improvement was as a rule the best that could be hoped for in the anxiety neurotics, even in the most recent and favourable; the continuing stresses of war, the threat of air-raids, etc., were sufficient, even if the patient was discharged to civilian life, to prevent the possibility of removing all anxiety feelings. Nevertheless, taking great improvement and recovery together, the anxiety neurotics and the depressives did better than the hysterics, who only score an average figure, all other diagnostic groups doing comparatively badly. It will be noted that the highest rates of return were obtained in the organic and head injury patients, in the anxiety neurotics, hysterics, and depressives, in that order; other groups showed a conspicuously low rate of return. Four per cent of the patients had to be transferred to other hospitals, though the figure is much higher in the schizophrenics and endogenous depressives, many of whom were too ill for treatment in our hospital and had to be removed to a neighbouring mental hospital. Nearly three quarters of the patients had to be invalided.

Follow-up records are available for 336 patients returned to duty, of whom approximately half later broke down again and had to be invalided any time from a few weeks or months to a year after discharge. The numbers are not big enough to provide significant differences in the individual groups, and for a detailed study of follow-up histories of neurotic soldiers the reader is referred to the paper by Lewis and Slater (1942). Later on in the history of the hospital, both the rate of return to duty and the follow-up statistics were greatly improved by new administrative arrangements for the Army as a whole. By this system it became possible to transfer a man from one unit to another on psychiatric grounds, to arrange his allotment to duties particularly suited to him, and to recommend him for a posting in the neighbourhood of his own home. At the time when the patients discussed here were discharged, they had either to go back to their own units to take pot luck in the duties that would be assigned to them, or to be boarded out of the army altogether.

TABLE 16.8. RESPONSE TO TREATMENT AND OUTCOME

	Improvement				Disposal			Follow-up		
	None	Slight	Great	Recovery	Returned to duty	Transfd.	Invalided	No.	Success	Failure
Diagnosis	%	%	%	%	%	%	%	Obsd.	%	%
1. Organic states	47.1*	25.5*	13.7*	13.7	30.6	8.2	61.2	11	36.4	63.4
2. Head injury	24.8	48.6	19.3	7.8	27.8	11.3	60.0	29	65.2	34.8
3. Epilepsy	54.3*	32.9	12.9*	0.0*	7.7*	4.6	87.7*	4	0.0	100.0
4. Schizophrenia	62.0*	22.0*	10.0*	6.0	8.3*	35.4*	56.2*	4	75.0	25.0
5. Endog. depression	21.6	35.3	27.5	15.7	22.9*	22.9	54.2*	9	66.7	33.3
6. Mental defect**	40.1*	43.1	10.9*	5.8	12.2*	4.1	83.7*	14	14.3	85.7
7. Psychopathic personality**	30.2*	45.7	18.2*	6.0*	10.0*	3.2	86.7*	23	34.8	65.2
8. Anxiety neurosis	14.6*	42.5	33.2*	9.7	26.5*	1.0*	72.5	122	52.5	47.5
9. Hysteria	17.7*	40.9	20.0*	15.4*	25.2	3.1	71.7	77	50.7	49.4
10. Reactive depression	16.6*	39.0	31.6	12.7	22.3	2.8	74.9	40	60.0	40.0
Total	23.5	41.2	25.2	10.0	21.5	4.3	74.1	336	50.3	49.7

* = significantly different from total percentage.

**Improvement and recovery are from presenting neurotic symptoms. The disposal figures in this table have suffered a systematic distortion, not now to be corrected; the rate of return was not 21.5 but 24.1 percent. This error, however, should have no effect on comparisons drawn between one diagnostic group and another.

These results in Table 16.8 are of course very disappointing. It seems that we are still very far from an effective, not to speak of a specific, method of treatment of the neuroses. The treatment of a neurotic patient resolves itself into two parts, the adjustment of the patient to his environment and the adjustment of the environment to the patient. That the latter is an effective method has been shown by our later results, when modification of the environment was possible along the lines outlined above. It is in the readaptation of the patient that psychiatric treatment breaks down. No matter what the main system of treatment employed, the results are always about the same. As Curran (1937) showed on a peace-time material, the results of a simple out-patient supervision are as good as those claimed by the exponents of intensive psychotherapy. And on a series of military neurotic patients very similar to ours, the results obtained at the 41st General (Neuropathic) Hospital, as reported by Hadfield (1942), by psychiatrists of strongly psychotherapeutic leanings are almost identical with ours — 20 per cent of men returned to the army, of whom 40 per cent broke down within three months. It would seem that what a man is by heredity and constitution is much more decisive for his future than any trifling alterations that can be brought about in him by psychotherapy and mental and physical rehabilitation.

THE DIAGNOSTIC GROUPS

We now come to consider the diagnostic groups as a whole. The main particulars in which the individual groups show significant deviations from the general average are illustrated in Table 16.9. We note that the organic syndromes score figures significantly lower than the average practically everywhere; they are constitutionally

TABLE 16.9. SIGNIFICANT ASSOCIATIONS BETWEEN PRECIPITATION BY STRESS, DIAGNOSIS AND OUTCOME, AND CLINICAL FEATURES

Diagnosis	Inhibited sex life	Poor intelligence	Bad early home life	Positive family history	Neurotic childhood	Previous nervous breakdown	Abnormal personality	Personality traits: Obsessional	Anxious	Hysterical	Unstable mood	Hypochondriacal	Paranoid	Impulsive	Unsociable	Anergic	No precipitation	Prolonged duration	Symptoms: Obsessional	Anxious	Hysterical	Depressive	Hypochondriacal	Paranoid	Specific
Military stress	−	−		−	−	−	−			−	−						−	−	−	−	+	+		−		−
Organic syndromes	−	−	−	−	−	−	−		−	−	−	−				−	−			−	−	−			+
Mental defect	+	+			−		−			−						−	+	+			+				+
Endogenous states																									
Epileptic		+			−		+	−		−	−		−		+		+	+	−			−	−		+
Schizophrenic						+	+	+		−		+		+	+		+			−	−			−	+
Affective	−			−	+	+		+	−	−	+						−					+			+
Reactive states																									
Depressive	−					+			−	+					−			−	+		−	+			
Anxious		+						+	−						−		−	−	−	+		+	+	−	−
Hysterical	+					−			+	−					−					+	−	+		−	−
Psychopathic personality	+		+	+	+		+	+	+	+	+	+	+	+	+	+	+	+	+	+	+	+		+	
Bad outcome		+	+	+	+		+	+	+				+				+	+	+	+				+	

a much more normal population, have less in the way of neurotic traits of personality and correspondingly less in neurotic symptomatology, but are on the other hand liable to their own specific symptoms. The same is to a lesser extent true of the epileptics, the mental defectives, the schizophrenics and the endogenous depressives, as far as neurosis is concerned. The mental defectives show an increased liability to hysteria, and they and the psychopaths are the only groups to show a special liability to a generally impoverished sexual life. The schizophrenics tend to be abnormal personalities, with marked tendencies towards a paranoid and unsociable attitude, but on the other hand show an absence of hysterical traits of personality and of neurotic symptomatology when ill. Relative freedom from constitutional hysterical tendencies also distinguished the anxiety neurotics, who show otherwise most importantly an association with illness of definite exogenic precipitation and of short duration. The hysterics show a positive association with subnormal intelligence, a negative association with obsessional traits of personality and instability of mood; when ill they tend to hypochondriasis and somatic fixation of symptoms. Persons diagnosed as psychopaths show a markedly increased liability to every sort of abnormal manifestation, with the few exceptions of poor intelligence, repeated breakdown, obsessional and hypochondriacal tendencies.

The endogenous and the reactive depressives are worth somewhat closer examination, particularly as there is frequent discussion on whether they should not be considered quantitatively different manifestations of what is fundamentally the same syndrome. We note that both groups show a negative association with poor intelligence and hysterical traits, a positive association with obsessional tendencies. On the other hand, whereas more than half the endogenous depressives were of pyknic constitution, reactive depressives showed this type of bodily habitus with hardly more than average frequency; childhood neurosis is rare in the endogenous depressives, of almost average frequency in the reactive group. When all the tables are gone through it will be found that the figures provided by the endogenous depressives do not occupy an intermediate position in among the figures provided by the reactive depressives, the anxiety neurotics and the hysterics, but rather lie at one extreme, now one and now another of the neurotic groups approaching them most closely. The question of the existence of a real difference can be put to a specific test, which yields a decisive result in its favour.

I have taken the records of 94 endogenous depressives, all that were accessible and sufficiently complete, and of 254 reactive depressives, and examined the frequencies of association of childhood neurosis, previous nervous breakdown, anxious and anergic traits of personality and pyknic habitus. If previous nervous breakdown and pyknic habitus can be regarded as "endogenous" signs, and the others as "reactive" signs, the findings can be divided into three groups: (1) endogenous outnumber reactive signs, 57 endogenous depressives, 54 reactive depressives; (2) endogenous and reactive signs are present in equal number, 31 and 104; (3) endogenous are outnumbered by reactive signs, 6 and 96. The χ^2 of this distribution is 57.4, indicating that the two groups certainly cannot be regarded as different samples of the same population. If it is not regarded as admissible to take any account of previous nervous breakdown, as a criterion which may have been used diagnostically, the frequencies in the three groups become: (1) 25, 31; (2) 52, 109; (3) 17, 114. The χ^2 of this distribution is 24.21, which is still far beyond even a 0.001 level of probability for two degrees of freedom.

BOARDING CATEGORY

Analysis by results is usually a most profitable method of attack. Unfortunately in this material analysis by follow-up record did not provide figures of interest, as the numbers in individual groupings were too small to give statistically significant differences. In any case a detailed attack along these lines has already been published (Lewis and Slater, 1942). Larger numbers were available for analysis by boarding category, i.e., mode of disposal. Nonconformity of confession, non-commissioned rank, normal childhood history, good school record, previous army service, satisfactory home life, breakdown occurring under military stress or with other adequate precipitation or with head injury, short duration of illness and treatment by psychotherapy are associated with a better than average chance of return to duty as shown in Table 16.10; whereas the opposite was true of asthenic habitus, positive family history, neurosis in childhood, certain abnormal personality traits, poor intelligence, unsatisfactory home circumstances, and a duration of illness exceeding two years.

It can justifiably be contended that the mode of disposal reflects rather the factors that influence the clinician than those that actually are of prognostic signifi-

TABLE 16.10. PERCENTAGE OF MEN RETURNED TO DUTY

	Better than average	Worse than average
General average	24.1	
Religion:		
Nonconformists	32.8	—
Rank:		
Non-commissioned officers	37.3	—
Habitus:		
Asthenic	—	18.7
Positive family history	—	19.6
Childhood:		
Neurotic	—	12.4
Normal	38.9	—
Personality:		
Abnormal	—	13.9
Traits:		
Obsessional	—	18.1
Anxious	—	15.2
Paranoid	—	16.5
Anergic	—	15.7
School record:		
Poor	—	18.7
Good	34.1	—
Poor intelligence	—	17.6
Previous army service	29.9	—
Bad early home life	—	15.7
Bad relationship to father	—	14.7
Present home life:		
Unsatisfactory	—	16.9
Satisfactory	28.1	—
Precipitation:		
Positive	31.4	—
Severe military stress	33.1	—
Head injury	30.7	—
Duration:		
Over 24 months	—	14.9
Less than 1 month	47.2	—
Symptoms:		
Obsessional	—	13.6
Treatment:		
Psychotherapy	39.5	—

In this table only significant differences are recorded.

cance. Such a criticism can, however, be pressed too far. The clinician judges a man on total impressions, rather than on items of information. Such a quality as, for instance, Nonconformist persuasion must correspond to an aspect of character and not be in itself a factor that influences a clinical view in any direction whatsoever. The fact that Nonconformists were returned to duty with a frequency significantly greater than the average is fairly surely due to a greater frequency among them of a type of personality that takes religion, and probably also personal and social duties, more seriously than the average man, and is perhaps more imbued with a degree of conscientiousness and dourness of personality. In the same way it is very unlikely that the occurrence of head injury at some time in the history has operated with clinicians as an indication of suitability of return to duty. Its association with a high rate of return is probably because in the presence of an organic factor there need not be the same degree of constitutional instability to bring about breakdown, and it is the clinical impression of the underlying instability that decides disposal.

It is of interest that patients treated by psychotherapy were more frequently returned to the army than others. *Post hoc sed non propter hoc.* The good rate of return is more likely to be connected with the type of patient chosen for psychotherapy than with the effects of the treatment itself. Very few would be chosen for psychotherapy who obviously had no chance of return to the army; this would not apply to other, less time-consuming methods.

The only other exogenic factor of prognostic importance is the circumstances of home life. It was frequently found that if there were difficulties or sources of worry here it was almost impossible to rid the patient of the notion that he would be better at home to look after affairs himself; only in rare cases was it possible to clear up the unfavourable home situation from the hospital. The nature of these home worries was seldom financial; illness of a relative, often the obviously neurotic illness of the wife, was more frequent. Other usual worries were damage to the home in air-raids and resulting dislocation of home life, and fears on the part of the soldier that his wife was being unfaithful to him.

In general, the factors which seem to be associated with eventual disposal are constitutional ones. Neurotic childhood, obsessional symptoms, abnormal personality are of particularly bad omen. It was possible to return to the army more than three times as many patients with normal childhood history as those with a neurotic childhood. Nearly half the patients whose illness had lasted less than a month could be returned to duty; where the illness had lasted longer than 24 months, only a seventh. The favourable and unfavourable features recorded here are very similar to those noted as of prognostic significance in a follow-up study of soldiers returned to duty. Lewis and Slater (1942) found that positive family history, unsatisfactory work record, psychopathic traits of personality, long duration of symptoms, lack of definite precipitating factor, resentment of army life, a paranoid attitude, querulous hypochondriasis, and the occurrence of fugue or amnesia, were all associated with an unfavourable follow-up history. This indicates that on the whole the actual symptoms manifested are of less prognostic significance than the indications of constitutional instability.

MILITARY STRESS

Table 16.11 classifies the patients into three groups of graded resistiveness to psychological and physical stress, and the usual signs of constitutional abnormality are associated with the least degree of resistance. It is a striking thing how the frequencies of different findings in the three groups make a graduated scale, severe, moderate and trifling degrees of stress balancing mild, moderate and severe degrees of constitutional abnormality. The relationship is clearly a quantitative one. Certain other points of interest also appear.

TABLE 16.11. MILITARY STRESS UNDERGONE

	Severe %	Moderate %	Trifling %
Number recorded	386	368	950
Occupation:			
Semi-skilled	44.3	43.8	35.6
Sedentary	14.0	16.6	21.3
Rank:			
N.C.O.'s	24.1	21.7	16.7
Habitus:			
Asthenic	37.5	41.9	54.9
Athletic	33.5	33.8	25.2
Pyknic	29.0	24.2	19.8
Inhibited sex life	33.1	34.6	47.8
Positive family history	45.1	56.0	57.2
Neurotic childhood	14.8	24.7	28.4
Previous nervous breakdown	16.6	23.4	25.6
Abnormal personality	33.9	42.4	48.9
Personality traits:			
Depressive	29.2	33.2	34.8
Hypochondriacal	3.6	7.6	8.0
Unsociable	26.4	26.6	33.8
Anergic	14.2	24.2	26.1
School record:			
Poor	19.9	26.1	32.0
Intelligence:			
Poor	25.0	28.1	38.8
Average	67.2	62.0	50.6
Good	7.8	9.9	10.5
Previous army service	53.9	44.6	31.7
Previous war service	17.4	12.8	11.6
Unsatisfactory home life	10.6	13.0	14.9
Symptoms:			
Obsessional	2.3	3.5	4.0
Anxiety	80.8	73.4	46.4
Hysteria	47.4	38.3	35.3
Amnesia	31.3	16.6	16.2
Hypochondriacal	37.6	35.6	44.4
Scrimshanking	3.4	4.9	18.6
Treatment:			
Non-specific	30.2	52.1	64.8
Physical measures	43.9	30.1	16.3
Psychotherapy	25.9	17.8	18.9
Result:			
Slight or no improvement	46.3	52.5	72.4
Great improvement	38.0	38.1	18.5
Recovery	15.8	9.4	9.1

Observations all show a significant difference between two at least of the groups.

The relationship of intelligence to stress needed for breakdown, and to outcome (Table 16.11), is peculiar. In the group of men who broke down under severe stress there is a preponderance of persons of average intelligence, whereas men of poor and of superior intelligence show a relative concentration in the no-stress group. Similarly men of the semi-skilled occupations broke down most frequently under severe stress, those of sedentary occupations under trifling stress. From Table 16.10 it can be seen that a poor school record and poor intelligence are unfavourable factors; a good school record is a favourable factor, but not superior intelligence. The interpretation seems to be that men of substantially better than average intelligence are not likely to be happily placed in the ranks, unless employed in a specialist capacity, or otherwise doing more intelligent work than falls to the lot of the ranker or even the lower grades of N.C.O. At the time when these patients were being dealt with there did not yet exist facilities for dealing with these "round pegs in square holes."

Interesting differences in symptomatology show themselves in the three groups of Table 16.11. Obsessional and hypochondriacal symptoms and the tendency to scrimshanking are found for preference in the no-stress group; military stress has a special tendency to produce anxiety symptoms, hysteria, and particularly amnesia. More active forms of therapy were necessary in the stress groups, and a better rate of return to duty was obtained; we are not in a position to know whether this better result was maintained on follow-up.

The men who went through severe stress represent a selection for greater constitutional stability, but the signs of a neurotic make-up are still to be found (e.g., 45 per cent had a positive family history). They had nearly all been involved in fighting and aerial bombardment in France, and had gone through a long retreat with prolonged physical exertion before reaching the beaches in the neighbourhood of Dunkirk. But only about half of them were admitted to this hospital immediately or shortly after this experience, and the rest dribbled into the wards through the succeeding months, some over a year later, having tried in the interval to carry on in their units under difficulties. These later cases proved difficult to treat and could seldom be returned to duty. By the time of their admission, their unpleasant symptoms had become so firmly connected in their minds with their life in the Army that treatment to be successful was hardly possible without a hopeful prospect of invaliding in view. These "conditioning" mechanisms were very frequent in our patients, but were not easily subjected to statistical analysis.

THE STRUCTURE OF THE NEUROSES

Table 16.9 represents in a highly compressed form the main results of our investigation. We note that the organic syndromes score figures significantly less than the average with great regularity, and in this respect show a parallel with states precipitated by military stress. This is presumably because both groups correspond more nearly than the average of our material to a normal, i.e., healthy, population, in the extent to which they are burdened with the signs of constitutional predisposition. At the other end of the table will be found the psychopaths and the patients whose illness had a bad eventual outcome, either in invaliding or a later repeated breakdown; both these groups show figures significantly greater than the average. They represent therefore the other extreme of greatest abnormality. These two associations provide ground for the hypothesis that the tendency towards failure and breakdown has to be regarded quantitatively. In some persons, though it exists, it is small and needs considerable stress for its manifestation; in others it is stronger, is manifested on slight stress, and is not so readily susceptible to treatment or manipulation of the environment.

Organic, endogenous, and neurotic states offer contrasts one with another. An organic disability depends on the nature, severity and site of incidence of the exogenic factor; its primary effects are to a large extent independent of the individual constitution. On the basis of the organic injury there may then be added a neurotic disability, whose nature will be largely predictable from knowledge of the constitution, gathered from previous and family history. But the organic and the neurotic symptoms will be clinically distinguishable one from another. Further, the organic injury may itself predispose to neurosis, which will occur in its presence with a lesser intensity of constitutional instability than otherwise necessary. In the endogenous states (schizophrenia, cyclothymia, idiopathic epilepsy, obsessional "neurosis"), the hereditary disposition is all-important; the manifest state does not occur in its absence, and none or only non-specific stimuli may be needed for its release. As with the organic states, neurotic features may be added but will be clinically distinguishable from the specific symptoms of the primary condition.

The neuroses and psychopathies show a more fluid state of affairs. The form of the exogenous stress is more important than in the endogenous states (e.g., military stress — anxiety), but far less so than in the organic states. But the form of the reaction is still principally determined by constitutional predisposition, and there are strong correlations between the make-up of the personality and the symptoms exhibited (see under). There are only a limited number of main types of reaction available — anxiety, hysteria, depression, hypochondriasis, etc. — and if neurotic breakdown occurs, it will be along one of these lines, or more than one simultaneously. In the neurotic states there are no symptoms that compare in specificity with the retardation or the phasic change of mood of the manic-depressive, with the primary delusion or the thought disorder of the schizophrenic, or the neurological manifestations of the epileptic. Whereas endogenous states, once initiated, run their course largely independently of environmental influences (other than such deeply reaching ones as insulin coma, convulsion and leucotomy), the neurotic states are comparatively readily reversible and recur as readily as they are relieved. The neurotic states appear indeed to be forms of behaviour, frequently mere exacerbations of a type of response characteristic of the individual.

It is of interest here to enquire into the degree of association of particular personality traits with their corresponding symptoms. Taking a random group of 400 of our case-records, the following tetrachoric correlation coefficients have been calculated.[3]

1. Obsessional. — *Trait:* Over-conscientiousness, caution, tendencies to doubt and re-checking, pernickety orderliness, devotion to duty, rigidity and unadaptability, etc. *Symptom:* Compulsive thoughts or actions, with insight, and resisted by the personality. $r = +0.76$

2. Hysterical. — *Trait:* Egocentricity, emotional dependence on others, excitability, superficial emotionality, self-satisfaction, demonstrativeness, desire for attention, vanity, love of show, etc. *Symptom:* Conversion symptoms, or a markedly hysterical attitude to the illness. $r = +0.51$

3. Paranoid. — *Trait:* Sensitiveness to imagined hostility, tendency to resentment and disgruntlement, self-consciousness, suspiciousness, etc. *Symptom:* Suspicion of or hostility to physician, ideas of reference or delusions. $r = +0.50$

[3] I am indebted to my brother, Patrick Slater, for much valuable advice on the statistical methods employed from here on.

4. Anxious. — *Trait:* Inferiority feelings, self-distrustfulness, fear of trouble, timidity, ready embarrassment, tendency to worry, etc. *Symptom:* Somatic anxiety, tremor, palpitation, tachycardia, sweating, tension, nightmares, prevailing mood of fear, etc.   r = +0.40

5. Depressive. — *Trait:* Ready pessimism or elation on trifling cause, moodiness, tendency for an upset in mood to persist unduly, etc. *Symptom:* Observed mood change of considerable duration.   r = +0.39

6. Hypochondriacal. — *Trait:* Preoccupation with bodily health, with bowel regularity, interest in physical exercises and get-fit schemes, fondness for patent medicines, etc. *Symptom:* Tendency towards somatic localisation of symptom and preoccupation with physical aspect of illness.   r = +0.19

These findings indicate that of all neurotic symptoms obsessional symptoms are most firmly rooted in a basis of specific predisposition, the next in order being hysterical and paranoid symptomatology. Depressive and anxious symptoms are distinctly less closely related to the endogenous predisposition, and hypochondriasis, at least as here defined, least of all. It is true that the constitutional disposition can nowhere be excluded, and its importance in anxiety and depressive states of all kinds is considerable. But hypochondriacal, depressive and anxious symptoms seem to be of all neurotic symptoms those most directly related to exogenic factors and those which can be most reasonably regarded as a general human weakness. The finding agrees with our preconceptions; under certain circumstances it would be abnormal not to be afraid, or depressed, or somewhat preoccupied with bodily processes.

It is to be admitted that this account of the structure of the neuroses leaves important factors out of the picture and provides a very inadequate theory for developmental purposes. It seems fairly clear that processes resembling conditioning occur in man as well as in experimental animals, and that neurotic states have their own dynamics. Our experience suggests that in the predisposed individual such reactive dispositions can be established with great rapidity. A man's experience of dive-bombing did not have to be very prolonged for the association in his mind of certain types of noise and a fear-producing situation to become firmly fixed; and for a long time after similar sounds, though recognized as harmless, would continue to produce the physiological and mental changes typical of fear. The disposition once established was difficult to break up, and even when it had apparently passed off was easily re-established. If this effect can occur so easily in the adult, there is plausibility in the view that the plastic mind of the child is even more susceptible.

The hypothesis presented here is, then, that neurosis represents a special case of a generalized type of behaviour, and signifies a failure of adaptation. The two primary reagents are the individual constitution and the environmental set-up of the moment. The individual constitution is in greater part determined by hereditary factors, to a lesser degree by environmental circumstances of the past producing their effects by organic lesion and psychological and physiological conditioning. These factors, especially the first, determine the form and the severity of the congeries of symptoms, which are the so-called neurotic states or neuroses. The momentary environment determines the time of manifestation, and to a lesser extent the severity and even the form of the symptoms (e.g., the association of military stress and anxiety). Other factors, such as physical illness or physiological upset and intellectual incapacity, can have an adjuvant effect, and may also influence the form of the reaction (e.g., mental defect in favouring hysterical manifestations, physical illness in favouring hypochondriasis).

213

On this view obsessional neurosis should be excluded from the other neuroses as more closely resembling in nature the endogenous psychoses. The syndrome called "psychopathic personality," on the other hand, though no doubt it includes types of abnormality of personality closely related to the psychoses, is otherwise an extremer form of the neurotic constitution, in which socially obnoxious or partially incapacitating symptoms are exhibited at all times, even when there is no perceptible degree of stress in the environment. There is little to be said for the convention by which certain traits, such as aggressiveness and asocial tendencies, are regarded as psychopathic, whereas tendencies towards anxiety, instability of mood, dissociation, etc., are regarded as neurotic. If we wish to introduce system and reason into our nomenclature it will be necessary to discover further traits showing the degree of specificity and independence that obsessionality seems to show, to work out their degree of specificity and independence from or association with other such traits, and then to rank personalities both horizontally and vertically by the specific traits they show and the degree to which they show them. The clinically convenient distinction as to whether an individual is subjectively and objectively ill or not appears to be only a crude quantitative measure, and of secondary biological importance.

We can now attempt a check on theory by observed fact. Positive family history, childhood neurosis, poor work record, repetition of nervous breakdown, abnormal personality make-up judged clinically, poor intelligence, are severally independent observations, touch different aspects of the life of the individual, have been shown to have relevance to outcome and prognosis, and can be taken as crude measures of the neurotic constitution and inadequate intellectual endowment. Neurotic constitution and inadequate intellectual endowment are held to be the two most important predisposing factors for the manifestation of neurotic breakdown. The frequencies of association in one and the same patient of these several observations have been counted in 1,600 records (i.e., omitting 400 records blemished by too many queries or unanswered questions), and the corresponding tetrachoric correlation coefficients are listed in Table 16.12.

TABLE 16.12. CORRELATIONS BETWEEN NEUROTIC CONSTITUTION AND
NEUROTIC BREAKDOWN

Diagnosis	Correlation coefficients						Factor loadings	
	1	2	3	4	5	6	Neurotic constitution	Inadequate intelligence
1. Positive family history		0.4521	0.1874	0.1716	0.4304	0.1368	0.5928	−0.0534
2. Childhood neurosis	0.0613		0.2870	0.0961	0.5644	0.1487	0.6617	0.0284
3. Poor work record	0.0375	0.0155		0.1212	0.4587	0.4061	0.4321	0.5857
4. Previous nervous breakdown	0.0302	−0.0542	0.0714		0.2245	−0.0578	0.2308	−0.0853
5. Abnormal personality	−0.0472	0.0215	0.0408	0.0458		0.1482	0.8157	0.1119
6. Poor intelligence	0.0816	0.0439	−0.0593	−0.0477	−0.0187		0.1374	0.4908

Observed correlation coefficients are given to the top and to the right; second residuals, after partialling out the first and second factor loadings, to the bottom and to the left.

From this table it can be calculated that 91.7 per cent of the total variance in the common factor space can be accounted for by the first factor loadings on 1–6

214

and the second factor loadings on 3 and 6; i.e., our double hypothesis of a neurotic constitution and poor intelligence as the main cause of the observations recorded accounts for all but 9.3 per cent of our observations. Within the limits of the statistical method employed and of the errors, which are probably considerable, of our original observations, this must be regarded as satisfactory agreement.

In Table 16.12 the factor loadings, which when multiplied by one another provide the individual correlation coefficients, indicate the extent to which the various findings are good tests of the underlying constitution. The best indicators of the neurotic constitution are, in order, clinically abnormal personality, neurosis in childhood, positive family history, poor work record; repeated nervous breakdown, a quality associated particularly with cyclothymia, and poor intelligence show but low correlations. A poor work record and poor intelligence as judged clinically are good tests of inadequate intelligence, but the other observations are no measures at all. Poor work record is, then, a good test of both types of inadequacy and should obviously have considerable attention paid to it clinically. The finding of greatest theoretical importance brought out by the table is that neurotic constitution and inadequate intelligence operate independently, and are clearly aetiological factors in their own right.

The neurotic constitution is then a useful hypothesis, and one which ranks with inadequate intelligence in accounting for social insufficiency, breakdown, and impairment of efficiency for military duties. It is interesting to compare these two biological handicaps one with the other. We know that intelligence is practically solely determined by genetic factors; our evidence suggests that the same may be true of the neurotic constitution. We know that the genetic determinants of intelligence must be numerous, and that they operate cumulatively, so that in a random sample of the community rated by measures of intelligence one finds a normal curve of frequency. There is no reason to think that the same would not be true of temperamental qualities, were we able to develop independent psychometric tests of the intensity of neurotic tendencies. It is clear that people can be more and less neurotic as they can be more and less intelligent. But there is an important practical difference. For whereas differences of degree of intelligence are much more striking than differences of quality, the opposite is true of neurosis, when we are more struck by differences of quality than of degree. Qualitative differences of intelligence and quantitative differences in neurosis have so far received little attention; the time will come when attack will have to be made along both these lines.

17

A HEURISTIC THEORY OF NEUROSIS

INTRODUCTION

In a recent communication (Slater, E., 24[1]), based on a statistical survey of two thousand neurotic soldiers, a hypothesis was developed to the effect that there was a generalized predisposition towards neurosis, which was in large part responsible for the appearance of neurotic symptoms in the individual when placed under stress. Evidence was adduced that this constitutional tendency, though it might be affected by such environmental factors as early processes of conditioning, was, at least in part, dependent on hereditary factors. Evidence was also brought that it could usefully be considered in a quantitative manner, and that so considered the intensity of the constitutional predisposition varied inversely with the degree of stress under which the individual was placed before breakdown occurred, i.e., the greater the intensity of the constitutional predisposition, the less was the degree of stress required to produce breakdown, and *vice versa*.

On this last point, strong confirmatory evidence has recently been supplied by Symonds (1943). He states "the incidence of neurosis in different tactical duties varies directly with the amount of hazard encountered, as measured by the casualty rates." He also provides a table correlating the degree of predisposition with the degree of stress in 2,200 neurotic casualties, which shows that the degree of flying stress falls steadily as predisposition increases. From his table a correlation coefficient between the two variables of -0.26 ± 0.02 can be calculated.

In the paper referred to no very detailed analysis of the nature of the neurotic predisposition was undertaken. Yet the frequency of various traits of personality

By Eliot Slater and Patrick Slater. Originally published in the *Journal of Neurology and Psychiatry* 7: 49–55 (1944).

[1] Paper 16 in this volume.

was shown to vary significantly in the several diagnostic groups, and significant and fairly high correlations were found between personality traits and eventual symptomatology. There was, therefore, evidence of constitutional heterogeneity in the population investigated. On the other hand all the neurotic personality traits were noted as being at least sometimes present in all the diagnostic groups, and the same was true of all the classes of symptoms observed, with the exception of obsessional compulsive symptoms and psychotic and organic symptoms. This means in effect that the different neurotic groups fade off into one another clinically, and do not form qualitatively distinct groups. This observation is one with which every clinician is in practice familiar.

This, then, is the starting point of the argument which is developed in the following pages. It is our purpose to reduce the hypothesis already propounded to precise terms which may be handled statistically, and made the basis of predictions which can be checked by further observations. What is involved is, in fact, a general theory of the nature of the neurotic constitution.

POSSIBLE THEORIES

The various theories which may be advanced to account for the phenomena of the neuroses seem capable of being divided into three classes. By the first of these, neurotic phenomena are regarded as a type of response to which all human beings are equally liable, such as, for instance, the general tendency to respond with fever to the occurrence of an infection. Differences between individuals would then be related solely, or at least to a preponderant extent, to environmental effects. This theory has been very commonly, even if implicitly, held in the past; but it has of late been found inadequate. If this were an adequate explanation of the phenomena we have to discuss we would expect, as indeed we find, that the intensity of the stress under which an individual was placed would be directly related to the frequency of nervous breakdown. But we would in addition expect to find a direct relationship, both qualitative and quantitative, between the type and intensity of the stress and the type and severity of the breakdown. This is true only to the most limited extent. In the survey referred to there was evidence that the terrifying stresses of war tended to provoke anxiety states to a significantly preferential extent, but they did so far from regularly. A more important determinant of the type of response was the constitution of the individual as shown by his family history, previous life, and personality. This theory, in fact, breaks down by not taking into account or explaining in any way the very large amount of evidence of the existence of constitutional differences between individuals in these respects, and especially of their genetic aspects. It would leave unexplained the results of investigations of personality differences and similarities in binovular and uniovular twins (Kranz, 1936; Lange, 1929; Newman, Freeman, and Holzinger, 1937; Stumpfl, 1936; etc.), and the evidence of the familial incidence of neuroses and psychopathy (von Baeyer, 1935; Berlit, 1931; Brown, 1942; Brugger, 1935; Curran and Mallinson, 1940; Gebbing, 1932; Kolle, 1932; Kraulis, 1931; Lewis, 1936; Pohlisch, 1934; Riedel, 1937; Ritter, 1937; Schröder, 1939; Slater, E., 24; etc.). In so far as early environmental differences might help to explain individual differences in disposition in later life, one would expect to find an association between the occurrence of neurosis and place in order of birth; the evidence is against this (Brown, 1942; Slater, E., 25). This theory must by rejected.

The second theory that engages our attention is that the neurotic constitution is of a unitary kind, but dependent on genetic factors. It is possible to consider this theory in two forms. By the first, the genetic basis would lie in a single abnormal gene, whose variations in expression could be accounted for by environmental differences and by differences in genetic modifying factors, the so-called genotypic milieu. Theories of this type provide a sufficient account of the relevant data in such psychiatric conditions as phenylpyruvic amentia (Jervis, 1939), juvenile amaurotic idiocy (Sjögren, 1931; Jervis, 1941), gargoylism (Halperin and Curtis, 1942), oxycephaly (Ferriman, 1941), epiloia (Gunther and Penrose, 1935), Huntington's chorea (Sjögren, 1935), cerebral dysrhythmia and epilepsy (Lennox, Gibbs, and Gibbs, 1939, 1940, 1942), manic-depressive psychoses (Kallmann, 1941; Slater, E., 4, 10), schizophrenia (Kallmann, 1938; Kallmann, 1941; Koller, 1939; Lenz, 1937; Luxenburger, 1937; Patzig, 1937; etc.). In all these conditions findings are made which are believed to be specific for the condition in question; and it is worth remarking that similar investigations of neurosis and psychopathy have not resulted in comparable findings. On the basis of the theory, transitional forms between the normal and abnormal may occur, but will either be relatively infrequent, or will be capable of resolution with more refined examination into character-bearers and normals. Where this is only doubtful, as, for instance, in manic-depressive psychosis, some doubt is thrown on the postulation of a single gene. If a single abnormal gene were postulated as the basis of neurosis, necessary consequences would be that neurotics would prove to be relatively homogeneous, and would show some highly discriminant characteristic which would differentiate them with fair certainty from the average population. As will later be shown, the evidence is against homogeneity, and no single discriminant characteristic has so far been discovered.

The alternative form of the second theory is that the neurotic predisposition, though still regarded as unitary, is dependent on a large number of separate genes of small but similar effect. This postulation would allow us to explain quantitative variation in the intensity of the neurotic predisposition, and would also permit the inclusion of neurotics within the limits of range of the general population. The outstanding example of a finding which is accounted for in this way is the distribution of intelligence in the general population. Fraser Roberts (1941), describing the situation, writes:

> General intelligence, in this sense, is a graded character and displays continuous variation from one extreme to the other . . . Over the great bulk of the range there is no discontinuity . . . A frequency curve is found to conform to the normal form. But at the extreme ends of the distribution, most certainly at one end, we find variations which are no longer continuous, and the curve is no longer normal . . . Without discontinuity anywhere we pass from the brilliant to the superior, the average, the dull, the very backward, and finally to the mentally defective. At the very lowest levels, however, we find not merely the very backward; we find gross deviations, the idiots, and the imbeciles . . . This portion of the curve is far from normal, for such individuals are far too numerous. The distinction, on the basis of measurement only, is not absolute . . . (but) is fundamental genetically . . . We have, on the one hand, multifactor inheritance, on the other hand, the transmission of single genes; on the one hand, the genes of individually small effect, on the other, the gene whose bearer is sharply distinguished from the rest of his fellows . . . It is not impossible to mark approximately the line of division between the two types of mental defective. On the Binet scale it may be drawn roughly at an I.Q. of about 45 . . . Feeble-minded persons must be regarded as abnormal, but this is probably true only against the background of our present complex civilization. They are merely the extreme minus end of the normal distribution of intelligence.

This theory is still capable of explaining all the important genetic data on mental defect, and long occupied a prominent position in the field of psychometric psychology. Hart and Spearman (1912) put forward the view that all mental processes belonged to a single class, and that the interrelations of all tests used to measure them could be accounted for in terms of a single common factor, g. More recently, however, this theory has been shown to be inadequate, and even when only cognitive tests are used, most tables of results indicate the operation of more than one common factor. A continuous variation from brilliance to defect is found in adequately measurable cognitive abilities other than intelligence (such as spatial judgment), and frequency distributions are of the normal form. Methods of assessing variations in temperamental characteristics have not been carried far enough at present to provide critical evidence, but there is no reason to suppose that the frequency distributions depart from normal. Thus the distribution of psychological characteristics is currently supposed to be of the multivariate normal form.

A necessary consequence of the unitary theory is the homogeneity of selected samples. If adding and subtracting depend on the same ability, men who add equally well are not likely to differ greatly in ability to subtract. Similarly if the neurotic predisposition is a unitary trait, variations in characteristics which differentiate neurotics from normals will be smaller among neurotics, who form a selected sample, than among an unselected normal population. The presence or absence of homogeneity among neurotic subjects is therefore a matter of crucial importance; if it fails to hold, as Roberts points out is the case in the lowest reaches of mental defect, the theory breaks down, and supplementary hypotheses have to be made.

But the heterogeneity of the neuroses is, actually, a commonplace of clinical experience. If it did not exist, we should not be tempted to diagnose one man as a hysteric, another as an anxiety neurotic, and a third as a depressive. In respect of purely qualitative findings the statistics already provided (Slater, E., 24) may be relied on. Further data of a quantitative and therefore more precise kind will be adduced later on. It is sufficient to state here that the evidence on this point is, in our opinion, sufficient to render the unitary hypothesis of the neurotic constitution unlikely and not suitable for use as a weapon of research.

We come, therefore, to the third of the possible hypotheses of the nature of the neurotic constitution. By this theory the constitutional basis of neurosis is still held to be, in part at least, genetic in nature, but due to the operation of factors not all of similar effect. This theory again may be presented in two forms. In the first of these the several genetic factors would be supposed to be each in itself sufficient, at least under suitable environmental circumstances, for the production of a neurosis, the type of the neurosis depending on the gene responsible.

Neurosis would then become a congeries of qualitatively distinct syndromes. With adequate knowledge of the differentiae of neurotics, we would be able to sort them out from the remainder of the population, who would be immune to neurosis; we would also be able to sort out the neurotics into their various classes. In the family histories of neurotics, we would expect to find that the specific forms of neurosis characteristic of the propositi occur with exceptional frequency, but that other forms of neurosis occur with no greater frequency than in the general population. We would also expect that the frequency with which neurotic abnormalities occur would bear no necessary relation to the extent to which these abnormalities deviate from the norms of the general population. The available evidence is against these expectations. Persistent search for characteristics which will clearly discriminate between different types of neurotics and between them and normals has so far proved fruitless. Not only specific, but also non-specific forms of neurosis are commoner among the relatives of neurotic propositi than in a control group. To substantiate this last point we may quote the evidence provided by Brown (1942).

This observer investigated the frequency of various types of psychiatric abnormality among the parents and sibs over the age of fifteen of different groups of neurotic propositi. From the data provided by him Table 17.1 can be constructed:

TABLE 17.1. PSYCHIATRIC ABNORMALITIES IN RELATIVES OF NEUROTICS
(After Brown, 1942)

Numbers of	Among Parents and Sibs of			
	Anxiety Neurotics	Hysterics	Obsessionals	Controls
Anxiety neurotics	55	7	3	—
Hysterics	7	12	—	2
Obsessionals	2	—	7	—
Depressives	9	—	4	—
Abnormal personalities	60	10	24	19
Other psychiatric abnormalities	22	9	2	4
Normal	199	69	56	160
Totals	354	107	96	185

We may observe, among the relatives of the three groups of propositi, the incidence of the non-specific anomalies, i.e., everything but anxiety neurosis among the relatives of the anxiety neurotics, everything but hysteria among the relatives of the hysterics, etc., and compare them with the corresponding incidences in the control group. In this way we obtain the figures in Table 17.2.

TABLE 17.2. COMPARISON OF NON-SPECIFIC ANOMALIES IN
RELATIVES VS. CONTROLS

	χ^2	Degrees of freedom	Probability
Anxiety group	26.363	5	$<.01$
Hysterical group	22.249	3	$<.01$
Obsessional group	30.418	5	$<.01$
Totals	79.030	13	$<.01$

In other words it may be asserted with a high degree of certainty that the relatives of all three neurotic groups of propositi distinguish themselves from normals by an excessive liability to other psychiatric abnormalities than the specific ones in question.

We are therefore led to consider an alternative form of the third hypothesis. According to this, the genetic determinants which produce a neurotic constitution are generally non-specific and additive in their effects. Each operates to produce a reduced resistance to some kind of stress; and in their endless combinations, they facilitate the occurrence of a wide variety of neurotic states, in which phenomena symptomatic of one type of diagnosis may overlap with those symptomatic of others. This theory again leads to a number of expectations, which can be compared with observed facts.

In summary, theories of neurosis seem capable of being classified in three main categories:

    i.   those which imply that the causes of neurosis are wholly exogenous;

ii. those which postulate a unitary endogenous factor determining variations in susceptibility to neurosis; it may be either:
    a. a single abnormal gene; or
    b. a large number of separate genes of small but similar effect; and

iii. those which assume more than one genetic factor, with dissimilar effects,
to account for the neurotic constitution. They may either:
    a. be specific to a particular type of neurosis; or
    b. overlap in their effects and produce predispositions to more than one
    type of neurosis.

Many of the phenomena of neurosis are compatible with more than one of these
hypotheses, and may be observed without provoking any explicit choice (though a
choice is often involved by implication in the interpretation placed on neurotic
phenomena). There may be advantages, however, in choosing a particularly promising hypothesis, even before it can be claimed to be the only possible one, and
seeing where it leads us. The one we have chosen belongs to class iii *b*. A general and
a precise formulation follow, together with evidence to explain our choice.

THE PROPOSED THEORY

A very large number of characteristics may be differentiated among men, each of
which plays a part in determining the success with which the individual adapts to
circumstances. We can define each of these characteristics in such a way that the
possession of it promotes success and lack of it promotes failure. In these terms our
theory is that the normal man possesses certain characteristics and lacks others in
roughly equal proportions; the man with neurotic tendencies, on the other hand,
lacks many and possesses few. Although he may not be found abnormally lacking in
any particular characteristic, the consequence of his being lacking in many is that he
is more than averagely prone to be unsuccessful in his adaptations, and to relapse in
consequence into neurotic symptoms. Thus a man with neurotic tendencies may be
no more lacking in characteristic A than many men whose adjustments are normal;
but he may also lack characteristics B, C, D, and E, of which men who lack A
normally lack only one or two. Another man with neurotic tendencies may not be
lacking in A or B, but may lack C, D, E, and F. Thus, although he falls into the same
broad class, of men prone to neurosis, his personality may present a different picture, and the conditions which induce him to break down and the symptoms he then
develops may all be different.

In more precise terms, every individual possesses characteristics variable in
strength which render him more or less liable to a neurosis of any kind. Whether he
succumbs to a neurosis of a particular kind or not depends on the extent to which
he is endowed with characteristics which help to confer immunity to that kind of
neurosis, and on the nature and the degree of the stresses to which he is exposed. We
do not wish to suggest that all these characteristics are entirely endogenous or
genetically determined.

In the general population each of these characteristics may be considered as
normally distributed, so that their collective distribution may be visualized as a
normal surface in many dimensions. This multivariate frequency ellipsoid is exposed
to a series of stresses of different degrees coming from different directions, which
have the effect of partitioning it in various ways. Each particular stress divides the
population into two classes — those who withstand it and those who succumb. The
apparent qualitative distinction between neurotics and normals is the resultant of a

balance between two quantitatively variable forces. When stress exceeds resistance, the man becomes classifiable as neurotic, when resistance exceeds stress, as normal. Both stress and resistance vary in degree.

But both vary also in kind. Some people may be so feebly endowed in all relevant characteristics that they may succumb to almost any stress, provided it is sufficient in degree. A particular stress, if sufficient, will produce symptoms of neurosis in these people, but may also find out the Achilles heel in others who would have been immune to any equally severe stress coming from a different direction.

We present this as a heuristic hypothesis, i.e., not as one which can be either finally proved or disproved on existing or readily accessible evidence, but as one which may prove useful for experimental purposes. Any satisfactory theory of neurosis is more likely to be reached rapidly and established soundly, we believe, if the implications of the proposed theory are explored than if they are ignored.

Why is it likely to be useful? Arising from genetic considerations, it offers an account of the relationship between normal and abnormal psychological phenomena and therefore extends the range of observations which students of either branch of psychology can take into account. In particular it relates the problems of psychiatry to the general concept of human variability which has been developed by psychometric psychology, and which again is related to the system of applied logic which has been found suitable for the biometric sciences as a whole. It therefore places at the disposal of psychiatry the scientific techniques, particularly those of statistical analysis which have been developed for the biometric sciences by Galton, Pearson, Fisher, and others. These practical advantages are sufficient, in our opinion, to justify asking for a trial of the theory.

Some of its corollaries may be suggested as suitable for study:

1. (Also reconcilable with theories of types i and ii b.) Neurotics, by hypothesis, are obtained from the normal population by a process of selective sampling, and are therefore a sub-class of normal men. If so, in the observation of any particular characteristic, neurotics will be found to fall within the limits of range of the general population, and will not occur in excessive numbers at a particular extreme.

2. (Also reconcilable with types i and ii b.) When unselected groups are submitted to environmental stress of varying degrees, the numbers of persons breaking down will increase with the intensity of the stress, and no final end-point will be found at which all have broken down who are ever liable to. The relationship between degree of stress and frequency of breakdown will be positive, but of limited extent because:

3. (Also reconcilable with iii a.) Certain types of stress will be particularly likely to produce breakdown among particular types of people, e.g., acute physical danger and uncertainty among persons liable to anxiety states, positions of grave responsibility among those of obsessional types, etc. This relationship will also be limited in extent, since people are affected by the degree of a given stress as well as the direction from which it comes.

4. Conversely, it should be possible to assess the liability of different individuals to neurosis generally and to neuroses of different kinds specifically. Those who break down under the least degrees of stress should be found the most heavily loaded with "negative" characteristics, as earlier defined.

5. (Also reconcilable with type i.) Mixtures of characteristics, and therefore mixtures of symptoms, will occur more frequently among neurotics than pure types.

6. (Also reconcilable with iii *a*.) Neurotics will be found heterogeneous.

7. Among relatives of propositi suffering from a given type of neurosis the incidence of neuroses of other kinds should be higher than among the normal population.

If satisfactory evidence can be adduced on all these points, we shall consider our theory confirmed, since, taken together, they are irreconcilable with a theory of any other type than iii *b*.

EVIDENCE RELEVANT TO THE CHOICE BETWEEN POSSIBLE THEORIES

Evidence has already been quoted from other sources in the discussion of possible theories above, which is sufficient, for instance, to exclude theories of type i; and other evidence published by Slater, E., (24) corroborates every expectation listed above except under 1, on which no data were available. Other sources might be cited. But investigations conducted at Sutton Emergency Hospital during 1942–44 provide fresh unpublished evidence which is presented and discussed below.

In one experiment, six tests used by the Army for selecting personnel were given to enough serial weekly intakes at the hospital to provide a sample of 200 men; four were tests of mental abilities (general intelligence, verbal, arithmetic, and mechanical abilities) and two of physical abilities (agility and auditory acuity). The patients proved to have the same average age as men in the serving army, and reached the same average scores on the tests of mental abilities. Their agility was found to be lower and their auditory acuity poorer. The correlation between their results on these two tests is +0.3307, which is significantly higher than the corresponding correlation in the normal serving army, +0.1004 (on 2,600 cases).

Several hypotheses might account for these findings, among them the hypothesis that neurotics tend to be constitutionally inferior. This belongs to type ii *b*; the fact that neurotics' agility is relatively poor is related hypothetically to the fact that their auditory acuity is also relatively poor, and a general common cause is supposed. If there is one, it should produce other effects, and appear, for instance, in other physical abilities. This was tested. The next 200 men in following intakes were given a test of visual acuity. They proved to have significantly poorer vision than men tested in the serving army, and significantly more of them wore glasses.

The hypothesis therefore appeared confirmed. It also agreed with previous results (Slater, E., 24) which showed by factor analysis that positive family history, childhood neurosis, poor work record, previous nervous breakdown and abnormal personality are all interrelated phenomena among neurotics, and that their interrelations can be accounted for as manifestations of a common underlying characteristic, the neurotic constitution.

But there is nothing in this evidence which excludes our proposed theory. If we take a random sample of the population, we shall expect not only to find some men deficient in auditory acuity, but also, among these, some who are deficient in agility, and finally, among these, some who are also deficient in visual acuity. Our theory, in this instance, is simply that those who happen to be deficient in two or three abilities are those most likely to find their way into a neurosis centre. This accounts for the observations as adequately as the hypothesis of a single common factor.

There is, moreover, a point at which the evidence accords only apparently with the single factor theory, and in fact conflicts with it; and where the consideration of our theory provokes a closer inspection of the evidence and reveals the importance of facts which might have been overlooked. This contradictory evidence is that the correlation between the auditory acuity and agility tests is higher among neurotics than among normals. If both defects are manifestations of a neurotic constitution, and this is a unitary trait, the neurotics, who are alike in respect of it, should also be relatively homogeneous as regards the defects. But homogeneity lowers the correlation between associated variables (Thomson, 1939); so the proportions of the two correlations should have been reversed.

This leads us to compare variances in performance on the two tests among neurotics and normals. The mean square variance on the agility test is 4.39 times as great among neurotics as among normals (5,000 cases), and on the auditory acuity test at least 1.19 times as great (2,600 cases; but this test is not so sensitive to degrees of acuity above average as below). Although neurotics are supposed alike as regards neurotic constitution, and this is supposed to affect their test results on both tests, they are found, in fact, abnormally heterogeneous. When the correlation between their results is corrected for heterogeneity (Thomson, 1939), it is reduced to +0.1676, which does not differ significantly from the normal value. Further corroboration is provided by the visual acuity test, on which the mean square variance of neurotics is 3.03 times that of normals (2,233 cases).

These observations suggested that further evidence on heterogeneity might be found if sought for. Qualitative findings differ in frequency among the different classes, as already shown (Slater, E., 24); but heterogeneity can also be demonstrated quantitatively. The alphabetically arranged card index of the admissions to all military neurotic wards of the Hospital from the beginning of the war until January 1944, were searched for persons with a diagnosis, or part diagnosis, of obsessional state: 113 of these were found. The next card lying to that of each of these was taken for a miscellaneous group, and the succeeding cards were searched for the nearest name with a diagnosis of anxiety state, hysteria, and reactive depressive state. Five groups, each of 113 persons, were so obtained by a strict method of random selection, and the relevant data are given in Table 17.3.

TABLE 17.3. MEAN AGE IN FIVE DIAGNOSTIC GROUPS

Diagnostic group	Mean age in years
Obsessionals	28.64
Miscellaneous	29.25
Anxiety neurotics	29.07
Hysterics	28.89
Reactive depressives	31.69

TABLE 17.4. ANALYSIS OF VARIANCE FOR AGE, DEPRESSIVES VS. OTHERS

Source of variance	Sum of squares	Degrees of freedom	Mean square
Total variance in age	25506.21	564	—
Variance between depressives and others	672.66	1	672.660[a]
Remaining variance between groups	23.05	3	7.683
Variance within groups (error)	24810.50	560	44.304

S.D. of age within groups = root mean square
variance = 6.656 years

[a]F = 15.183 P < 0.01

As shown in Table 17.4, the reactive depressives appear older than the others. A precise test shows that the difference is significant. The remaining groups do not differ significantly from one another, nor, for that matter, from the larger group of which they form a sample.

Scores of many of these patients on intelligence tests are kept, and were inspected for evidence of heterogeneity: the same procedure was followed. Different tests were in use at different periods. Records were sufficient to enable 300 patients to be classified in 12 groups of 25 according to diagnosis and test given. The diagnoses were the first four given above, and the tests used, Progressive Matrices, Shipley Vocabulary, and Cattell Intelligence Tests II, a. They show that obsessionals score significantly higher on intelligence than others, but that anxiety neurotics and hysterics do not differ significantly from each other or from the miscellaneous group [Slater, P., 1945a].

Other data collected at the hospital by Miss E. Bennett, but not published, show that psychopaths are heterogeneous in their reaction times under free-association tests (2,400 times recorded).

Thus when age is considered, the heterogeneity of neurotics is demonstrated by the difference between reactive depressives and others; when intelligence is considered, heterogeneity is demonstrated by the difference between obsessionals and others; and heterogeneity is found among psychopaths when reaction times are measured. The accumulation of evidence demonstrating the heterogeneity of neurotics is considerable, and might be held sufficient to exclude theories of type i or ii.

Evidence of a different kind is required to differentiate between theories of type iii a and iii b. If the former is correct, neurotics must be treated as qualitatively distinct from normals; this would become necessary if it could be shown that some characteristics are present among neurotics which are entirely absent among normals, or that the absolute frequency with which abnormal degrees of certain characteristics occur among neurotics is too great to be treated as a random deviation from norms appropriate to the general population.

It is therefore important to arrive at the best possible estimate of the incidence of neurosis under the circumstances with which we have to deal at present. From the most complete information available, we estimate that the odds are about 65:1 against a man being referred to hospital for the treatment of a neurosis during a year's service in the army.

Let us apply this estimate to another criterion of neurotic tendency. In an experiment carried out by Miss Elizabeth Bennett at Sutton Emergency Hospital, lists were prepared of 100 things men might disapprove of, 100 that might make them nervous or afraid, and 100 that they might enjoy. This is an adaptation of the Pressey Cross-Out Test. It was given to 80 normal men and to 160 patients from the neurotic wards, of whom 80 were classified as neurotic and 80 as psychopathic. It was found that neurotics and psychopaths alike tended to disapprove of more, to be afraid of more, and to enjoy fewer things than the normals. An analysis of the answers suggests that the test functions as a measure of inadequacy. When the separate sections are appropriately weighted, neurotics and psychopaths tend to obtain negative scores, and normals positive ones. The overlap between the two groups is 26 per cent. We can estimate that the correlation between test result and neurotic tendency is +0.5, and this is about as high as we can expect to obtain with any single test.

How much use is such a test as a diagnostic instrument? If neurotics and normals were two divergent types, and occurred in equal numbers, like males and females, we could differentiate them from each other correctly in 74 per cent of our cases. But we have estimated that the odds against an unknown man developing a neurosis within a year are 65:1. So even if his score is an unusual one for a normal man, and a common one for a neurotic, the odds may still be in favour of his being normal, at least for an operationally effective period. In point of fact, if a man obtains the average score for a neurotic, the odds against his developing a neurosis are 13:1. Even if his score is so low that only 1 per cent of neurotics score lower, the odds are only even that he will develop a neurosis within a year. The whole neurotic group falls within the normal group (i.e., those in an apparently normal state at a given time), when we take into account the relative sizes of the two groups.

As another instance, we might consider the use of the electroencephalogram as an index of abnormality. This test is ordinarily used to supplement a diagnostic opinion which carries its own independent weight. In treating the evidence of the test in isolation, we do not wish to be taken as implying any criticism of diagnostic opinions it has been used to supplement. In the average population the incidence of abnormality of EEG is believed, on estimates available, to be approximately 10 per cent. In various types of the psychiatrically abnormal this frequency rises to any figure up to 90 per cent; for a general neurotic group it has been given as approximately 25 per cent. Then if one man in 66 is liable to neurosis within a year, one in 79 of those with normal EEGs is so liable, and one in 26 of those with abnormal EEGs. Let us, however, take a much larger estimate of the frequency of "neurosis." It has been suggested that about 10 per cent of the population exhibit neurotic or psychopathic traits (that they exhibit them in some degree is readily admissible on our hypothesis). Then of those with normal EEGs one in twelve will be neurotic, and of those with abnormal EEGs one in four. In this case, as in the foregoing, one of a psychological test, the range of the neurotic group falls within the range of the normal, and no clear-cut qualitative distinction appears.

This evidence is only sufficient to illustrate the difficulties that are likely to be encountered in attempting to establish a theory of type iii *a*, and the necessity of carrying out adequate control experiments among normals before any criteria are accepted as valid for differentiating neurotics. Ideally, if a theory of type iii *a* can be established, an exact classification of cases should be possible, into normals and neurotics of different varieties. If we prefer a theory of type iii *b*, we are not obliged to suppose that neurotics cannot be differentiated from normals or from one another. But our approach to this problem and our method of formulating conclusions will be different. By selecting a fairly large number of characteristics for measurement which are relatively independent of one another and which are more noticeable among neurotics than normals, and applying methods of weighted summation (e.g., by computing discriminant functions) we may be able to measure the probability that an individual may develop a neurosis, and grade people for relative liability of immunity (which may approach certainty of one kind or another in certain cases). Our main reason for preferring a theory of this type is that we believe it provides the more promising approach at the present time. A weighted summation of ten tests tried out by Miss Bennett, including the three sections of the adapted Pressey X-O test already mentioned, provides a range of scores on which the probability of neurosis rises from less than 0.001 to over 0.99 (taking into account the estimate of the incidence of neurosis already given). Up to 20 per cent of the

226

population can be classed in the former category; while a bottom 2.2 per cent can be differentiated, amongst whom 61.4 per cent of the neuroses can be expected to occur [Bennett, 1945; Slater, P. 1945b]. The interpretation of observations according to our theory has therefore led to promising results.

SUMMARY

Possible theories of the nature of the neurotic constitution are considered, together with their consequences in statistical expectations of various kinds. A theory is proposed, which is held to accord best with the relevant data available at present, and which has heuristic value in providing a scheme of attack on the genetic problems of psychopathy, and in rendering available to psychiatry the techniques of statistical analysis which have been found suitable to the biometric sciences. According to this theory, the neurotic constitution is preponderantly determined by a very large number of genes of small effect. The effects of these genes, at least in so far as they are qualitatively similar, may be additive; and they become manifest by producing a reduced resistance to some form of environmental stress, and so facilitate the appearance of a neurosis. In so far as the effects of the genes are qualitatively dissimilar, the types of stress effective in producing breakdown, and the neurotic symptoms produced, will tend to differ. The neurotically predisposed man is then to be regarded as a man who has a more than average susceptibility to environmental stresses of one or a number of kinds; he represents one of the extremes of normal human variation.

18

NEUROSIS AND SEXUALITY

INTRODUCTION

Neurotic men have been found to differ from normal men in a number of particulars, in the frequency with which they show qualitative findings, and in the degree to which they show quantitative findings. In addition they have been found to be abnormally heterogeneous. In respect of graded characters we may expect them at times to vary from normals at both ends of the scale. If we choose a single criterion for the distinguishing of neurotics from normals, we cannot expect it to be of value over more than part of the range; it may be useful in distinguishing some neurotics but not all. For instance, Rees and Eysenck (1945) have shown that an index relating stature to transverse chest diameter (1) exhibited greater variability in the neurotic than in the normal, (2) was associated at one end of the scale with symptoms of anxiety, depression, effort syndrome, etc., (3) at the other extreme was associated with hysterical symptoms. Attention is rightly being paid to the physical correlates of psychological qualities. For physical characteristics are often capable of preciser definition and more exact measurement than any psychological characteristic with which they may be associated; and the discovery of an association between a physical and mental trait may give us a clue to causal relationship. For this purpose it is desirable to examine the neurotic and the normal subject particularly in respect of those physical and psychological qualities where deviations might be expected to have an effect in reducing good health, adaptability, or emotional stability.

In the psycho-analytic theory of the development of the neuroses it has always been maintained that the eventual neurotic adaptation of the adult is determined by disturbances of one kind or another in early psycho-sexual development. This theory has been supported by a wealth of individual observations, but by no general evidence that the sexual activity of neurotics differs in any way from that of the

Originally published in the *Journal of Neurology, Neurosurgery and Psychiatry* 8: 12–14 (1945).

normal. A certain amount of evidence of this kind has, however, been forthcoming from other sources. Billings *et al.* (1943) made a comparison between 100 U.S. Army psychiatric patients and 100 enlisted men. Of the psychiatric patients 54 were neurotic or showed psychopathic personality, while the remainder showed schizophrenic or affective symptoms or were feeble-minded. They state that 44 per cent more of the enlisted men than of the patients showed an average sexual development, 30 per cent had regular girl friends, 41 per cent more had intentions to marry. Absolute figures are not given. Also in the U.S.A., Steinberg and Wittman (1943) have reported on their findings on 267 men from the Services. Of these 158 formed a control group, 22 were predominantly neurotic, and 87 predominantly psychotic. As tested by the Elgin developmental history, the psychotic subjects (of whom 76 per cent were schizophrenic) made a less satisfactory early sex adjustment than the controls, but the difference between the neurotic patients and the controls was negligible; the same was largely true for adult sex adjustment. As far as the female is concerned, it is worth noting that Bernard (1935), working with a group of married couples, found significant positive correlation coefficients between (1) marital dissatisfaction of wife and neuroticism of wife, (2) marital dissatisfaction of husband and neuroticism of wife, and (3) days since last coitus and neuroticism of wife; there was, however, no significant correlation between days since last coitus and neuroticism of husband. It cannot be asserted that any of this evidence is very precise or takes us very far.

In a previous communication (Slater, 24), dealing with the statistical analysis of the clinical records of two thousand neurotic soldiers, it was observed that a considerable proportion (45 per cent) had led lives in which sexual activity had played a surprisingly minor role. In these men "sexual relations began at a late age, occurred with unusual rarity and were associated with little interest or satisfaction." The question whether the sexual activity of an individual patient was to be regarded as inadequate or normal in degree was decided by the doctor in charge of the case. No doubt standards of judgment varied from clinician to clinician. But as each doctor would be consistent with his own standard, the division of the case material into two classes in this way does represent a real though crude distinction. From here on the one group will be referred to as "inadequate" and the other as "average" in respect of sex life. The statistical material was analysed, using this criterion for classification, but consideration of the findings was postponed as it was hoped to combine the data with those obtained from a biochemical and genetical investigation which was then in progress. Unfortunately, these latter investigations had to be interrupted, and are not likely to be completed in the near future. The results of the statistical investigation are, however, so interesting that it is thought that they merit publication on their own account. In the table below are listed all and only those findings in which there was a statistically significant difference between the frequencies observed in the two groups of men with "inadequate" and with "average" sex lives.[1]

[1] It is to be noted that there was a small but significant difference between the mean ages of the "inadequate" and "average" groups. This indicated that the clinicians, in forming their judgment, had not been able to allow sufficiently for the effects of age. For the young must of necessity have had as a rule a less abundant sex life than their seniors. It was therefore thought desirable to make allowance for this adventitious factor. The necessary corrections for age, which all proved to be very small, have therefore been made throughout the table, a process which though laborious was quite simple as the material had been classified by age groups as well as by sex life in the primary card counts.

RESULTS

Several interesting points appear from Table 18.1. The first is that the group of under-sexed men are clearly a more abnormal group than the others. In them, with few exceptions, the positive psychiatric findings are more frequent. The exceptions are themselves interesting. Head injury is more frequent in the group of men with "average" sexuality; it is a finding which has already been shown (Slater, 24) to be

TABLE 18.1. FREQUENCIES OF VARIOUS OBSERVATIONS AMONG
NEUROTIC MILITARY PATIENTS, CLASSIFIED BY SEX LIFE

| | Sex Life | | | | | |
| | Inadequate | | Average | | | P |
Observation	N	%	N	%	CR	less than
Childhood:						
Neurosis*	487	33.4	701	28.7	—	—
Neurotic traits	—	38.3	—	37.1	—	—
Normal	—	28.3	—	34.2	2.2	0.05
Home life:						
Unsatisfactory*	419	24.3	637	14.4	3.9	0.001
School record:						
Poor*	499	31.0	690	26.6	—	—
Average	—	50.1	—	57.9	2.6	0.01
Good	—	18.7	—	15.5	—	—
Occupation:						
Semi-skilled manual*	501	35.9	695	44.8	3.1	0.01
Sedentary*	—	13.3	—	6.5	3.8	0.001
Army rank:						
N.C.O.'s*	516	15.6	717	20.9	2.4	0.02
Previously:						
Head injury	516	11.3	717	20.5	4.5	0.001
Military stress	—	38.8	—	50.9	4.3	0.001
Precipitation	—	41.4	—	54.4	4.6	0.001
Bodily habitus:						
Asthenic*	353	53.3	538	44.5	—	—
Athletic*	—	23.5	—	34.4	3.5	0.001
Pyknic	—	23.3	—	21.1	—	—
Intelligence:						
Poor*	456	34.1	658	26.9	—	—
Average*	—	53.4	—	64.1	3.6	0.001
Good*	—	12.5	—	9.0	—	—
Personality:						
Anxious	516	25.3	717	19.1	2.5	0.02
Hysterical	—	16.7	—	11.7	2.5	0.02
Impulsive, aggressive	—	15.5	—	21.7	2.8	0.01
Unsociable	—	40.2	—	30.1	3.7	0.001
Anergic	—	29.1	—	22.4	2.7	0.01
Generally abnormal	—	51.6	—	41.4	3.5	0.001
Symptom:						
Amnesia*	516	13.6	717	19.2	2.8	0.01
Outcome:						
Unimproved*	516	26.0	717	18.8	2.9	0.01

N = number of persons on which relevant observations made
CR = critical ratio, i.e., ratio of difference between percentages to its standard error
P   = probability of such a ratio being obtained by chance.
*   = comparable finding made when patients classified by degree of military stress undergone (see Table 11, Slater, 1942 [Table 16.11]).

associated with lesser rather than greater degrees of constitutional predisposition. The amnesic symptoms are also more frequent in the averagely sexed group; these symptoms are particularly frequent among men who break down in battle (Sargant and Slater, 1941). The only abnormal personality trait which is more frequent among the averagely sexed are the qualities of impulsiveness or aggressiveness. This can be related to the finding by Denis Hill that patients suffering from the clinical electro-encephalographic syndrome which he has termed "dysrhythmic aggressive behaviour" (Hill, 1944) are very commonly troubled by a quite excessive libido (personal communication).

The second point of interest is that where a graded characteristic is being considered, the sexually inadequate tend to be found in excess at one or other extreme. Compared with men of average sexuality, they are more likely to have either a poor or a good school record, to be either of poor or of good intelligence, and to be relatively infrequently average in these respects. They are more likely to have an asthenic or a pyknic physique and are less likely to be of athletic habitus. Exactly parallel findings have recently been reported from comparisons of neurotics as a whole with normal controls. Eysenck (1943) has found that neurotics were less frequently average in respect of intelligence, and Rees and Eysenck (1945) have found that they were less frequently average in respect of bodily habitus than were the normal men with whom they were compared.

The third point is that the table that is published here bears a very remarkable resemblance to Table 11 [Table 16.11] in my previous communication (Slater, 24), where the same clinical material was classified by degree of military stress undergone. All the findings marked by an asterisk in the present table were found to be associated with degree of military stress, and in every case the association is of the same kind; i.e., a finding which is more frequent among the sexually inadequate than among the average, is more frequent among those who have not undergone military stress than among those who have. Breakdown in the absence of military stress and inadequate sexuality are themselves positively associated; and it might be supposed that this association might by itself explain their common associations with other psychiatric findings. This suggestion, however, cannot be supported. For, if these associations are expressed in the form of correlation coefficients, the coefficients are all of the order of 0.2; that is, they are so low that partial correlation coefficients corrected for their communalities would be very little smaller. The several associations of these two findings, degree of stress undergone and degree of sexual activity, must be regarded as having independent validity.

DISCUSSION

We must conclude therefore that the factors which predispose to neurotic breakdown are related to those which tend to bring about a reduction of normal sexuality. This is entirely consonant with the hypothesis of Freud. There are, however, other ways of looking at the matter, two of which particularly suggest themselves. We might suppose that the relationship between tendency to neurosis and tendency to sexual inhibition might be in either of two directions. It is possible that the listlessness and inadequacy of personality, which shows itself in so many neurotics, was also expressed to some extent in their sex lives. This would imply that impoverished sexuality was an almost accidental by-product of the general tendency to failure and defeat. On the other hand, it is possible that constitutional factors, such as minor degrees of endocrine insufficiency of various kinds, which result in deficient sexuality, were so impairing the personality as to increase the liability to nervous breakdown. Both hypotheses seem plausible; there is no reason why both should not be to some extent true; and we have no present evidence which would lead us to favour either at the expense of the other. Nevertheless, it may be pointed out that the former hypothesis does not lend itself to translation into any very precise terms, and cannot be subjected to any simple test. The second hypothesis suggests the advisability of investigating the endocrine balance of neurotics, and even provides a hint that the results of such an investigation might eventually prove to be not only of aetiological but also of therapeutic significance.

SUMMARY

The clinical records of 1,233 neurotic soldiers were classified by the degree of sexual activity they had shown and the frequencies of various psychiatric findings were analysed in the two groups of the sexually inadequate and the sexually average. Sexual inadequacy was found to have significant associations with neurosis in childhood, unsatisfactoriness of home life, school record, occupation, rank in Army, past head injury, degree of military stress undergone, bodily habitus, intelligence, various personality traits, amnesic symptoms, outcome of illness. In nearly every case sexual inadequacy was found to be positively associated with a higher frequency of the abnormal finding. Where a graded characteristic is in question, such as in intelligence and bodily habitus, sexual inadequacy was more frequent at the extremes of the distribution. The findings are closely paralleled by a similar analysis of the same clinical material by degree of military stress undergone. It is concluded that the factors which tend to bring about neurotic breakdown and those which predispose to sexual inadequacy are related. Various hypothetical bases for this observation are discussed. One which appears to be particularly favourable for further investigation suggests that the common factors are to be sought in an imbalance of the endocrine system.

19

THE THIRTY-FIFTH MAUDSLEY LECTURE:
"HYSTERIA 311"

Permit me to begin by saying how pleased and proud I am to have received the invitation to deliver this year's Maudsley lecture. This is, I think, one of the highest honours that our psychiatric confraternity can confer on any of its members, and is something that the recipient will treasure as an enduring reward.

Henry Maudsley, whom we commemorate today, advanced the psychiatry of his time by applying philosophical ways of thought to clinical observations on individual patients. Experimental and statistical techniques in his day were little understood, and psychiatry itself was not yet ripe for their application. The situation is now a very different one; and we have reached the stage where work which does not rely on one or more of the powerful techniques now available is likely to be received both by editors and by the generality of readers in a spirit of no enthusiasm.

It is, therefore, with some trepidation that I venture to offer you a discourse which is based on observational data of a solely clinical type. These data have, indeed, been accumulated on a genetical principle, the hypothesis that monozygotic twins offer a controlled experiment set up by nature. But the limitations which apply to all purely clinical studies still obtain. However, there are certain rather primitive questions for which clinical studies are still the appropriate instrument. Controlled experiment and delimited statistical survey are the methods needed for problems which can be isolated and precisely defined. Until we can say just what it is we want to know, exploration along a wide front is still the most promising approach. This is, I submit, still the case with the neuroses; and of all the neuroses perhaps to the greatest degree in hysteria. If I have to trouble you with case presentations, which will lend an anecdotal air to my remarks, I must ask for your indulgence; I know no other way to make my points.

Originally published in the *Journal of Mental Science* 107: 359–81 (1961). Case histories omitted. Table added.

COLLECTION OF MATERIAL

The twins which are the subject of this report were collected, as part of a systematized unselected series of all twins with a neurotic or psychopathic diagnosis, from the in-patient and out-patient material of the Bethlem and Maudsley Hospitals between 1 March, 1948 and 31 December, 1958, and from Belmont Hospital between 1 November, 1950 and 30 June, 1953. The Bethlem-Maudsley group in the present study includes all those and only those twins, with a twin partner of the same sex who had survived into adult life, who in the records were at any time allotted the diagnostic classification number 311 of the W.H.O. International List of Diseases (1957), "Hysterical reaction without mention of anxiety reaction", with one further case (DZ 5) who had been given the number 320.7, "Pathological personality NOS" and specified as "hysterical". The Belmont diagnoses which were accepted for inclusion were those of "hysteria" and "anxiety-hysteria".

I would like here to express the gratitude of our Unit to both of these hospitals, and to all the many colleagues whose ungrudging co-operation has made this work possible. If at times I suggest corrections of their views, such as a revision of diagnosis, it must be understood that all I claim is the easy advantage of the observer who can be wise after the event.

The preliminary case-work on these cases was largely carried out by Mr. James Shields, my colleague in the Genetics Unit at the Maudsley. But for the last three years Miss M. Malherbe has undertaken a complete review of all the data obtainable on the neurotic twins, filling in gaps in our information and securing interviews with the surviving patients and their twins. Diagnosis of zygosity has been made on the basis of history, physical comparison, bloodgroups, finger-prints and the P.T.C. test. In the series reported there is only one case (DZ 5) in which there is any material doubt that this diagnosis might be incorrect.

CONCORDANCE

The most striking of our findings is that, in the 12 MZ and the 12 DZ pairs, there is no single twin partner of all the 24 probands who has at any time received a formal diagnosis of hysteria. [The author's diagnoses on follow-up of probands and co-twins are given in Table 19.1.] The nearest approach to such a diagnosis is found in one of the dizygotic pairs (DZ 9).

> The family background of this pair was a curious one. The father was a manic-depressive with several hospital admissions, and in addition a crank who ran an unsuccessful campaign for the revival of craftsmanship among country blacksmiths. The mother was his first cousin, with further manic-depressive illness on her own side of the family, and must have been as cranky as he was. When the Proband was taken to the Child Guidance Clinic at the age of 11, the psychiatrist noted that the little girl prattled to him about coprophilia and of her twin sister's inferiority complex and infantile attachment to the father. She was regarded as an anxious self-dramatizing girl, but was not then diagnosed as a hysteric. However, it was the Twin who was first taken to the C.G.C. some months before her sister at the age of 11, and again later between 13 and 16. She was then regarded as "an unstable adolescent with hysterical and depressive traits, reacting to an abnormal environment"; but the depressive aspect was thought more important than the hysterical one.
>
> The Proband was diagnosed as a hysteric when she was treated in the Maudsley at the age of 18. She had become depressed and unable to go on with her studies at the university, and was self-reproachful and agitated, picking her hands and biting her nails. Several suicidal attempts were thought to be histrionic. Her illness was put down to a romantic attachment to a psychopathic criminal, who was shortly expecting release from prison. She was treated with psychotherapy and improved, but two years later was back again, now four months pregnant

by a Ghanaian student. There is a suggestion in the case record that the earlier depression had been succeeded by a mildly hypomanic state, involving the patient in her pregnancy. If that is so the whole cycle may have been a cyclothymic one.

TABLE 19.1. DIAGNOSTIC SUMMARY[a]

Case No.	Sex	Age (last info.)	Author's Diagnosis on Follow-up	
			"Hysteria" Proband	Co-twin
Z 1	f	52	Hysterical psychopath, hysteria (320.3)	Normal
2	m	40	Endog. depression, hyst. sympts. (301.1)	Psychoneurosis, unspecified (318.5)
3	f	51	Hysterical hypochondriasis reactive to physical illness (318.0)	Normal
4	m	40	Endog. depression (301.1)	Normal
5	f	28	Hysterical psychopath (320.3)	Normal
6	m	45	Anxiety state (310)	Anxiety state (310)
7	f	44	Epilepsy, hysterical personality (353)	Normal
8	m	45	Hysteria (compensation neurosis), anxious personality (311)	Normal
9	f	26	Vasovagal instability (315)	Normal
10	m	43	Hysterical psychopath (320.3)	Hysterical psychopath (320.3)
11	m	25	Schizophrenia, low intelligence (300)	Schizophrenia, low intelligence (300)
12	m	21	Psychopath (hyst. sympts., delinquency, low intelligence) (320.5)	Psychopathic personality with amoral trend (320.5)
Z 1	f	28	Psychopathic personality, mainly hysterical (320.3)	Depression (301.1)
2	f	39	Chronic primary tension state (310)	Normal
3	f	38	Anxiety tension state (310)	Recurrent depression (301)
4	f	43	Hysterical psychopath (320.3)	Normal
5	f	41	Psychopathic personality, mainly hysterical (320.3)	Normal
6	f	27	Hysteria on basis of anxious personality (310)	Normal
7	f	31	Epilepsy (atypical), secondary hyst. & obsess. symptoms (353)	Normal
8	f	37	Temporal lobe abscess (342)	Mental defect (325.2)
9	f	21	Cyclothymia (depressive and hypomanic phases), hyst., personality traits (301.0)	Inadequate personality (320.3)
10	f	28	Depressive illness, prob. on basis of epilepsy (353)	Normal
11	m	34	Psychopathic personality, hysterical sympts. (320.3)	Asocial personality (320.5)
12	f	41	Organic brain disease, anxiety tension state (309)	Normal

[a]This table has, with the author's permission, been incorporated by the editors as a substitute for some of the omitted information included only in the appendix of the original paper. The formal diagnoses shown and the code numbers of the International Classification of Diseases are those made by Slater for the purposes of a subsequent paper, "Diagnostic Similarity in Twins", which appears in the present volume as Paper 21.

If we can accept this pair as a concordant one, we must calculate the concordance rate for hysteria as 0 per cent in the MZ pairs, 8 per cent in the DZ pairs, which is far from impressive evidence of any specific genetical causation. We may, however, cast our net somewhat wider, and consider whether there are further cases of neurosis among the twins. In fact, three of the MZ and one of the DZ twins have come under psychiatric observation for this cause (MZ 2, 10, 12, DZ 1). One of these (MZ 2) may be taken as an illustration.

> This pair, also, comes from a family in which endogenous depressions have occurred. From the beginning the Proband was a little behind his twin in development and vigour, but they were both forward children. They won scholarships to grammar school and university, and were on the point of starting at their universities in 1939 when the war came. Both registered as conscientious objectors, and were assigned to such duties as land drainage and civil defence. This was too much for the Twin, who according to his mother, decided he must get out and organized himself a medical discharge on grounds of psychoneurosis. The patient might have had more cause for this. He had had a mild depression at the age of 16 after the death of his father, and another depression lasting three months in 1943. However, he stuck it out, and served his time.
>
> After the war both returned to their universities. The Twin completed his three years, got his B.A., and through a varied and adventurous career, till recently in the theatrical world, has never had any later neurotic episode. The Proband, however, got behindhand with his studies, and as the finals approached began to fear he would not even get a good pass and would be left without means or profession. He could not concentrate, had difficulty even in talking, and had symptoms of depersonalization such as the feeling he was doing everything "second-hand." On the day of the finals he did not present himself, but had an amnesic fugue lasting six hours. A few days later he was admitted to the Maudsley, underweight and depressed, but without other abnormality. Psychotherapy and a modified insulin treatment brought improvement. After discharge he was recommended to come up for further psychotherapy, but did not, and improved to recovery without further aid. He went back to his studies for a time, but eventually gave up without taking his finals. Ever since he has been perfectly well.

In this case the hysterical dissociation seems to have occurred under psychogenic pressure, but also at a time when powers of adjustment were impaired by a state of depression. Dealing very briefly with the three remaining pairs in which there is technical concordance in respect of neurosis, we have (MZ 10) a pair of psychopaths with numerous hysterical personality features, of which the Proband has a long history of hospital attendances, the twin a single episode when he was invalided out of the Army for psychoneurosis, having lost his memory after a fall. The second (MZ 12) is a pair of boys, now 21, who from earliest years have been of dull intelligence, enuretic, truants, subject to a number of neurotic traits, and with long records of delinquency, and with hysterical symptoms such as faints, falls, and visual hallucinations. Characterologically they are almost mirror images of one another, but it is only one who achieved a psychiatric diagnosis of hysteria. The third case (DZ 1) is one in which the Proband is a severely psychopathic woman, her twin much more normal with a single illness, with symptoms of an anxious and depressive type, from which she recovered spontaneously in four months.

So far, then, we have 3 MZ pairs and 2 DZ pairs concordant for neurosis, giving us concordance rates of 25 per cent and 17 per cent. Neurotic states, however, are not infrequently handled entirely by the family doctor, with or without referral to general hospitals, and never reach the psychiatrist at all. In this series there are four cases in which this has occurred (MZ 6, 8, DZ 2, 3). In the first of these the Proband is a higher civil servant who, after many years of work and war service in the Far East, found himself at the age of 38 reacting badly to the stresses of a very responsible post. He complained of headaches, depression, inability to concentrate and a head that seemed full of cotton wool. He worried about a sister-in-law who had been under treatment for cerebral tumour, and the psychiatrist considered his illness hysterical, presumably on the basis that it was the product of suggestion. He arranged, himself, to get psychotherapy, but despite it remained ill for four years, having to be off work for 6 months three years after the first onset. Eventually he made a fair recovery. His less brilliant twin found himself a much easier and less ambitious life, but also had an unexplained illness which started about a year later than that of his brother. The main symptom was lassitude, but after a time he also complained of an unpleasant smell in the nose. Moving in less sophisticated circles than the Proband, he was satisfied with treatment along ordinary medical lines; but he remained ill until an antropuncture a year after the onset put an end to the smell in his nose.

The other monozygotic pair which falls into this group (MZ 8) is one in which the Proband had an industrial neurosis with difficulty in walking, which lasted about 2 years, and kept him off work for a year. His twin was a bus-driver, who was unable to walk for a fortnight after a road accident in which a man was killed.

If we are to include these cases also in our concordance figures, we have 5 concordant pairs among the MZ twins, and 4 concordant pairs among the DZ. The difference is still negligible, and again we are driven towards the conclusion that specific hereditary factors are not manifesting their presence. We have not entirely covered all the psychiatric abnormalities among the twins of our probands; the list is complete with mention of a schizophrenic (MZ 11), a mental defective (DZ 8), and a ne'er-do-well with a criminal record (DZ 11).

FAMILY HISTORY

Our effort, then, to track down one type of aetiological factor, the genetical one, through the aid of concordance figures, appears to have taken us very little distance. Similarities of personality are often far-reaching, but are rather seldom brought to the fore in symptomatology. Furthermore, despite the totally different genetical situation in MZ and DZ twins, in this group there is little difference between the two kinds of twins, whatever the criteria we employ. There is one further step we can take along genetical lines, and that is an examination of the family history.

In his valuable monograph on Hysteria, Ljungberg (1957) calculated that the incidence of hysteria in the fathers, brothers, and sons of hysterics was approximately 2, 3, and 5 per cent and in their mothers, sisters, and daughters 7, 6, and 7 per cent. For the general population he gives a morbidity risk of 0.5 per cent. The findings, he thought, supported the view that polygenic factors were responsible.

Ljungberg provides a life-table showing the distribution of morbidity risk of hysteria with age. Using this, we can calculate that in the 23 fathers, 24 mothers, 43 brothers and 29 sisters of our probands we have observed the equivalent of 96.31 life-times of risk. Among these first-degree relatives there is no single individual who has ever been diagnosed as having a hysterical illness. However, two mothers can be written down as having abnormal personalities of a hysterical kind, and one brother is an abnormal socially poorly adjusted individual who, I think, would have been classified by Ljungberg as a hysteric. The incidence of hysteria, on these criteria, is then approximately 3 per cent. This fits in fairly well with Ljungberg's own figures. Another way of putting it is to calculate that, if the incidence of hysteria among the relatives of my probands had been the same as in Ljungberg's group, I could have expected to find 4.2 hysterics among them, with which the observed 3 agrees fairly well.

Ljungberg found no significant increase in the incidence of other psychiatric disorders among the relatives of his propositi, but there was such an increase in the propositi themselves. Among his male hysterics he found 3 who were schizophrenic, and among the females 5. The incidence of schizophrenia in the propositi themselves was, therefore, 3.1 per cent. In addition there were 1 male and 4 female manic-depressives, i.e., 2.4 per cent; and 4 male and 8 female epileptics (3.3 per cent). All these figures are high, and although individually they are not very significant, together they are impressive. Ljungberg states that the total incidence of psychoses among his propositi, that is including schizophrenia, manic-depressive psychosis, presenile and senile psychoses, psychogenic psychosis and undiagnosed psychosis, is 9.9 per cent for men, 9.5 per cent for women, diverging significantly from the expectation for the general population of 3.1 and 3.2 per cent.

Among the relatives of my probands I found no schizophrenics, and only two epileptics, a brother and a sister. There was, however, a noteworthy number of manic-depressive and typically endogenous affective psychoses. There were no fewer than 5 well-established cases, 3 fathers and 2 mothers; and in addition one mother and one brother are of cyclothymic personality, one sister possibly had a depressive illness, and one mother had a depression diagnosed as reactive, but quite probably predominantly endogenous. If we take the risk period as lying from 20 to 65 in the male and 20 to 60 in the female, we may calculate that 69.5 risk-lifetimes have been observed, against which 5 sure cases represents an incidence of 7 per cent.

Among his propositi Ljungberg found that nearly half of both the men and the women had shown abnormal personalities, hysterical, asthenic and psycho-infantile types predominating. However, among the first-degree relatives there was no great incidence of psychopathy, as judged by fairly strict criteria, 4.9 per cent among parents and 2.6 per cent in siblings against an expectation of approximately 3 per cent. Among the relatives of my probands 2 fathers, 4 mothers and 1 brother were personalities abnormal to the point of psychopathy; but 3 of these individuals have already been classified as hysterics, so that we are left with an approximately 4 per cent incidence of non-hysterical psychopathy among the parents. In addition, one each of the fathers, brothers and sisters, and 3 of the mothers, could be regarded as showing hysterical traits of personality within normal limits.

The findings are, therefore, largely what might have been expected on the basis of Ljungberg's work, with the single exception that in this series the cyclothymic constitution shows up in a remarkable way. There is no indication that hysteria (or 'hysteria 311') can claim the autonomy of a genetical syndrome.

EARLY ENVIRONMENT

Let us then turn to the environmental determinants, beginning with those that arise in infancy. There are two findings here which are interesting. In the dizygotic pairs, in all 8 cases where a difference in birth weight is known, it was the proband who was the lighter; and of the 6 cases where there was a noteworthy difference in health in childhood, in 5 cases it was the proband who was at a disadvantage. No such systematic difference shows in the MZ pairs. Both these findings suggest the significance of physical factors operating in early life; but as the differences between proband and twin are confined to the DZ pairs, we cannot exclude the possibility that these physical factors may have a genetical basis. Finally, a striking finding is that where there was a difference in handedness, in 3 MZ and 3 DZ pairs, it was the proband who was left-handed or ambidextrous. The probability of such a finding arising by chance is one in 64. This, too, is a feature which may be speculatively connected with an organic predisposition.

Sometimes, in the individual case, it is possible to be a little more precise. Thus in one of the DZ pairs (DZ 6), the proband at the age of 13 was away from school for a year, and in hospital for 4 months, with an illness involving jerky movements, provisionally diagnosed as chorea and finally as habit spasm. Recovery was very gradual when she was taken to the seaside to live with an aunt. The mother does not remember nervous traits before this illness; but according to another source both twins had neurotic symptoms before this age. In the Proband anxiety attacks started at the age of 19. A feature of her illness was that whenever she became emotionally upset, numbers of jerky and tic-like movements would appear. The development of the illness was most unfavourable, the patient ruthlessly exploiting her symptoms to dominate her environment, but it seems to me by no means out of the question that a post-choreic personality change of an organic type partly laid the ground for her hysterical disposition.

A diligent search for other factors which might have played a part, such as birth order, birth difficulties, differences in breast feeding, in early development, and in parental attitude, and twin leadership, etc., have brought no quantitative differences between proband and twin to light.

BODILY HEALTH IN ADULT LIFE

We receive an indication that this may be of moment in the observation that in the MZ pairs 5 of the twins enjoyed rather better health than the proband, the opposite being seen only once. In the DZ pairs the difference is more striking; in 9 cases the twin had the generally better health, and there is no case where the proband had the advantage. One way in which physical illness may predispose to hysterical symptoms is illustrated by MZ 3. The only noteworthy difference between the twins in this case is the amount of illness suffered by the Proband, gastric and intestinal trouble, cystitis, etc., which seems to have had a genuine physical basis; when her physical health improved, the hysterical symptoms passed off. However, differences are more quantitative than qualitative, and there is only one case (DZ 8) in which a physical factor played a recognizably decisive role.

In this case the Twin, who is a mental defective, has stayed at home and has had no physical illness. The Proband had otitis media and later mastoid disease. She had in all six mastoid operations, then a labyrinthotomy, and finally in 1953 at the age of 35 an operation for drainage of a tempero-sphenoidal brain abscess. There was delay in healing, and she was suspected of interfering with the ear and stirring up infection whenever her work as a nursing sister got beyond her. Her matron regarded her as having exhibitionist tendencies. She did her work well, but had too much sick leave. On one occasion she was found to have "large quantities" of barbiturate drugs in her possession, and was thought to be taking them to excess. Her neurosurgeon referred her to a psychiatrist with a note that "although she recently had a brain infection with B. coli abscess in the brain, I think there is no doubt that many of her symptoms are not organic in origin." The psychiatrist thought she showed organic intellectual deterioration, with indications of a nominal dysphasia, also an absence of insight not wholly explained as a hysterical reaction. Psychometry confirmed impairment of memory, learning difficulties and some nominal dysphasia.

She was admitted to hospital in an excitable, talkative, emotionally labile, and rather euphoric state. She felt that her condition had been neglected and was "selfrighteous and sanctimonious, naïve, and exhibitionistic." She rejected any suggestion of self-injury. The

239

diagnosis was "Hysteria,? self-injury." Two weeks after admission her ear began to discharge, and for an interim of a fortnight she was transferred to an E.N.T. hospital. After her return she continued to run an intermittent temperature. At times she seemed little bothered by her own illness, at other times she would complain of pain in the ear, and hint that more investigations should be done.

Perhaps the poor girl was right. She went home in September 1953, and died a year later, the post-mortem revealing that a large abscess in the left temporal lobe had ruptured into the ventricles. There was very little infection in the middle ear.

In this tragic case there can now be little doubt that the whole of the illness was attributable to the chronic cerebral abscess, which was never effectively treated. The hysterical colouring to the case, which led to unworthy suspicions of the Proband's integrity both as a patient and as nurse, was presumably derived from the personality. Before her illness she was a rather over-enthusiastic humourless person, attracted into nursing by a genuine idealism. Brain changes in the temporal lobe probably made her more labile, sensitive, and difficult. The bad relations which developed between the patient and her medical advisers seem a not unnatural result of pressure on her side to get more effective treatment, and despair on theirs about how that could be provided.

EPILEPSY

Among his group of hysterics Ljungberg found 3 per cent were epileptic. The suspicion that epilepsy has provided the basis of a hysterical predisposition arises in a number of cases in the present material. One of the most interesting is MZ 7, in which the Proband suffered from faints from adolescence onwards. One is tempted to regard them as having been vaso-vagal, since low blood-pressure runs in the family, and the Proband's blood-pressure has always been very low, when taken in hospital 80/50, as against her twin's 115/70. Her psychiatric history is long and complex, with hysterical symptoms such as aphonia, talking in sleep and a trance state at different times. However, at the age of 44 at last follow-up, she was having attacks occurring almost entirely at night in her sleep, with bladder incontinence, and was being treated with epanutin.

Two of our probands had epileptic siblings. In one of these (DZ 1) the patient suffered from attacks of giddiness and faintness, but showed nothing else to suggest epilepsy. In the other (DZ 7) the patient had atypical fits at the age of 11, leading to an examination at the National Hospital and the conclusion that they were not epileptic. At 25 she had a severe anorexia nervosa, so intractable that after 3 years she had an anterior leucotomy. After this the fits recurred and persisted despite anticonvulsants. EEGs showed numerous slow and fast waves, but nothing specific of epilepsy. Some attacks were observed, and regarded as tetanic and produced by over-breathing. At the age of 31 she had a second leucotomy. At follow-up this year, aged 38, she is once again having fits about once a month. She has a walking disability of the grossest hysterical kind, but also a mass of obsessional rituals. Her state suggests a progressive cerebral process.

Apart from these cases, blackouts, attacks of going limp, dizzy attacks, faints, falling attacks, short lapses of memory, have been observed in 6 MZ cases (1, 4, 5, 8, 9, 12) and in 4 DZ cases (2, 4, 5, 10). In one of these (DZ 2), the patient was found to have a very unstable EEG, and metrazol produced a burst of typical spike and wave suggestive of epilepsy. In another case (DZ 10) the patient's illness, which was depressive in form, was preceded some months previously by the occurrence of two epileptiform attacks on the same night. The general practitioner was sent for, and found her semi-conscious, having bitten her tongue.

Not very many of these patients have had any EEG examination, and those that have showed only non-specific anomalies. However, considering how atypical a temporal lobe attack can be, and how much EEG investigation is often required to demonstrate a temporal lobe focus, it seems to me far from improbable that more thorough and systematic examination would have brought to light some unmistakably positive findings. One of the probands (DZ 12) was under my own care in the National Hospital with a state of agitation and depression, in which she complained of overwhelming sexual feelings and the continual recurrence of spontaneous orgasms. Though I was unaware of it at the time, the symptoms were very similar to those of the well-known case of Erickson (1945) of angioma of the paracentral lobule; and the temporal lobe epileptics of Van Reeth *et al.* (1958) had comparable sexual experiences.

SCHIZOPHRENIA

Among his 381 propositi, Ljungberg found 3 males and 5 females who were schizophrenic. In the present material there is also a schizophrenic (MZ 11). These twins were dull and backward boys who became schizophrenic within a year of one another between the ages of 22 and 23, in 1957. They are now both chronic patients in mental hospitals. When the Proband was admitted to the Maudsley Hospital he had shown a personality change and catatonic symptoms for three months, and had had delusions, such as that the sound of passing cars was that of aerial activity indicating the imminence of war. However, such symptoms were to some extent in abeyance while he was in the Maudsley, and the foreground of the picture was taken up by a hysterical pseudodementia. Asked in digit retention to repeat 246, he gave 358. He said 2 + 3 = 6, 3 + 3 = 5, 4 + 2 = 7, that there were 13d. in 1s. and 21s. in £1. On a later occasion he denied all knowledge of his home address, his brother and his previous career, and even said he did not know his own name; but he now said there were 12d. in 1s. and 20s. in £1. Asked why he had got the answers wrong before, he said "Joking, doctor, just for a joke." Asked why he had been walking round with an empty wheelbarrow, he said, "An empty wheelbarrow is easier than a full one; I don't like heavy work." In short, the picture, which was of very temporary duration, was that of a Ganser state or buffoonery syndrome. These states have attracted much psychiatric attention from time to time, and have been found to be of very various aetiology, schizophrenia accounting for a certain number.

ENDOGENOUS DEPRESSION

Ljungberg found 5 manic-depressives in his group, and in the first two case histories I quoted there are grounds for thinking that hysterical symptoms arose in the course of an endogenous depression. These are not the only ones. The illness of the proband in MZ 6, already quoted, was depressive in symptomatology, and the principal justification for a diagnosis of hysteria was the belief that the patient's headaches were the product of suggestion. A fourth case is that of DZ 10, whose illness, depressive in form, came on in the puerperium shortly after a stillbirth. A fifth case is that of MZ 4.

241

In this case, the patient attended the Maudsley out-patient department at the age of 34 with the complaint that every three or four months he would have 7 to 10 days in which he was dizzy, irritable and taciturn. The attacks came without precipitating cause, and between whiles he would be all right. His wife thought they had started after hearing that an acquaintance had been found to have cancer. Three weeks before attending, the patient had gone to work, had felt bad, and had collapsed at the First Aid post. He had had several slight turns of weakness almost daily since. He slept well, but woke tired, was constipated, got very depressed, and had fears of cancer. On examination, though he looked pale and ill, nothing abnormal was found but a numbness of the shoulder thought to be hysterical. He soon ceased to attend the out-patient department, but follow-up six years later shows that he made a spontaneous recovery and has remained well ever since; in the interview he showed nothing hysterical. The father of this man was admitted to Bexley Hospital with a depression at the age of 62, dying there five years later.

PERSONALITY

In his study, Ljungberg assigns a principal aetiological role in hysteria to deviations of personality, and in this he follows excellent precedents. Nevertheless he found that more than half of his propositi had shown no marked deviation of the premorbid personality. The commonest deviant types were the hysterical 21 per cent, the psycho-infantile 10 per cent, and the psychasthenic 8 per cent. Ljungberg further defines these types as follows. The hysterical type shows the suggestibility and distractibility postulated by Janet; he is quick to learn and to forget, with enthusiasm easily aroused but endurance limited; he has a pressing need of variety, and of being the centre of attention; he is subjective and egocentric.

The psycho-infantile type has a strong affective fixation and dependence on his relatives, and needs guidance and help; he shows traits of childishness, is credulous and easily led; under external pressures he is apt to react with a state of insufficiency.

The psychasthenic type easily becomes tired and suffers from anxiety. In order to compensate for a reduced supply of energy, the psychasthenic tends to avoid surprises and choice situations, and often subjects himself to a routine. He is shy, withdrawn, meticulous, dutiful, irresolute and vacillating.

In the present study, I have not subjected these cases to the same analysis. I have not attempted, in fact, to estimate any deviation from an imagined norm. Instead I have tried only to note the particular ways in which probands differed in personality from their twins. Nevertheless the results agree fairly well with those of Ljungberg, with the proviso that the main differences between proband and twin were along the psychasthenic and the psycho-infantile dimensions rather than the hysterical dimension.

The commonest and most consistent difference was for the proband to be the more anxious, worrying and tense of the pair, this difference being shown in 9 pairs in the one direction. It may be quite marked, even in MZ pairs, and then of course is not genetically caused. In one pair (MZ 6) the difference arises as the result of a polar development of the twins; in the rivalry in which they were involved the one who excelled became increasingly ambitious, serious and tense, while his brother gave up all lofty ambition and relaxed into a humdrum career. The important role which tendencies to tension and anxiety have played, not only in the personalities but also in the illnesses of these patients, is illustrated by the fact that two of them have each been submitted not to one but to two leucotomy operations.

Related to the anxiety tendencies, minor perfectionist and obsessional features were shown in 7 probands and in 2 twins; and there was greater social timidity and shyness in 11 probands to 1 twin. Differences in energy and initiative also showed a preponderance, the twin having the advantage over the proband in 11 cases to 4.

Traits which I should call hysterical — excitability, suggestibility, shallow affects, selfishness and self-will, histrionic traits — were about as common as in Ljungberg's material, and were more marked in the proband than the twin in a quarter of the cases (MZ 1, 10, 12; DZ 1, 6, 9). Some degree of hysterical disposition is, however, shown by 4 twins (MZ 2, 5; DZ 3, 10).

From the historical point of view, it was as a rule the proband who was the more neurotic in childhood, and who had more changes of occupation. There were also striking features about their sex lives which to some extent support Ljungberg's emphasis of psycho-infantile traits.

Taking the probands, there are only 3 men and 1 woman who have had fairly normal lives, with marriage to normal partners. Two male and 6 female patients have probably never had any sex relationship at all. Two other women have had difficulties in marriage, one being separated from her husband for a time. All the remainder have chosen odd partners. Of the men, MZ 2 married a wife who had been hysterectomized; MZ 4 married a woman who was a chronic neurotic and hypochondriac; MZ 10 married a neurotic woman who later had a paranoid psychosis. Of the women, MZ 3 first got engaged to a Canadian soldier who proved to have a wife already, and later married a man who had been in hospital with a schizophrenic illness. MZ 5 married a man who later went to prison for car frauds. Since her divorce she has cohabited with a man she refuses to marry, though she has twice been pregnant by him. One of these pregnancies was aborted on psychiatric grounds; after the other she arranged to have the child adopted.

In the dizygotic series, DZ 2 married a man who had been deaf since childhood, and who later left her perhaps owing to her illness; this woman was also sterilized; DZ 3 married a man with chronic nephritis who soon became impotent; DZ 7 found her husband through a marriage bureau, a shy and nervous man who dotes on her; DZ 9 fell in love with a criminal psychopath twenty years older than herself, and later had an illegitimate baby by a black man; and DZ 12 married an unsociable rigid man, who is both vegetarian and valetudinarian.

The twins have been more fortunate, but in them too, sex interest which is late or feeble, and failure to marry is found in 10 cases; and two marriages have ended in divorce.

PSYCHOGENESIS

It is not easy to exclude the operation of psychogenic factors in any of our cases; but in about half of them it is difficult to put one's finger on anything very particular. If the proband has come under one form or another of psychological stress, the same has been no less true of the twin, and a differential incidence cannot be discerned. In a further 5 cases (MZ 2, 4, 6; DZ 3, 12), we find psychogenic factors obtruding, but with some doubt about the extent to which they have been effective. These stresses are of a banal kind; examination anxiety, an extravagant wife, responsibilities of an exacting post, an impotent husband, a rather unimportant love affair. In two further cases the psychogenic factor exercised a decisive role, but one which would hardly have been effective save for the pre-existing hysterical disposition. Thus the illness in MZ 8 was essentially in the nature of a compensation neurosis; and the repeated fugues of DZ 11 were precipitated by the most trivial embarrassments.

243

In one case (MZ 5) there was a stress situation of a truly drastic kind. The patient married a man of whom her parents disapproved, and even after the marriage they waged a long, ruthless and eventually successful campaign to part her from him. When she was in the Maudsley, the patient complained she felt in the middle of a battle that was tearing her apart, and that she was being asked to make decisions which were too difficult for her. However, the case was an exceedingly complex one. Both the patient and her unstressed monozygotic twin developed Graves' disease and had to undergo thyroidectomies; the Proband showed an EEG abnormality not shown by her twin; and during her illness she exhibited a depression with diurnal variation of endogenous type, obsessional features and depersonalization. Her after-history was very psychopathic for years after the solution of the acute conflict by divorce.

Four of the cases show a psychogenic situation of a particularly interesting kind, what one might call a form of folie à deux, since two people share the same delusion. We see, as it were, the sick patient on the obverse of a medal, on the reverse side of which is the face of a fellow-conspirator. This figure is that of a member of the family who is busily employed in fostering the illness. Where the patient is female, this individual is commonly a father or husband. Thus in MZ 1 the hysterical development of the Proband's personality can be traced to the father, who preferred her to her twin and after an appendix operation gave orders she was to do no more heavy work. In DZ 4 we find a husband who is dominated by the Proband's complaints, has to come home to comfort her in the middle of the day and is never allowed out in the evening. In DZ 6 the Proband suffers from attacks of breathless-ness, and has had almost continuous psychotherapeutic support for 9 years; the situation is made almost unmanageable by the fact that her father panics if she has one of her attacks, and feels he must be able to give her, at once, all the sedative tablets she wants. In the fourth case (DZ 7) the husband not only works for a living but also runs the house for the patient, looking after her in every way. He is repeating the pattern of behaviour of the Proband's own parents, since her father also did all the work for his supposedly crippled wife.

This situation is one which is commonly met in the cases one calls hysterical, though it is less frequently recognized. The supporting partner, when seen, makes a normal impression, and his attitude to the patient seems, at first glance, to be everything that is proper. The patient and her partner, however, make a closed circuit with one another, isolating them from other relationships, each supplying the other's needs. The effect tends to be very malign; the four cases quoted have periods of continuous and still continuing illness of 15 years, 7 years, 9 years and 11 years.

COURSE AND OUTCOME

Such long illnesses are seen in only a minority of cases, but they are not uncom-mon. Ljungberg regards hysteria as a relatively benign condition, and reports that after 1 year only 38 per cent of patients were still suffering from symptoms, after 5 years 23 per cent, and after 15 years 20 per cent. Looked at in another way, these results are not so encouraging: if 62 per cent of patients recover within the year, less than half the remainder can ever be expected to recover at all. The follow-up results in the present series are a good deal worse. Five of the probands recovered within a year, and a further 7 in periods of 2 to 7 years. To the present time half the patients are still suffering from symptoms, at a mean duration of 5½ years after the critical diagnosis was made.

It is often made a subject for wonder that the psychiatrist does not frequently see patients in middle life who have had hysterical symptoms for many years; and the comforting conclusion has been proposed that this is because the youthful hysteric nearly always gets better. Both Ljungberg's material and the present series show that this is not so. If the psychiatrist does not see these patients in later life, it is because the patients themselves have found out the hollowness of the hopes that he can offer. They have given up attendance at psychiatric clinics, and have learned to rely on the medicines they can get from their family doctors.

Perhaps the most surprising feature of the follow-up statistics is their lack of uniformity. Some patients do well, others very badly indeed; and good or bad outcome bears little relation to the nature, the amount or the severity of the hysterical symptoms. To get a clue to the prognosis, we have to look, not at the hysterical mechanisms exposed, but to their aetiological basis, whether this is a brain lesion, an endogenous psychosis, a deviation in personality development, a temporary stress situation, or a built-in self-perpetuating mechanism.

CONCLUSION

We have now reached the position when we are compelled to ask, what is the justification for regarding hysteria as a syndrome? The aetiology appears to be very various; and the hypothesis of a genetical basis of a specific or indeed important kind has had to be discarded. Among the hysterics of the present series we have found patients suffering from a focal brain lesion, also probably from epilepsy, from schizophrenia, from endogenous depression, and from anxiety states falling more easily into the category of affective than hysterical illnesses. Comparative analysis of personalities shows the affected twin not so much more hysterical as more anxious than his partner. Both psychogenic and physical factors play a role in aetiology; but with some interesting exceptions they are of a varied and non-specific kind. The clinical picture is equally various; and the hysterical symptoms which are relied on for diagnosis are always accompanied by others of a different nature. No particular method of treatment seems to be of more general application than any other. Drug therapy, psychotherapy, E.C.T. and leucotomy have been tried, none showing any sign of being a specific remedy; patients get well or remain ill for reasons which are individual and often far from clear.

The one thing which is common to a large majority of the cases we have investigated is that they were very difficult problems clinically; even after prolonged follow-up many remain complicated and obscure. It is certain that some clinicians make the diagnosis of hysteria more readily than others. In some sense it is true to say that "hysteria" is a label assigned to a particular relationship between observer and observed; it appears on the case-sheet most readily if the doctor has found himself at a loss, if the case is obscure and if treatment has been unsuccessful. Of all diagnoses it is that which is least likely to be made in a spirit of detachment. There is a temptation to shelve further enquiry along aetiological lines, if the clinician sees or thinks he can see a histrionic quality in the patient's complaints, if some symptoms can be regarded as lacking genuineness, and if the patient demands rather than accepts treatment.

To be sure, the dissociative mechanisms of hysteria are known of old, and can lead to symptoms which deserve no other name. But the diagnosis of an illness as hysterical goes much further than the recognition of a symptom. The unreliability of the diagnosis indicates the unsatisfactoriness of a psychopathology which is based solely on a mental mechanism. In the past, delimited studies of such conditions as Ganser states and anorexia nervosa have repeatedly shown their heterogeneous nature. It seems permissible to suggest that this principle might be of wider application. The mere manifestation of a mental mechanism within the range of normal potentialities tells us little of consequence. If in our patient we find the signs of hysteria and no more, then these are signs that we have not yet looked deeply enough.

20

A FOLLOW-UP OF PATIENTS DIAGNOSED AS SUFFERING FROM "HYSTERIA"

In 1962 we tried to follow up all the patients who had gone through the wards of the National Hospital during the years 1951, 1953 and 1955, and had been given a diagnosis of "hysteria." We tried to contact 99 patients, and actually succeeded in finding out the after-histories of 85 of them, 32 men and 53 women. One third of the women and one quarter of the men had been diagnosed as hysterical by one or other of the Hospital's psychiatrists; in the remainder the diagnosis had been made on the neurological side. In the course of the follow-up 5 patients were admitted to the National for re-assessment, 35 came up and were seen in an out-patient capacity, 30 were visited (by E. G.) at home, and in 15 cases we depended for information on relatives, doctors, letters and records. In 12 cases the patient had died.

One does not expect patients suffering from hysteria to die in considerable numbers after a relatively short interval, and you will ask for some further explanation. Our patients were mainly a middle-aged group, with mean age for the men of 42 years and 37 years for the women. Three men and one woman committed suicide at intervals of 3 to 6 years after their illness in the National Hospital. Eight patients were aged 31 to 57 years on admission, and died of natural causes at a mean interval of 3 years after the diagnosis of hysteria was made. We can be reasonably sure that all the conditions which eventually proved fatal had been present at the time when the diagnosis of "hysteria" had been made. In some cases one might say, either that the clinician was aware of the existence of the killing disease, or that, as with two patients who later had coronary thromboses, the cause of death was related somewhat indirectly with the presenting symptoms. In other cases the effective cause, both of the presenting symptoms and of eventual death, was present but overlooked. These include a case of generalised vascular disease, a case of old brain injury and epilepsy, and two neoplasms, a renal carcinoma and an angioma of the brainstem.

By E. Slater and E. Glithero. Originally published in the *Journal of Psychosomatic Research* 9: 9–13 (1965).

The four suicides also make an interesting group, and it is unfortunate that we know practically nothing about the one woman among them. One of the three men was in the National for "barbiturate intoxication and hysteria," and committed suicide by gas three years later. The second was a man admitted to the National at the age of 52 years with unsteadiness of gait, pain in the legs, urgency of micturition and impotence. There were no abnormal physical signs and both neurologist and psychiatrist agreed in a diagnosis of "hysteria." He gassed himself four years later; but in the interval had twice been in the Maudsley Hospital, where on each occasion a diagnosis of disseminated sclerosis with hysterical elaboration was made. The last case is that of a man of 38 years who came into hospital complaining of weakness of the legs and abdominal cramps. In an amytal interview he confessed that he was an exhibitionist, and that the present symptoms had begun after an episode in which he had been chased and nearly caught by a park-keeper. He was diagnosed as suffering from "hysteria," and his symptoms of weakness were thought to be without organic basis. However, five years later he was re-admitted to the National, and was then found to have an atypical myopathy. He was a man who was subject to depressions, and more than once had been in psychiatric hospitals. It was in a recurrence of depression that he finally killed himself. To summarise, in this group also we see organic disease, a myopathy and disseminated sclerosis, eluding diagnosis; but we also get a hint that cyclothymic mood changes may underlie hysterical manifestations or hysterical appearances.

After we have eliminated the patients who died, we can classify the remaining 73 patients into three groups. First are those for whom the diagnosis of "hysteria" was coupled with an organic diagnosis. Second are those who were regarded as purely hysterical at the time, but whose subsequent history indicates that organic illness was present and undetected all along. Third are those who, even now, are free from any evidence of organic disease.

In the first group we have eight men and eleven women. These are the cases in which the clinician is inclined to talk of a "hysterical overlay," or to regard some symptoms as not determined by the known physical disorder. Typical examples of this group are the epileptics some of whose fits are thought to be hysterical; and the sufferers from disseminated sclerosis, multiple disc lesions, etc., whose pains, or anaesthesia, or disturbance of gait, do not fit the expected picture. From a prognostic point of view, the addition of "hysteria" to the diagnosis seems to make little difference. The hysterical admixture is of temporary duration, and in the long run the course of the illness is that of the basic organic process.

The second group, in which an organic basis for the symptoms was eventually disclosed, though it had been missed at the time of admission to the National, includes eight men and fourteen women. In most of these cases what follow-up has brought is a changed interpretation of medical facts that have not changed. But in some cases the observations on which the diagnosis of hysteria was made were incomplete. Examples of the pathology which has since been uncovered are, duodenal and gallbladder disease, Takayashu's syndrome, meningitis serosa circumscripta, and three cases of generalized brain disease — a young woman with cortical atrophy and two men who have steadily deteriorated into presenile dementia.

We are finally left with the third group of 8 men and 24 women in whose cases no evidence for organic illness has yet been found. Two of these patients have developed into unambiguously schizophrenic states. No fewer than eight of them have shown themselves as liable to cyclothymic depression.

These are instructive cases, since it seems probable that the patients were in a depressed state at the time that the diagnosis of "hysteria" was made, even though the mood change was not recognised. The complaints these patients made were rather nebulous and usually included weakness and exhaustion. Physical symptoms included giddiness, pains and paraesthesiae, and faints or black-outs. Specifically depressive symptoms, other than insomnia, could hardly be expected and are not mentioned in the records. All but two of these patients were quite well at the time of follow-up, although recovery in one case was not achieved until after a leucotomy, and in another is only maintained with the aid of imipramine. Several of these patients have had recurrences of affective illness in the interval. One woman had had clear cut depressive illnesses at the age of 18, 30, and 48, in the last of which conversion symptoms appeared. She has had two further hospital admissions since for the same hysterical difficulties in walking; and it seems that in her case any relapse into depression potentiates the tendency to dissociation.

The aetiological breakdown of the material finally leaves us with 21 patients, less than a quarter of the group with which we started, in which no underlying pathology can be traced. Among them are seven patients whose illnesses were in the nature of acute psychogenic reactions. These patients were very young, and included children of 9, 11 and 13, two young men of 18 and 21, and only two adults aged 35 and · 45. There was definite psychogenesis in every case, but in two cases it was never discovered in hospital. All these patients had typical conversion syndromes; all of them were well on follow-up, but three of them have shown tendencies to develop symptoms when stressed.

More chronic states were shown by 14 patients, 3 men and 11 women. The long-term course of these illnesses has not been encouraging. One girl came into the National at the age of 15, with a very short history of two weeks' pain behind the ear and double vision for two days. We didn't do her any good, and she went on to the Maudsley Adolescent Unit. Since then she has attended about twenty-five different hospitals; and though she is now married with two children, she spends much of her time in hospital.

Not all have done so badly. One woman is virtually symptom-free after 28 years of periodic attacks of weakness. One woman, who never forgave us for diagnosing as "hysterical" her right facial pain of eighteen years' duration, has forsworn hospitals ever since, and rarely even goes to see her G.P. When she gets the pain, as she does, for instance, after exposure to cold, she puts up with it. Another woman of 55 years, who had suffered from weakness of the legs all her life, was eventually persuaded to put up with her trouble when she was advised that it was due to "sixth sense nervousness." "If only I had known that all along!" she said.

All the other patients in this group are attending hospitals or doctors. Four of them are partially disabled and three are totally disabled, one of them after a disastrous prefrontal leucotomy. These severe and chronic states remain an unsolved mystery. In some cases one can content oneself by regarding the patients as invalids of choice; in other cases one cannot do so with conviction. With these last one has the impression that at any time might emerge some physical factor, on which the whole tremendous hysterical superstructure had grown up. But one may wait for this in vain.

What have we to learn from this enquiry about the bodily conditions which may predispose to states liable to be called hysterical? Organic disease appears capable of doing this in two principal ways. The less interesting is by the production of a local lesion or disorder of function which is liable to be misunderstood, for instance, because the symptoms are atypical, because there is no evidence of a physical basis, or because the symptoms could be understood as a conversion reaction. Naturally, in the National Hospital material, these local lesions are predominantly neurological. Thus we have three cases of minor damage to an eye which caused a defect of vision thought to be hysterical, three cases of facial pain, two of them later successfully dealt with by the neurosurgeon, four cases of local spinal lesions, two cases of minor damage to the vestibular system, a basilar vessel migraine, etc.

Alternatively organic disease may bring about a general disturbance involving the personality. This personality change may then be a basis for hysterical conversion reactions, or by causing affective lability, hypochondriasis, attention-seeking, self-concern, suggestibility, variability of symptoms, etc., lead directly to an unfavourable reaction on the part of the clinician. In 1961 (94), I wrote, "In some sense it is true to say that "hysteria" is a label assigned to a particular relationship between observer and observed; it appears on the case-sheet most readily if the doctor has found himself at a loss, if the case is obscure and if treatment is unsuccessful." These are conditions which are especially likely to be fulfilled if the patient has a personality disorder.

Conditions which were noted as producing effects in this way included six cases of epilepsy, four cases of cerebral vascular disease, three cases of brain damage in childhood, and cases of damage done by head injury, subarachnoid haemorrhage, encephalitis, meningitis, polyneuritis and pre-frontal leucotomy. Disseminated sclerosis is particularly frequently associated with a diagnosis of "hysteria" since it operates at two levels. It both produces an organic personality change, and also causes focal symptoms which are variable, of temporary duration, and likely to be highly unpleasant to the patient while still difficult to confirm by objective methods. Despite the alertness on the part of the clinician which this condition inspires, two cases found their way into the National Hospital material.

Among the functional syndromes which especially predispose to hysterical manifestations, endogenous depression occupies a place of importance, with schizophrenia also playing a part.

It is not easy to generalise about the nature of the organic noxa nor its site of impact. But it does seem as if frontal and central sites of impact, possibly classifiable as parts of the visceral brain, are the most likely ones. At least one, and probably more than one of our epileptics had a temporal lobe epilepsy; and our material included two lesions of the brain-stem. All the other disorders found are such as cause widespread effects.

SUMMARY

In 1962 an attempt was made to follow up 99 patients who in the years 1951, 1953, and 1955, had left the in-patient department of the National Hospital, including the psychiatric ward, with a diagnosis of "hysteria." Of these patients it was possible to contact 85 (32 men and 53 women).

Since leaving hospital, 4 patients (3 men and 1 woman) had committed suicide and 8 patients had died of organic disease which must have been present at the time when the diagnosis of "hysteria" had been made.

Of the 73 living patients, 19 (8 men and 11 women) had received in hospital the diagnosis of "hysteria" coupled with an organic diagnosis. In 22 cases (8 men and 14

women) the subsequent history indicates that organic illness was present but undetected when the diagnosis of "hysteria" was made. Finally, there remain 32 patients
(8 men and 24 women) who still show no evidence of organic disease. The last group
comprise 2 patients who have developed clear-cut schizophrenia, 8 who have shown
themselves liable to cyclothymic depression, 1 woman whose conversion symptoms
appeared in the course of a severe depressive illness, and 21 patients who still have
no demonstrable underlying pathology. Of the patients "without pathology," 8 are
severely disabled (5 partly and 3 totally).

Organic disease appears to predispose to conditions liable to the risk of diagnosis
as hysterical, mainly in two ways. It may cause a lesion with accompanying
symptoms which at one stage are atypical or without demonstrable evidence of a
physical basis, but which could be understood as a conversion reaction. Alternatively
organic disease may bring about a general disturbance involving the personality
which results in modes of behaviour (exaggeration, attention-seeking, etc.) which we
naturally think of as the typical manifestations of "the hysterical personality."

21

DIAGNOSTIC SIMILARITY IN TWINS WITH NEUROSES AND PERSONALITY DISORDERS

For some decades it has been fashionable in Anglo-Saxon psychiatry to belittle the contribution which attention to diagnostic aspects of the individual case can make to its understanding. This has not been a prominent fault of French psychiatry; and Paul Guiraud, to whom this article is dedicated, consistently taught the value of clinical observation for the purposes of diagnosis and the significance of exact diagnostic appreciations for the advance of clinical knowledge. The paper which we now present attempts to relate these basic concepts with the biological substrate of psychiatric illness, as evidenced in twins.

We have followed up an uninterrupted series of patients admitted to the adult in- and out-patient psychiatric services of the Maudsley and Bethlem Royal Joint Hospital between 1948 and 1958 (and over a period of 31 months, 1950 – 1953, to Belmont Hospital), who were notified as having a twin of the same sex still alive or older than 15 years. The portion of this case material which will be discussed here is that of the 192 index cases who had an official Hospital diagnosis other than epilepsy, brain tumour or psychosis. However, it is not the Maudsley or Belmont diagnosis which has been used in this research, since with repeated readmissions and admissions to other hospitals, this often varied from time to time. Instead, the following procedure was adopted. All the hospital case material and all the follow-up information in each case was condensed (by J.S.) into a single case summary, from which all reference to the psychiatric state or zygosity of the patient's twin was excluded. These case summaries were then presented to the co-author, (E.S.), who was called on to make a diagnosis according to the schema of the International Classification of Diseases and Causes of Death (W.H.O., 1957). The only exceptions to this procedure involved the 24 twin cases, with official diagnosis of "311. Hysteri-

By James Shields and Eliot Slater. Original English version. First published in French as "La Similarité du Diagnostic chez les Jumeaux et le Problème de la Spécificité Biologique dans les Névroses et les Troubles de la Personnalité" in *L'Évolution Psychiatrique* 31: 441-51 (1966). Title shortened.

cal reaction without mention of anxiety reaction", which were reported by Slater in 1961 (94). [See Table 19.1.]

This process of re-diagnosis involved a considerable number of changes from the original Maudsley diagnoses. In the original Maudsley diagnoses 144 probands were diagnosed as suffering from neuroses (diagnostic code 310–18), 43 as suffering from disorders of character, etc. (320–26), and 5 others, non-psychotic, non-organic. In the re-diagnoses neuroses (310–18) covered 78 probands, disorders of character (320–26) 68, and no fewer than 46 patients were found to be suffering from schizophrenia, manic-depressive reaction or other states covered by the psychotic and organic codes. Much of this re-diagnosis was, of course, determined by the large amount of information about the later course of the illness brought in by the follow-up investigations.

GENERAL FEATURES OF THE CASE MATERIAL

The 192 index cases came from 185 twin pairs, 7 pairs being represented by both twins, each having entered the series as an index case. It is obviously necessary to deal with these pairs twice over, as the two twins could and sometimes did have different diagnoses. Patients and their twins were seen, examined and interviewed by a member of the staff of our Genetics Unit (most usually by J.S.) whenever possible, and often on more than one occasion over the years; in all 170 probands and 133 co-twins were personally seen in this way. The mean length of follow-up was 7 years, 6 months, and the mean age of the subjects on last information was 40 years. The examination included measures for determining the zygosity of the twinship, e.g., blood-grouping, finger-prints. There were 80 monozygotic (MZ) and 112 same-sexed dizygotic (DZ) pairs, and in terms of sex 86 male pairs and 106 female pairs; 38 of the male pairs and 42 of the female pairs were MZ. Representation of the diagnostic groupings by zygosity of twinship was much what might be expected; but it is interesting that diagnostic groupings were not distributed randomly with regard to sex, as may be seen from Table 21.1. Taking both probands and co-twins together,

TABLE 21.1. DISTRIBUTION OF PROBANDS AND CO-TWINS BY SEX AND DIAGNOSIS

Code	Diagnoses	Probands			Co-twins		
		m	f	total	m	f	total
310–318	Neuroses	27	51	78	7	19	26
320–326	Personality disorders	44	24	68	13	15	28
	Other	15	31	46	9	10	19
	Total	86	106	192	29	44	73

the diagnoses most frequently made (by E.S.) were: anxiety state 61, inadequate personality 48, endogenous affective disorder 35, neurotic depression 33, schizophrenia 19, sexual deviation 8, chronic alcoholism 7, epilepsy 6, cyclothymic personality 6. Twenty-seven other diagnoses were made between 1 and 5 times, and account for 42 cases.

From Table 21.1 it will be seen that out of the 192 co-twins of our probands 73 have themselves been given psychiatric diagnoses, the remainder being diagnosed as within normal limits. We shall now examine the extent to which conformity between diagnosis of proband and diagnosis of twin varies from one diagnostic category to another. There would be reasons for regarding diagnostic categories in which there was close agreement between members of twin pairs as having some biological foundation; while if there were diagnostic categories in which there was no resemblance (concordance) within MZ twin pairs, these categories might be based on criteria with relatively little biological foundation. The fact that there was so little diagnostic concordance within twin pairs, of which one member had been diagnosed as suffering from "hysteria", led Slater (94) to question the validity of this diagnosis, a sceptical attitude which was later reinforced by a follow-up study of neurological case material (Slater, 109).

NEUROTIC DIAGNOSES

The diagnostic groups 310–18 of the International Classification may be grouped for the purposes of this study into two classes: 310 anxiety reactions; and 311–18 others. The reason for this is two-fold; the anxiety reactions are much more numerous than other neurotic states, and they are the only ones to show a marked degree of concordance. This may be seen from Table 21.2.

TABLE 21.2. NUMBERS OF CONCORDANT PAIRS BY DIAGNOSIS AND ZYGOSITY

| | | Concordance in | | | | | |
| | | MZ pairs | | | DZ pairs | | |
Code	Diagnosis	N	a*	b*	N	a*	b*
310	Anxiety state	17	7	8	28	1	5
311–18	Other neuroses	12	–	3	21	–	5
320–26	Personality disorders	33	11	18	35	2	10
300	Schizophrenia	6	2	4	7	–	2
301	Endogenous depression	11	3	7	14	1	8
	Other (organic)	1	–	–	7	–	3
	Total	80	23	40	112	4	33

*Concordance (a) means agreement within the pair in allocation to the same code number, (b) agreement in allocation to a psychiatric code number of whatever kind.

It will be seen that there is a higher proportion of concordant pairs in the MZ than in the DZ series, and also that the contrast between MZ and DZ pairs is much more marked when we demand the same diagnosis (a), than if we take presence of any psychiatric diagnosis (b). The concordance in the MZ series in pairs where the proband was given a diagnosis of anxiety state becomes even more impressive when we consider the technically discordant pairs. The only co-twin to have a psychiatric diagnosis other than 310 was a man coded 320.3 but characterized "anxious personality". Three of the 9 co-twins regarded as within normal limits were described (by E.S. on the summary prepared by J.S.) as (1) anxious disposition, mild anxiety reaction; (2) anxious-obsessional personality, mild chronic tension state; (3) anxious and obsessional traits. Among the DZ co-twins of the anxiety probands were observed one anxiety state, two reactive depressions, one recurrent depression (manic-depressive), one case of imbecility (possibility due to birth trauma) with psychotic episodes.

Neuroses other than the anxiety states showed very much less concordance. Among the MZ co-twins of probands diagnosed as suffering from reactive depression, there were 3 who were psychiatrically abnormal, two of them diagnosed as suffering from "inadequate personality 320.3" and one from "alcoholism 322.0"; the co-twins diagnosed as having inadequate personalities showed much resemblance in personality to their probands. The psychiatrically abnormal DZ co-twins had all sorts of diagnoses: anxiety state 310, recurrent endogenous depression 301, schizophrenia 300, epilepsy 353, inadequate personality 320.

DIAGNOSES OF PERSONALITY DISORDERS

In this group of diagnoses, "disorders of character, behaviour and intelligence", there were 44 male and 24 female probands, the male preponderance contrasting sharply with the female preponderance in the neurotic diagnoses. There were 33 MZ and 35 DZ pairs, relatively more MZ than in the other groups. Of the 68 probands 47 were diagnosed as suffering from "pathological personality 320" and a further 5 "immature personality 321." Other diagnostic groupings were sparsely represented, though there were 6 in the class "alcoholism, chronic, 322.1." In the large 320 class 35 out of the 47 were classified "inadequate personality 320.3." The inadequacies were very various, including anxious, hypochondriacal, obsessional, sensitive, emotionally labile and sexually inadequate traits, but commonest of all were traits of a hysterical kind. Although the 8 subdivisions of the 320 class of diagnoses (schizoid, paranoid, cyclothymic, inadequate, antisocial, asocial, sexual deviation, other) reflect what might well be regarded as clinical niceties, it is interesting that both members of 8 MZ pairs were placed in the same decimal code. A further 3 MZ pairs received the same whole number. Of the DZ pairs only two achieved the same code number, one of them matching 320.3 hysterical with 320.5 delinquency, the other pair being both homosexuals 320.6.

DIAGNOSES OUTSIDE NEUROSIS AND PERSONALITY DISORDER

Although all the probands discussed in this paper had at some time presented with symptoms which led at the Maudsley Hospital to an official diagnosis within the 310–18 or 320–28 groups, some were rediagnosed on later attendances at the Maudsley or elsewhere, and some cases caused differences of opinion among the clinicians handling these patients at the time. It is not surprising that a total of 46 probands had their diagnoses changed (by E.S.) in the light of follow-up information up to 16 years after the first admission.

These cases included 15 males and 31 females from 18 MZ and 28 DZ pairs. Twenty-five (including 20 females) were coded under 301 endogenous affective disorders, 13 under 300 schizophrenia, one 306 cerebral arterio-sclerotic psychosis, two 309 psychosis with organic brain disease, three 353 epilepsy, one 342 temporal lobe abscess, one 856.9 post-traumatic personality change.

From Table 21.2 it will be seen that there is a substantial level of concordance within MZ pairs in this group of diagnoses. It is interesting that this should have been the case when the diagnostician was deprived of all knowledge of the history and psychiatric state of the twin partner. It is tempting to re-examine the diagnosis of proband and co-twin in the light of information about the partner; and if this is done a number of further concordances emerge. Thus one proband diagnosed as having an affective psychosis had a co-twin who was regarded as within normal limits but "emotionally unstable, possibly on a cyclothymic basis"; and a non-concordant 309:300 DZ pair could easily turn out to be both schizophrenics.

255

TOTAL MATERIAL: GENERAL CONSIDERATIONS

A point of interest, which we have not yet touched on, is the question whether either sex, male or female, tends to be more concordant than the other. In a study of neurotic and psychopathic patients and their first degree relatives, Coppen, Cowie, and Slater (1965) found that pairs of male relatives were more alike than pairs of female relatives. On the other hand, Rosenthal (1962b), reviewing the literature, found a general tendency for females to be more alike than males in respect of psychoses and normal personality measures. In the present material there was no difference between the sexes. Concordance in having the same code number was shown by 29% of the male MZ pairs and 29% of the female MZ pairs; among DZ pairs by 4% of the male and 3% of the female pairs. The corresponding figures for concordance in having any psychiatric diagnosis were in the MZ pairs 47% in males, 52% in females; in DZ pairs 23% in males, 34% in females.

By far the most striking result which emerges from this study is the extent to which the difference between MZ and DZ pairs is connected with particularity of diagnosis. If presence or absence of psychiatric abnormality or illness is the matter under consideration, there is no very strong contrast between the MZ and the DZ pairs: 50% of the former and 29% of the latter are concordant. But if we confine ourselves to resemblances of a more exact degree, such as to require the same code number in the International Classification, then 29% of the MZ pairs but only 4% of the DZ pairs achieve this level of similarity.

DISCUSSION

The International Classification of Diseases was used solely because it is the official classification of mental disorder used in the Maudsley Hospital and in the U.K. generally. According to Stengel (1959) it is used also in Finland, New Zealand and Peru and Thailand. The French Standard Classification of 1943 was made convertible into the ICD in 1948. The many schemes of classification in use are confusingly variable and none is entirely satisfactory. Nevertheless, they have many features in common; and we believe that this paper shows that shortcomings of a classification are not a sufficient reason for giving up an attempt at diagnosis.

The earlier genetic studies of the neuroses have been reviewed by Slater (101, 105); and later twin studies by Ihda (1960), Braconi (1961) and Tienari (1963) support evidence of specific genetic factors particularly in anxiety, phobic and obsessional states. Ihda finds concordance for neurosis in 10 out of 20 Japanese MZ twins; classification of the neurosis is the same in all concordant pairs. Braconi finds concordance for neurosis in 18 out of 20 Italian MZ pairs; cases were predominantly anxiety states in children and young people. Tienari reports concordance for any kind of neurosis in 12 out of 21 Finnish MZ male pairs; in respect of phobic and obsessional symptoms 11 out of 12 pairs are concordant. Tienari (1963) has also studied 15 pairs where one twin shows "unmistakable psychopathic behaviour"; in 10 cases the other twin shows resemblance in respect of "basic characterology". Studies of normal twins on psychometric lines by Gottesman (1962) or using physiological measures of anxiety (Lader and Wing, 1966) may also be interpreted as supporting this position.

It might be objected that in the above clinically investigated series knowledge of zygosity and of the diagnosis in one twin could have influenced the investigator in diagnosing the other twin. Such an objection does not hold in the series reported here.

It might also be asked whether resemblance of MZ twins is not biologically determined but due entirely to imitation or to psychological difficulties of growing up as one of a twin pair. Zazzo (1960, 1961), among others, has drawn attention to difficulties of this kind and is sceptical of the traditional use of the twin method in studies of heredity and environment. It must, however, be pointed out that no evidence has been adduced to show that twins as such or MZ twins in particular have a higher incidence of psychiatric disorder than non-twins. The frequency with which twins of both kinds are admitted to the Maudsley Hospital is not higher than would be expected from the frequency of twins in the general population. The evidence of MZ twins brought up apart (Shields, 1962; Juel-Nielsen, 1965) shows that considerable resemblance in personality occurs in such pairs too.

Our findings in respect of diagnostic similarity seem to us to underline in the most emphatic way the desirability of making every effort in coming to the most exact diagnosis possible when dealing with individual psychiatric cases, whether this be for scientific or for purely medical and clinical purposes. By this work on twins it seems to us that new support of a biological kind is given to the view, which has been such an inspiration in both British and French psychiatry, that the problems of diagnostic classification are of fundamental importance.

SUMMARY

All same-sexed twins admitted to the Maudsley Hospital over an 11-year period with an original diagnosis of neurosis or personality disorder were followed up. Diagnosis of the 192 index cases and their co-twins was made independently according to the International Classification of Diseases. 50% of 80 MZ co-twins and 29% of 112 DZ co-twins were diagnosed as psychiatrically abnormal. 29% of MZ co-twins had the same diagnosis as the index case compared with only 4% of DZ co-twins. Anxiety states showed higher concordance than other neuroses. It is concluded that support is given to the view that diagnostic classification is of biological significance in psychiatry.

V

METHODOLOGY

EDITORS' COMMENTS: In his very first publication (1) Slater showed his inclination for devising a new method of data analysis when those already known to him appeared inadequate. Further examples have been given in Part II. Perhaps the most outstanding example in this collection of papers so far has been his calculation of the disease expectancy for relatives of schizophrenics under monogenic inheritance intermediate between complete dominance and complete recessivity, as shown in the curves of the figure in Paper 10. Earlier, with his brother, he was concerned with a very different kind of problem, that of deriving a masculinity-femininity scale in the form of a vocabulary test which at the same time controls for level of intelligence (45).

This section contains three papers. The first describes an original formula expressing in the form of a coefficient the place in the sibship for an individual from any size of family except an only child. It can be applied in a wide variety of fields. Here it is applied to male homosexuality. The paper is included more for the sake of the birth order formula than for the conclusions about homosexuality. The latter are open to more than one interpretation, as subsequent correspondence columns in the *Lancet* showed. With Slater's encouragement the data have now been re-analysed by Abe and Moran (1969), taking other variables into account. It appears that the late age of the mothers of the homosexuals may be secondary to late paternal age — a finding which, if confirmed, may also allow more than one interpretation. As for the birth order method, Tsuang (1966) has applied it along with other methods to Maudsley Hospital patients with a wide variety of diagnoses.

Methods for establishing whether a pair of twins is monozygotic or dizygotic are a practical concern for all twin investigators. As already seen in Paper 9, Slater worked out his own method for using fingerprints to this end. Paper 23 presents a later attempt at getting the best information from the data in a way that does not involve tedious computation. The method was an empirical one. In a later paper (107) a more rigorous mathematical analysis was carried out. Correlation between the two methods pair by pair was very high and for practical purposes the one republished here is probably adequate and certainly easier to apply. In his forthcoming book with Valerie Cowie (142), Slater shows how his fingerprint method can be incorporated with the Smith and Penrose (1955) method of zygosity determination, using blood group data.

The final paper in the section tackles a problem which the professional mathematical geneticists have themselves not yet attempted — a test for discriminating between dominant inheritance with low manifestation rate and polygenic inheritance, using an index derived from the relative numbers of similarly affected cases on the paternal and maternal sides of the family. In a more recent companion paper (127) Slater and Tsuang (1968) applied the method to an unselected series of Maudsley patients. Their findings, on which they do not place any great reliance, suggested the presence of a major dominant gene in schizophrenia, while polygenic inheritance seemed more likely in the manic-depressive psychoses.

BIRTH ORDER AND MATERNAL AGE OF HOMOSEXUALS

In a communication to the *Symposium on Nuclear Sex* (80), I reported that male homosexuals tended to be born late in sibship order; the estimate of birth order — 0.58 — unfortunately was misprinted in the published proceedings as 0.68. Since then the material available has been enlarged, and is here reported in detail. As comparative data, the observations on a large group of epileptics of both sexes are reported.

MATERIAL AND METHODS

A total of 401 males admitted to the outpatient or inpatient departments of the Bethlem Royal and Maudsley Hospitals between January 1, 1949, and December 31, 1960, were diagnosed as suffering from "320.6 pathological personality, sexual deviation, homosexuality." Data relating to birth order were available in 389 cases, and data relating to maternal age in 355. A total of 338 epileptics were admitted to the same hospitals between January 1, 1949, and December 31, 1959. Data relating to birth order were available in 296 cases, and data relating to maternal age in 289.

When an individual comes mth in order in a sibship of n individuals — i.e., in the total of children borne by his mother — his ordinal position may conveniently be designated by the figure $\frac{m-1}{n-1}$. This expression varies in value between limits of 0 and 1, with a mean value which in a random collection of individuals tends towards 0.5. Within sibships of a stated size the values are not normally distributed, since each ordinal position is equally probable; but the means of values obtained on a series of individuals will tend to be normally distributed. The variance of values of this expression is easily calculated, so that the probability of a deviation from the expected mean of 0.5 can be reliably estimated. Not only the expected mean but also the expected variance of a series of observations may be calculated; for it is

---

Originally published in the *Lancet* 1: 69–71 (1962).

readily shown that the average theoretical contribution of each single observation to the total variance is $\dfrac{n + 1}{12(n - 1)}$, an expression which takes high values in small sibships and approximates to 1/12 as the sibship size increases.

Late birth order in a sibship is closely correlated with maternal age. As a general rule, its biological significance resides in that fact. However, to quote Penrose (1961), "there are conditions in which association with maternal age can be residual to a birth order effect, as in maternal immunisation by the foetus and in lateral placenta praevia." Even when we are primarily interested in maternal age, we may find that birth order supplies more reliable information. People are usually more certain of their ordinal position in a sibship than they are of their mother's age at the time of inquiry or at the time when they were born. Furthermore, maternal age is sensitive to such influences as social traditions affecting age at marriage, so that it may not be safe to compare maternal age for groups derived from different regions, different social classes, or different epochs. The subject's own sibship provides the control data which can be relied on to equalise such adventitious differences, if the datum taken is birth order.

The unsatisfactory nature of data on maternal age, when not accompanied by data relating to the maternal age in the general population from which the material under investigation was drawn, is shown by work on the relation between maternal age and twinning. Much work has been published on this subject, but this rarely includes an estimate of mean maternal age. McArthur (1953) cited the distribution of maternal age in monozygotic and dizygotic twins, on a material of Negro twin births from the U.S.A.; but this is clearly not comparable with twin data from other national and racial groups. Dahlberg (1926) cited national data from France for 1907–10, from which the mean maternal age for twin births in towns may be calculated as 28.98 — i.e., little higher than the figure for the general population cited by Penrose. However, the mean maternal age for all births in towns in France was at that time only 27.10.

FINDINGS

Table 22.1 shows the distribution of birth order of 389 male homosexuals, and Table 22.2 shows how the mean birth order, the variance, and the standard error of

TABLE 22.1 ORDER OF BIRTH OF 389 MALE HOMOSEXUALS

Sibship size	Order in sibship																
	1	2	3	4	5	6	7	8	9	10	11	12	13	14	15	16	17
1	52																
2	46½	42½															
3	24	18½	31½														
4	10	14	14	21													
5	4	3	4	8½	13½												
6	5	3	2	3½	3	9½											
7	3	1	1	2	4	1	4										
8	1	2	1	—	1	1	—	1									
9	1	—	—	1	1	—	2	4	9								
10	—	—	—	—	—	—	1	1	2	1							
11	—	—	—	—	—	—	—	1	—	1	—						
12	—	—	—	—	—	—	—	—	—	2	1	3					
14	—	—	—	—	—	—	—	—	—	—	—	—	—	1			
17	—	—	—	—	—	—	—	—	—	—	—	—	—	—	1	—	—

Patients who were one of a pair of twins are allotted as one-half to the birth order of the first-born of the pair, one-half to the birth order of the second-born.

TABLE 22.2. CALCULATION OF MEAN BIRTH ORDER OF 337 MALE
HOMOSEXUALS FROM SIBSHIPS OF TWO OR MORE
AND OF STANDARD ERROR OF MEAN

	No.	Sum of values	Sum of squares
Sibship:			
2	89	42.5000	42.5000
3	74	40.7500	36.1250
4	59	35.0000	28.7778
5	33	22.6250	19.4625
6	26	15.4000	13.1200
7	16	9.0000	7.1111
8	7	2.8571	1.9592
9	18	14.8750	13.5781
10	5	4.2222	3.6296
11	2	1.6000	1.3000
12	6	5.5455	5.1653
14	1	1.0000	1.0000
17	1	0.8750	0.7656
Totals	337	196.2498	174.4942
Mean	–	0.5823	–
Correction term	–	–	114.2847
Total variance	–	–	60.2095
Mean variance	–	–	0.1792
S.E. of mean	–	0.0231	–

the mean have been calculated. The total variance observed – 60.21 – corresponds closely with the theoretically expected value, which is 55.83. The theoretical variance also allows an improved estimate of the standard error of the mean (0.0222). One might have anticipated that the observed variance would be less than the expected, since a shift of the mean value from the expected 0.5 might well have been accompanied by some diminution of total variance. That this is not so suggests that the male homosexuals reported constitute a heterogeneous material. As will be seen, the variance of maternal age is also high. The principal conclusion is, however, that the mean birth order of 0.5823 represents a deviation from the expected mean by 0.0823, which is more than three times as great as its standard error. A similar deviation was observed in the small group of female homosexuals; there were 32 of these with known birth order, the mean value being 0.625. In contrast, the mean birth order of the epileptics was 0.5091, with standard error 0.0219 – a value well within the expected span.

The distribution of maternal ages of the male homosexuals is shown in Table 22.3, with Penrose's data for the general population and for mongols entered for

TABLE 22.3. MATERNAL AGE FOR EPILEPTICS AND FOR MALE HOMOSEXUALS, WITH
COMPARATIVE DATA FOR THE GENERAL POPULATION AND FOR
MONGOLS FROM PENROSE (1961)

Age-class years	General population (%)	Epileptics		Homosexuals		Mongols (%)
		No.	%	No.	%	
15–19	3.9	7	2.4	12	3.4	1.0
20–24	22.3	58	20.1	54	15.2	6.1
25–29	32.8	94	32.5	79	22.2	10.8
30–34	23.8	63	21.8	99	27.9	14.1
35–39	12.8	44	15.2	62	17.5	27.3
40–44	4.0	20	6.9	36	10.1	31.9
45–49	0.4	3	1.0	13	3.7	8.8
Totals	100.0	289	99.9	355	100.0	100.0

comparison. These distributions are also shown in Figure 22.1. Table 22.4 shows the means and variances of maternal age for these and a variety of other groups, some of which are quoted from Penrose (1961). As might have been expected from the data on birth order, the homosexuals show a late mean maternal age, and in the distribution of maternal ages show a shift from the standard of the general population towards the distribution shown by mongols. The difference between the mean maternal age of male homosexuals and that of epileptics — 1.7 years — is more than three times its standard error.

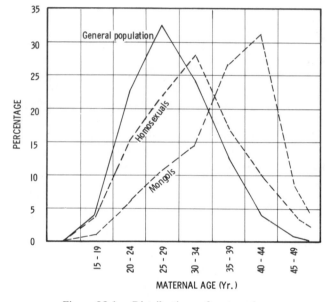

Figure 22.1 — Distributions of maternal ages.

TABLE 22.4. BIRTH ORDER AND MATERNAL AGE FOR A VARIETY OF
CONDITIONS, INCLUDING DATA FROM PENROSE

Group	No.	Birth order	Maternal age (yrs.) Mean	Variance
General population	632,408	0.50*	28.5	37.1
Epileptics	338	0.51	29.6	41.2
Exhibitionists	116	0.47	28.7	–
Transvestites	36	0.46	29.2	32.8
Male homosexuals	401	0.58	31.3	50.8
Female homosexuals	53	0.62	30.3	40.3
Turner's syndrome	40	–	29.0	56.2
Klinefelter's syndrome	25	–	30.8	61.0
Psychiatric twins, MZ	68	0.67	–	–
Psychiatric twins, DZ	221	0.69	–	–
Mongols	545	0.79	36.7	49.9

*Theoretical value.

DISCUSSION

These findings are suggestive. A distribution curve for maternal age, which was obtained from a mixed group of individuals consisting of one-third mongols and two-thirds general population, closely approximated to the distribution curve of the male homosexuals. A hypothesis of heterogeneity, in fact, goes far to explain the findings. This is supported by the high variance of maternal age for male homosexuals — actually greater than that for mongols and approaching the figures given by Penrose for Turner's syndrome and Klinefelter's syndrome. Furthermore the clinician would expect male homosexuals to prove to be aetiologically a heterogeneous group, including persons of notably feminised constitution with others of more normal make-up who had become homosexual in sexual attitude from social and psychological causes. Although investigations — for instance, by Pare (1956) — have failed to show anomalies of nuclear sex in male homosexuals, the possibility that some members of this clinical group are the subjects of some chromosomal anomaly such as might be connected with late maternal age seems worth investigating further.

SUMMARY

A numerical expression for designating birth order is proposed, with expected mean of 0.5 and with limits of 0 and 1. The expression permits easy calculation of its theoretical and observed variances.

Comparative data on 401 consecutive admissions of males diagnosed as homosexual, and on 338 epileptics, are reported. The homosexuals had a mean birth order of 0.58±0.02, showing a significant shift to the right. The birth order of the epileptics did not differ significantly from the expected mean of 0.5.

The maternal age of the male homosexuals also showed a significant shift to the right. The variance of maternal age of homosexuals was as great as that of mongols, approached the figures obtained with the small numbers of Turner's syndrome and Klinefelter's syndrome which have been reported by other workers, and differed widely from that of the general population.

The findings are regarded as supporting a hypothesis of heterogeneity in the aetiology of homosexuality in the male, and as suggesting that a chromosomal anomaly, such as might be associated with late maternal age, may play a part in causation.

23

DIAGNOSIS OF ZYGOSITY BY FINGERPRINTS

In 1953 the present author described a method of using ridge-counts of finger-prints for the diagnosis of zygosity of twin pairs. Since then contributions to the subject have been made by Smith and Penrose (1955), Wendt (1955), Nixon (1956), Lamy *et al.* (1957), Allen (1960), Richter and Geisser (1960), and Dencker *et al.* (1961). In an article on a more general theme Holt (1961) has also reviewed this particular field. However, the relevance of these papers to the present communication is restricted. Richter and Geisser have described a statistical model which is not used here, and has not so far been applied in any practical study. The paper by Wendt provides data based on a classification of pattern types rather than ridge-counts. With the exception of the reports by Slater and by Nixon from this Unit, all the other communications deal with total ridge-count differences (TRCDs) which are obtained by making only one count on each digit. This is a method of enumeration which gratuitously sacrifices information; and it leads to some loss of efficiency, as will be seen from Table 23.1, in which data from 180 MZ and 90 DZ pairs are presented. Using the single count, with a total of 10 observations on each individual, the highest observed TRCD in the MZ pairs was 48, which was exceeded by 28 of the DZ pairs. When two counts are made on every digit, including the smaller of the two available counts even when it is zero, a total of 20 observations is made on every individual, with a consequently greater range of variation. With this method the highest observed TRCD in the MZ pairs was 69, which was exceeded by 36 of the DZ pairs. Discrimination between MZ and DZ pairs is also better when TRCDs are very small, as may be seen from the top lines of the table. It does not seem justifiable to abandon useful information, by using the single count method; and the discussion which follows is confined to work done by making two counts on each digit.

The method of making these counts is that described by Holt, and consists in counting "the number of ridges which cut or touch a straight line running from the

---

Originally published in *Acta Psychiatrica Scandinavica* 39: 78–84 (1963).

TABLE 23.1. DISTRIBUTION OF INTRA-PAIR TRCDs WHEN ONE
AND WHEN TWO COUNTS ARE MADE ON EACH DIGIT

| | Total ridge-count differences | | | |
| | Single count | | Double count | |
	MZ	DZ	MZ	DZ
0	9	1	6	—
1– 4	39	4	32	4
5– 9	49	9	34	2
10–19	54	13	49	8
20–29	16	17	34	12
30–39	12	11	11	8
40–49	1	9	9	11
50–59	—	5	3	3
60–69	—	4	2	6
70 +	—	17	—	36
Totals	180	90	180	90

triradius to the core or centre of the pattern." To this statement Holt adds the words "with the exception of the two terminal points." My own method of enumeration has not been subjected to this proviso, but involves including one of the two terminal points; this is on the principle that informs us that from Tuesday to Thursday of the same week it is two days and not one. Thus in the whorl depicted by Holt in her Fig. 8, her two counts of 9 and 22 would by my enumeration be 10 and 23. With the single count method, the smaller of these two numbers is omitted from further consideration; with the double count method, both are included in the analysis.

In 1953 the method I proposed for using ridge-counts to diagnose twin zygosity involved calculating five characteristics of which three were correlation coefficients, between the twins, between their right and left hands, and the crossed correlation between the right hand of one twin and the left hand of the other. Nixon pointed out the disadvantages of the method, in that the five characteristics were to some extent intercorrelated, and that computation was tedious. He proposed a method involving only two characteristics, S and T. To quote from his paper:

Each of the 20 possible ridge-count values for a single individual is associated with a particular digital locus (that is, with either the radial or the ulnar margin of a particular finger on either the right or the left hand); each such locus may be given an index-number i between 1 and 20. For a twin-pair, then, there are 20 ridge-count differences to be taken into account, one for each locus; each single difference may be expressed logarithmically in the form $d_i = |\log_{10}a_i - \log_{10}b_i|$ where a_i is the ridge-count at the ith locus for twin A, and b_i is twin B's ridge-count at the same locus — in both cases increased by unity before taking logarithms, so that a_i (or b_i) is 1 when the actual count is 0, and the anomalous expression 'log 0' is avoided. Clearly d_i is zero when $a_i = b_i$. The twin-pair is then characterised in respect of its overall dissimilarity by a single value of S, the simple sum of the 20 values of d_i, from d_1 to d_{20}. Now d_i is the numerical logarithmic difference at a locus (that is, it is always taken as positive whichever twin has the larger count there), so that successive values of d_i reinforce one another in contributing to the sum S, instead of tending to cancel one another out if they happen to be in opposite senses. . . .

T . . . is calculated from the total (double) ridge-counts of the twin pair exactly as d_i is calculated from their single ridge-counts: that is $T = |\log_{10}A - \log_{10}B|$ where A is the simple sum of the 20 single ridge-counts a_i for twin A, and similarly for B from twin B — again after each single count has been increased by 1. It will be clear that for T, as for S, it does not matter which member of the pair be labelled 'A', as T, like the d_i, is a numerical, i.e. positive, difference. In the formation of T, single differences are this time permitted to cancel one another if they happen to be in opposite senses, and T is always much smaller than S (the correlation between S and T is +0.34 . . .).

267

Nixon proposed as a discriminant the expression $L = S + 12T - 6$. Since the publication of his paper, work on twins has continued in our Unit, and we now have available for the setting up of a standard the finger-prints of 180 MZ and 90 DZ twin pairs. A word of explanation for the large excess of MZ pairs is needed. Part of the material was derived from a special source.

In a BBC television programme in 1953 on the subject of twins, volunteers were invited to submit themselves for study, especially "identical" twins who had been brought up apart. They were asked to fill in a form in the current *Radio Times,* which enquired among other things whether the twins had been so alike as to be mistaken for one another by other members of their families and by acquaintances. The names of volunteer twins who had been brought up apart were made available to this unit; and they have been specially studied by my colleague, Mr. James Shields (1962). These pairs provided 75 double sets of finger-prints; and of them 69 were monozygotic, 6 dizygotic.

When this material is subtracted we are still left with a small preponderance of MZ pairs, i.e. 111 MZ to 84 DZ. This preponderance is due to the necessity of making more thorough zygosity investigations of pairs who could possibly prove to be monozygotic, than of those who from the history are undoubtedly dizygotic, e.g. because of markedly different eye colour. Furthermore, we have omitted from the

TABLE 23.2 OBSERVED AND EXPECTED DISTRIBUTIONS OF 180 MZ AND 90 DZ PAIRS

MZ Pairs			DZ Pairs		
Z	Obs.	Exp.	Z	Obs.	Exp.
−0.25			+0.50		
	7	5.22		5	6.35
+0.20			0.65		
	7	8.30		7	6.81
0.30			0.75		
	5	6.85		13	10.52
0.35			0.85		
	9	9.03		18	13.70
0.40			0.95		
	7	11.29		13	14.93
0.45			1.05		
	17	13.34		12	13.72
0.50			1.15		
	11	15.09		6	10.63
0.55			1.25		
	13	16.14		8	6.89
0.60			1.35		
	17	16.39		8	6.46
0.65			1.65		
	20	15.72			
0.70					
	17	14.45			
0.75					
	16	12.54			
0.80					
	15	10.34			
0.85					
	5	8.08			
0.90					
	5	5.98			
0.95					
	9	11.23			
1.10					

Expectations for the number of pairs between stated values of Z are calculated on the basis of normal distributions, with means MZ 0.61444 DZ 1.00111, standard deviations MZ 0.21855 DZ 0.23847. Observed and expected numbers are shown lying between the Z values which are their limits.

material used here all twin pairs who though diagnosed dizygotic have had the same blood groups.

All these 270 pairs have been blood-grouped; all the MZ pairs have the same blood groups, and all the DZ pairs differ in at least one group. The groups used have been ABO, MNS, P, Rhesus, Lutheran, Kell, Lewis and Duffy; and the grouping has been carried out by Dr. R. R. Race and his colleagues at the Lister Institute. Diagnosis of zygosity in these two series is also consistent with all other available data, such as information obtained from anthropometric examination and from the history.

TABLE 23.3. PROBABILITIES OF MONOZYGOSITY OR DIZYGOSITY
AS A FUNCTION OF Z

P_{MZ}	P_{DZ}	Z	Ser. 1 MZ	Ser. 1 DZ	Ser. 2 MZ	Ser. 2 DZ
—	—	-0.25	—	—	—	—
—	—	0.20	1	—	—	—
—	—	0.15	—	—	—	—
—	.0047	0.10	—	—	—	—
—	.0061	0.05	2	—	—	—
—	.0076	0.00	1	—	—	—
—	.0098	+0.05	—	—	—	—
—	.0125	0.10	1	—	—	—
—	.0161	0.15	2	—	1	—
—	.0209	0.20	2	—	—	—
—	.0274	0.25	5	—	—	—
—	.0360	0.30	5	—	3	—
—	.0477	0.35	9	—	—	—
—	.0632	0.40	7	—	2	—
—	.0842	0.45	17	—	4	1
—	.1121	0.50	11	2	2	—
—	.1485	0.55	13	2	6	—
—	.1959	0.60	17	1	8	1
—	.2554	0.65	20	1	4	4
—	.3271	0.70	17	6	5	5
.5896	.4104	0.75	16	4	7	6
.4987	.5013	0.80	15	9	3	7
.4059	—	0.85	5	8	1	1
.3177	—	0.90	5	10	1	7
.2395	—	0.95	5	8	1	10
.1743	—	1.00	3	5	—	12
.1229	—	1.05	1	4	—	8
.0845	—	1.10	—	8	—	9
.0568	—	1.15	—	3	—	6
.0377	—	1.20	—	3	—	5
.0245	—	1.25	—	6	—	6
.0157	—	1.30	—	2	—	3
.0100	—	1.35	—	3	—	5
.0063	—	1.40	—	1	—	3
.0041	—	1.45	—	1	—	—
—	—	1.50	—	1	—	—
—	—	1.55	—	1	—	—
—	—	1.60	—	1	—	—
—	—	1.65	—	1	—	—

The values of $Z = \log_{10} (S + 30T)$ are shown in the third column. In the first and second columns to the left are shown the corresponding probabilities of monozygosity or dizygosity. In the four columns to the right are the observed distributions of two series of MZ and DZ pairs, lying between the Z values which are their limits. Series 1 constituted the standard on which P_{MZ} and P_{DZ} were calculated; Series 2 is independent.

On the basis of this material it was desired to calculate the distribution of values of Nixon's L in MZ and DZ pairs, so that a scale of values of probability of dizygosity could be associated with given values of L. This proved a harder task than was at first anticipated. Whereas values of L were fairly normally distributed in the MZ pairs, the distribution was seriously skewed in the DZ pairs. Neither a logarithmic nor a square root transformation of L succeeded in normalising both distributions at the same time. As Nixon's L had been empirically derived, an alternative was looked for. Individual values of S, T were plotted on graph paper and tried against a straight edge. It was found not only that the expression $S + 30T$ gave good discrimination between MZ and DZ pairs, especially at low values; but also that in the form $Z = \log_{10}(S + 30T)$ Z was normally distributed in both MZ and DZ pairs, as may be seen from Table 23.2. A χ^2 test gives for the MZ pairs a value of 12.13, 15 d.f., $0.70 > P > 0.50$; and for the DZ pairs a value of 5.25, 8 d.f., $0.80 > P > 0.70$. The parameters used for calculating the expected normal distributions were:

means, MZ 0.61444, DZ 1.00111;

standard deviations, MZ 0.21855, DZ 0.23847.

The means and standard deviations of the two distributions can now be used to calculate the heights of the ordinates of the corresponding normal curves at different values of Z; and the relative heights of these ordinates give the relative probabilities of monozygosity or dizygosity. These values are entered in Table 23.3.

Finally, it was decided to validate the discriminant for 48 MZ and 99 DZ pairs who had not been blood-grouped. Their distribution is shown in the final columns of Table 23.3. In this material the means are respectively 0.630 and 1.029, which do not differ significantly from those of the standard material.

TABLE 23.4. EXAMPLE OF WORKING OUT OF DISCRIMINANT

Hand	Digit	Twin A Pattern type	Twin A Ridge count	Twin B Pattern type	Twin B Ridge count	S
Right	1	Whorl	24	Ulnar loop	23	.0177
			20		—	1.3222
	2	Radial loop	—	Ulnar loop	10	1.0414
			25		—	1.4150
	3	Ulnar loop	15	Ulnar loop	15	—
			—		—	—
	4	Radial loop	—	Ulnar loop	14	1.1761
			23		—	1.3802
	5	Whorl	26	Ulnar loop	7	.5283
			14		—	1.1761
Left	1	Double loop	26	Ulnar loop	23	.0512
			13		—	1.1461
	2	Whorl	23	Ulnar loop	23	—
			24		—	1.3979
	3	Ulnar loop	16	Ulnar loop	8	.2762
			—		—	—
	4	Ulnar loop	18	Ulnar loop	16	.0484
			—		—	—
	5	Ulnar loop	18	Ulnar loop	14	.1027
Sums			285		153	11.0795

Pattern type differences = 6. Total ridge count differences, by double count = 132, by single count = 62. $I = \log 305 - \log 173 = 0.2463$. S = sum of $(\log 25 - \log 24)$, etc. = 11.0795. $Z = \log(7.389 + 11.0795) = 1.2664$. $P_{MZ} = 0.022$.

SUMMARY AND CONCLUSIONS

Fingerprints obtained from 180 MZ and 90 DZ twin pairs have been used to calculate a discriminant, based on the work of Nixon, for the diagnosis of zygosity.

A scale is provided relating values of the discriminant with probability values of monozygosity or dizygosity. In Table 23.4, the working of the data from a single case is shown.

The work of Torsten Sjögren has been in essence the work of discovery. While it has enlarged and enriched the fields of neurology, psychiatry and human genetics, it has always had an intensely practical orientation. In such an approach, the investigation of twins finds a legitimate place. The foregoing article is offered to the great pioneer in affectionate dedication, as a practical if make-shift tool for the field-worker.

ACKNOWLEDGMENTS: The Psychiatric Genetics Unit is deeply indebted to Dr. Race and his colleagues for invaluable help. The author also wishes to thank Mr. James Shields for his assistance.

24

EXPECTATION OF
ABNORMALITY ON PATERNAL AND MATERNAL SIDES:
A COMPUTATIONAL MODEL

Edwards (1960, 1963) has recently pointed out that conditions which have been attributed to the effects of a single major gene of diminished penetrance are also capable of being explained as the result of polygenic factors, if the condition in question is not very infrequent. It is only necessary to suppose that polygenic factors bring about a predisposition which expresses itself in a recognizable apparently qualitative deviation, once it has passed a given threshold. There is, for instance, evidence that the presence or absence of the harelip/cleft palate syndrome is due to polygenic factors (Carter, 1965). It is supposed that there is a critical stage in development by which time the embryonic layers involved must have united; a delay in union short of this point is without effect, but beyond it leaves an incomplete state which is never made good.

Edwards has also pointed out that the two alternative hypotheses are very alike in their effects, so that it is difficult to devise tests to distinguish between them. Nevertheless, it is important to make such a distinction if possible, since they are not equivalent. It has been said that the penetrance of every gene is complete, given the right test of its biochemical action. A hypothesis of major gene action, therefore, suggests investigation along biochemical lines. The polygenic hypothesis is of less heuristic value.

It occurred to the writer that it should be possible to distinguish between polygenic inheritance and the effects of a single dominant major gene with diminished penetrance, by noting the distribution of secondary cases among the relatives on the paternal and maternal sides of the ascendance of affected individuals. On the single gene hypothesis one would expect, in the cases where two or more affected relatives were known, that these would be either on the paternal or the maternal side, but not on both. Relatives coming in question would include uncles and aunts, grandparents, and cousins. If polygenic inheritance was operative, the author imagined that a more even distribution between paternal and maternal sides would be found. It was,

Originally published in the *Journal of Medical Genetics* 3: 159-61 (1966).

however, by no means easy to prove this; and when mathematical geneticists, to whom the problem was offered, showed some disinclination to tackle it along rigorous lines, the attempt was made to find an approximate answer by computation carried out on a simplified model.

It is supposed that the many genes predisposing to a condition A are additive in their action; the predisposition to A, measured quantitatively, will accordingly be normally distributed. It is also supposed that any individual exceeding $+2\sigma$ above the population mean is liable to pass the threshold and become recognizable as an A-deviant. Whether he actually did so or not, might or might not depend on some additional, possibly accidental, factor.

We now classify fathers and mothers in classes, each class covering a span of 0.5σ, and its frequency corresponding to the area of the normal curve between the limiting ordinates. Supposing that mating is at random, we are able to calculate the frequency of any given mating as the product of the frequencies of the maternal and paternal classes severally. As a simplifying hypothesis we may then suppose that the children of this mating are distributed normally about the mid-parental value. We take an example from the Table and consider the cell where mothers between the values of $+1.5$ and $+2.0\sigma$ have mated with fathers between $+2.5$ and $+3.0\sigma$. The log maternal frequency is $\bar{2}.6440159$, the log paternal frequency is $\bar{3}.6866184$, and the mating frequency is $\bar{4}.3306343$. The children of this mating are distributed about a mean of $\frac{1}{2}(1.75+2.75) = 2.25\sigma$, and the proportion of them who will deviate from the population mean by 2σ or more will correspond to the area of the normal curve to the positive side of -0.25σ, the log frequency being $\bar{1}.7772139$. The contribution of this mating to our observed propositi may, therefore, be estimated, in comparison with the contributions of all other cells, as $\bar{4}.1078482$.

We now have to make some rough-and-ready assumptions about the paternal and maternal relatives. Uncles and aunts will tend to be distributed about means of $+0.875$ on the maternal and $+1.375$ on the paternal side; mothers and fathers, of course, deviate by twice those margins, but more distant relatives by a lesser amount. At this point we may treat all relatives as if they were sibs of the parents. Maternal relatives will accordingly need to exceed their expected mean by 1.125σ, and paternal relatives by 0.625σ, to attain the critical value of $+2.0\sigma$. We may call the probabilities of these deviations respectively m and p, with log values in this case of $\bar{1}.1149360$ and $\bar{1}.4248623$, respectively.

We now consider the relative probabilities of finding two affected relatives on the paternal side, of finding one paternal and one maternal affected relative, and of finding two affected maternal relatives. Supposing that n relatives are examined on each side, these probabilities reduce to being proportionally $(n - 1)p^2 (1 - m)^2$, $2npm (1 - p) (1 - m)$, and $(n - 1)m^2(1 - p)^2$. Omitting coefficients in terms of n they are in the cell we have instanced in log form $\bar{2}.7284660$, $\bar{2}.6459025$, and $\bar{3}.9612790$, respectively. Adding to these the log of the cell probability, $\bar{4}.1078482$, we get figures whose antilogs are respectively 6.9, 5.7, and 1.2×10^{-6}. The Table has been so prepared as to include all matings which gave a value for the log cell probability added to the log of $p^2(1 - m)^2$ in excess of $\bar{7}.0$, stretching over three orders of magnitude. The probabilities of one paternal and one maternal relative affected, and for two maternal relatives affected, are entered also, where they exceed this figure.

We may now use this Table to compute the relative expectations of finding two paternal relatives affected, two maternal relatives, or one of each. The section of the

TABLE 24.1. RELATIVE EXPECTATIONS OF FINDING TWO PATERNAL, TWO MATERNAL OR ONE OF EACH AFFECTED RELATIVES AS A FUNCTION OF PARENTAL DEVIATION (SIGMA UNITS)

	−2.5	−2.0	−1.5	−1.0	−0.5	0.0	+0.5	+1.0	+1.5	+2.0	+2.5	+3.0	+3.5
−0.5													
0.0						1 / 2 / 1							
+0.5				1 / — / —	3 / 2 / —	7 / 8 / 2	9 / 18 / 9						
+1.0			1 / — / —	5 / — / —	14 / 4 / —	30 / 19 / 3	49 / 56 / 16	58 / 116 / 58					
+1.5		1 / — / —	4 / — / —	14 / 1 / —	39 / 7 / —	81 / 54 / 9	125 / 84 / 14	140 / 165 / 49	112 / 224 / 112				
+2.0		2 / — / —	7 / — / —	27 / 1 / —	74 / 9 / —	146 / 33 / 2	193 / 85 / 9	228 / 167 / 31	174 / 216 / 68	100 / 200 / 100			
+2.5		3 / — / —	11 / — / —	37 / 1 / —	94 / 7 / —	176 / 26 / —	245 / 65 / 4	250 / 117 / 14	182 / 144 / 29	100 / 127 / 41	39 / 78 / 39		
+3.0		1 / — / —	10 / — / —	20 / — / —	80 / 4 / —	144 / 14 / —	191 / 33 / 1	186 / 66 / 4	129 / 67 / 9	69 / 57 / 12	26 / 34 / 11	7 / 14 / 7	
+3.5		1 / — / —	6 / — / —	8 / — / —	64 / — / —	80 / 3 / —	101 / 12 / —	94 / 19 / —	63 / 22 / 2	32 / 18 / 2	12 / 10 / 2	3 / 4 / 1	1 / — / 1
+4.0			3 / — / —	8 / — / —	19 / — / —	30 / 1 / —	37 / 3 / —	33 / 4 / —	21 / 5 / —	10 / 4 / —	4 / 2 / —		
+4.5			2 / — / —	2 / — / —	5 / — / —	8 / — / —	9 / — / —	8 / — / —	5 / — / —	2 / — / —			
+5.0						1 / — / —	1 / — / —	1 / — / —					

Note: Each cell defines the limits of deviation, in standard deviations, of the two parents from the population mean. The numbers in the cells represent from above downwards the relative probabilities of an individual of such parentage, himself deviating from the population by 2 σ or more, having respectively two sibs of a father, one sib of a father and one sib of a mother, and two sibs of a mother, and both deviating from the population mean by 2 σ or more.

bivariate expanse shown in the Table should have been extended symmetrically on the other side of the diagonal marked in heavy outlines, so that paternal figures become maternal ones and vice versa. Adding up the figures for the entire area so described we obtain the numbers 4675:4193:4675, or approximately 11:10:11.

A similar computation was made on the basis that all relatives were equivalent to mothers or fathers. This produced the proportions 31233:12454:31233, or approximately 5:2:5. It was not thought necessary to make yet another computation, to take care of the cases in which information was obtained about more remote relatives. In their case, the proportion of cases in which both a paternal and a maternal relative were ascertained should exceed the proportion of cases in which two paternal, alternatively maternal, relatives were ascertained.

We now have to take account of the value we set on n. In the limiting case, in which n is large, n and $(n - 1)$ approach equality, and the proportions above noted remain undisturbed. At the other limit, where $n = 2$, the expected proportion of cases in which one paternal and one maternal relative are ascertained has to be doubled relatively to unilateral distributions. In practical application, one could make an estimate of the mean number of paternal and maternal relatives per family, on which information was available, in the course of collecting the information designed to test the alternative hypotheses of polygenic or monogenic inheritance. This empirically found value of n could then be used to adjust the expectations against which comparison was to be made.

SUMMARY

It is difficult to distinguish the effects of inheritance by a dominant major gene with diminished penetrance from polygenic inheritance. Nevertheless, it seems to be worth while making the distinction in the case of genetically determined abnormalities, if this is practicable. The possibility has been considered that, if families are sought for in which relatives on the paternal or maternal side include two or more secondary cases of the condition under investigation, single gene inheritance might be exhibited in a preponderance of cases on either the paternal or maternal side, while polygenic inheritance might tend to go with a more even distribution of secondary cases between the two sides of the ascendance. A computational model, making use of some simplifying hypotheses, has been set up to test this possibility. It is found that, in the cases of near relatives such as parents or sibs of parents, even with polygenic inheritance, one expects a unilateral preponderance of secondary cases, rather than a more even distribution. This does not exclude the possibility of distinguishing between the consequences of the two alternative hypotheses, if reliable accounts of more distant relatives are available, or if use can be made of families with three or more secondary cases.

VI

SOCIETY AND THE INDIVIDUAL

EDITORS' COMMENTS: The nine miscellaneous papers in the final part of this selection can be grouped broadly into those dealing with eugenics, psychiatry and the law, and pathography. Despite the variety of topics sampled thus far in the book, our selection does not do full justice to the wide range of interests on which Slater has published something worth saying. These include the inheritance of twinning in man (18, 50), psychosomatic (31, 40, 97) and somatopsychic (22, 35, 51) medicine, the fear of (81) and acceptance of death (138), his sceptical view of ESP (126) and his application of statistical method to the game of chess (62, 74). In concentrating on the genetic aspects of psychiatry, we have even been unable to find room for papers evaluating the effects of insulin, ECT and leucotomy (58, 70, 75, 83); and among papers related to genetics we have not included any of those, usually written in collaboration with Valerie Cowie, which deal with mongolism or other chromosomal abnormalities (103, 116, 122, 129).

The four of Slater's papers on eugenics reprinted here span the years 1936–67. Paper 25 is the first detailed and informed critique of the operation of the sterilization law in Germany by one who, while interested in the possible advantages of voluntary sterilization, abhorred German eugenic practice as an attack on personal and physical liberty, quite apart from its racist aspects. Slater's own views as expressed, for instance, in his paper (30) published in 1945 in a symposium on rebuilding family life after the war, led him to the conclusion that, as to whether a couple has a large family or none at all, "we may safely leave people to be judges in their own case." Paper 26 was written in collaboration with Dr. J. A. Fraser Roberts, F.R.S., a pioneer in the development of the quantitative genetic analysis of intelligence and later of the associations between blood groups and disease. Until 1964 he was Director of the Medical Research Council's Clinical Genetics Research Unit at Great Ormond Street Hospital. It is one of the earlier attempts at a discussion of the eugenic implications of polygenically determined characteristics. Much of it is still relevant. However, the differential birth rate with respect to intelligence is generally no longer thought to entail the dire consequences of a drop in the intellectual level of the community which was then feared. It has been shown (Higgins, Reed, and Reed, 1962) that the high fertility of some parents of low intelligence is balanced by the fact that many other persons of even lower intelligence remain unmarried. However, the recent evidence that the trend of differential fertility may now be reversed, as the authors hoped, can only be welcomed, and geneticists are now cautiously suggesting that the intellectual level of the population may be slowly rising.

Galton's Heritage, delivered as the Galton Lecture in 1960, might have been classed as pathography, along with Paper 33 on Schumann, since it relates Galton's deviant traits of character to his creativity. It is more appropriate to place it with the papers on eugenics, the science of which he was the founder. Slater criticized Galton's preoccupation with the elite, while attempting at the same time to understand it. As in Paper 26, he emphasized the importance of the whole community: "all mankind is in one boat together." Next is a vote of thanks to the Galton lecturer seven years later in which the theme of the proper relationship between sociology and biology is once again taken up, albeit briefly, and in which a model of genetic-environmental interaction is put forward in which no genotype and no environment need be consistently disadvantageous.

The next two Papers, 29 and 30, are of sociological as much as genetic interest. In his *Retrospect,* Slater has some additional comments to make on the ideas put forward in the paper on anti-Semitism. Part of this last paper derived from work at Sutton when the religious affiliation of psychiatric and non-psychiatric patients was compared (43). The next paper is taken from the book reporting the wartime investigation of the backgrounds of married patients from the Sutton Emergency Hospital and their wives, to which we alluded in our introduction to Part IV. Moya Woodside, co-author of *Patterns of Marriage,* is currently a research psychiatric social worker at the Royal Edinburgh Hospital. The important topic of assortative mating in respect of personality has not subsequently received the practical attention it merits, whether from the genetic or purely social point of view. Garrison *et al.* (1968), however, have recently studied assortative mating and educational level, while Kreitman (1968) has stressed how overt neurotic illness in both partners of a married couple can result from personal interaction as well as from assortative mating.

The sometimes conflicting points of view of lawyer and psychiatrist as they affect the notion of responsibility and the criteria of what is acceptable evidence are discussed in Papers 31 and 32 as well as in the *Retrospect.* Slater's interest in forensic psychiatry and in the rights of the individual and of society was sharpened by his being called as expert witness and by his membership of the Royal Commission on Capital Punishment, 1949–53. Among recent research projects in which he has been involved is that which he carried out with John and Valerie Cowie into the backgrounds and after-histories of young female delinquents (130). Their book stresses the advantages of an individual psychiatric approach to criminology over a purely sociological one. In its analysis of data it also provides further evidence of Slater's methodological ingenuity and clarity of reasoning.

The final paper illustrates Slater's interest in the problems of pathography and creativity. Furthermore, his discussion of Schumann's mental illness, based inevitably on documentary evidence, reveals the importance he lays on accurate clinical observation as opposed to speculation. The joint author is Alfred Meyer, Professor Emeritus of Neuropathology at the Institute of Psychiatry, University of London, who at one time nearly embarked on a career as concert pianist. In their second paper on the pathography of the German composers (89), they discussed the possible neuropsychiatric illnesses of Handel (cyclothymic depression), Gluck (arteriosclerotic dementia), Mozart (mild symptomatic psychosis associated with terminal uraemia) and, in greater detail, Hugo Wolf (abnormal personality, general paresis). In his unpublished inaugural address as President of the Psychiatric Section of the Royal Society of Medicine in 1958 on *The Creative Personality* and again in the paper written for Erik Essen-Möller's *Festschrift* (139), Slater has, on the evidence described in the introduction to the paper on Schumann, argued forcefully against the popular idea that genius is allied to madness. The great majority of creative artists and scientists were mentally normal and highly endowed with energy derived from healthy elements in their personality. As a further example of his application of scientific method to the problems of creativity, we may mention his contribution to the *Festschrift* for Manfred Bleuler (102). Slater, himself a poet (133) and Shakespeare scholar (134), chose to report the result of his counting the frequency with which English poets used words describing different colours: each tended to have his individual colour preferences. Only just completed is Slater's sensitive discussion of Shakespeare's sonnets (141), written in honour of another distinguished European psychiatrist, Barahona Fernandes. Here Slater discusses the age of the poet, and his tendency to depression and homosexuality. Slater doubts that the poet who wrote the Sonnets was "William of Stratford."

25

GERMAN EUGENICS IN PRACTICE

According to figures quoted from *Deutsche Justiz* on page 90 of the July 1935 issue of the *Eugenics Review*, some 56,000 people were sterilized in Germany in the first twelve months after the introduction of the sterilization law. If this figure may be taken as correct, it does not follow that the first year of sterilization will be typical of the following ones, or that this rate of sterilization will be kept up. The operation of the law is likely with time to improve in efficiency, leading one to expect an increased number of sterilizations per year. On the other hand, in the first year the standing population of defectives, schizophrenics, etc., will be attacked, the operations of subsequent years being more confined to the yearly increment. Could, however, this figure of 56,000 be taken as a probable yearly average, it would imply about two per thousand of the fertile population being sterilized every year, with a total expectation of sterilization for the average individual in the neighbourhood of 4 per cent.

PUBLIC REACTION TO STERILIZATION LAW

It is not easy to discover the reaction of the population to this very definite attack on their personal and physical liberty. My information, from a well-informed source, is that there is much resentment throughout Germany among the common people, particularly directed against its compulsory nature. Compulsion itself is not liked, and as a police affair is doubly objectionable. The nature of the operation does not improve matters. An attack on the sexual organs is calculated to arouse more resentment than any operation of corresponding severity on another part. Among women there is a definite mortality, not entirely to be eliminated in any double laparotomy, and this mortality tends to be exaggerated and associated with both sexes. Lastly, the nature of the operation is still misunderstood and thought to have

Originally published in the *Eugenics Review* 27: 285–95 (1936).

a castrating effect. Some of these grounds for objection will disappear in the course of time; others will always be felt.

Patients to be sterilized seldom protest; they know that if they did it would have no effect. Physical resistance must be extremely rare. The law provides for the use of direct force, but this has not yet been necessary. Resistance to sterilization by appeal is statutory and frequent. There have indeed been attempts to organize this resistance. In Bavaria pamphlets were printed and found in Catholic hands recommending all patients to appeal in every case. This was, of course, an attempt to make the law unworkable. The pamphlet was seized and destroyed. The frequency of appeal has varied much from time to time and from place to place, in some areas being as low as 1 per cent, in others as high as two-thirds of all cases where the order was made.

In many scientific and more liberal circles there is a strong objection to the compulsory aspect of the law, partly as a matter of principle, partly based on reasoned argument. In support of this view are quoted the calculations of Haldane and others, which go to show that sterilization operates extremely slowly towards the removal of characteristics dependent on infrequent recessive genes, and the findings of one scientific worker, that practically all the children of schizophrenics are born before the manifestation of the disease. One authority, with whom I discussed the matter, was of the opinion that the law would operate at least as well if sterilization were made voluntary — that in fact one would get as good results by propaganda as by compulsion. Against this one must put the opinion of such a well-informed authority as Sjögren of Sweden, who told me that in his opinion the reverse would be the case. Apparently the experience in Sweden with voluntary sterilization has been very disappointing, only a few hundreds having been sterilized since the introduction of the law a few years ago.

Practising doctors in general are inclined to object to the law, and to the increase in their duties, and to the increasedly police nature of these duties which the law entails. The doctor must notify all cases of the hereditary disorders named in the law, as far as these become known to him through the practice of his profession. For instance, were he, on a professional visit, to see the patient's brother have an epileptic fit, he would not be bound to notify him, though he could do so if he wished. If the patient himself were to have the fit, and it could not be referred to definite exogenous causes, then he must notify. If, on the other hand, the doctor passing casually along the street were to see a patient of his having a fit, he would not be bound to report him. Presumably, however, if he were to proceed to his assistance, the duty to notify would reappear.

The keenness with which doctors carry out their duties varies greatly from place to place. In small country villages, with only one doctor, he generally does it satisfactorily, because he neither loses nor gains by it. In places with two or more doctors they usually notify only where it is obviously unavoidable. The doctor slackest in notifying will tend to profit at the expense of the others. On the other hand in Thuringia and Baden these duties were carried out with the greatest enthusiasm. In the latter place, the doctors seemed possessed of the notion that the more cases they notified, the better pleased would they be in high quarters. At length a circular had to be sent round, telling them that they were only to notify cases properly capable of reproduction.

In clinics, the duty of notification is carried out conscientiously, and proceeds for the most part automatically. The chief difficulties are those of diagnosis. The diagnosis should be of such a degree of certainty that the clinician would be prepared to back it in a court of law, or alternatively for the Professor to be able to demonstrate the case as such to a class of students. Many authorities find difficulty in fitting their cases into the official scheme of classification — particularly, for instance, Kleist. According to Kleist's classification there are a number of separate syndromes, for instance — motility and confusion psychoses, which would by most clinicians be considered schizophrenic, but which he treats as separate entities. As in these cases his researches into the heredity have shown no connection with schizophrenia, he does not hold them to be schizophrenic, nor covered by the law, nor in his clinic are they notified.

Difficulties of diagnosis must necessarily occur, and may have unfortunate effects. The following is such a case.

> The daughter of a doctor had had in childhood an obscure febrile complaint, accompanied by some minor neurological signs. At puberty she developed periodical but rare and slight "absences"; but with the years these increased in frequency and severity until they were major epileptic fits. In the course of treatment her father was informed she would have to be notified for sterilization. He objected very much, and took her from doctor to doctor in the vain attempt to get her recognized as a case of fits of exogenous origin. At last she was seen by one of the best-known neurological surgeons of the country, who after an encephalography operated on her and removed a large cyst from the brain, with complete recovery and cessation of the fits.

Such cases cannot be published, owing to the disrepute into which they might bring the law, if they were at all frequent.

In the first few months after the law was passed, there was a considerable amount of overcrowding in clinics and hospitals, because cases of recovery from schizophrenia and manic-depressive psychosis had to be held pending decision on the matter of sterilization. This is the case no longer. Once the case is notified, he may be discharged and wait at home for the notice of reception into a surgical clinic, or alternatively conduct his appeal before the court from home. Only cases where the danger of procreation is really serious, e.g., men in a mild hypomanic state with much sexual desire, should be held till the question of sterilization is finally settled and they can be directly transferred to the surgical clinic. In all other cases it suffices for the law to have been set in motion, and patients are subjected to a minimum of delay and inconvenience.

Cases for sterilization are notified to the "Bezirksarzt" [district health officer]. He would correspond to some degree to the English local medical officer of health, though his activities are being more and more confined to the operation of the eugenic laws. He draws up a document, the "Antrag," which summarizes all available data to enable a decision to be reached as to sterilization or not. To obtain sufficient information he is entitled to order the patient's admission to a psychiatric clinic for a period not longer than six weeks for examination and report. The "Antrag" is laid before the local eugenic court ("Erbgesundheitsgericht"), which consists of a jurist as president, a "Bezirksarzt," and a specialist in medical genetics, and they reach the decision on sterilization. If the patient is dissatisfied with the decision he may appeal to a higher court, the "Erbgesundheitsobergericht."

If the "Bezirksarzt" is a Catholic, difficulties of conscience are likely to appear. Catholic general practitioners are allowed by their Church to make the notification, because it does not necessarily follow that the patient will be sterilized. Also such notifications have an unrelated statistical significance. The actual order to sterilize is another matter, and a Catholic "Bezirksarzt" is forbidden by his Church, and compelled by the State, to make such sterilization orders. In districts where there are two such doctors, one of whom is a Catholic, it has sometimes been arranged that the Catholic hands over the whole of these duties to his colleague. Presumably the whole matter could be settled by an agreement between Church and State.

The order for admission to a psychiatric clinic for examination and report is made in quite a fair proportion of cases where the original notification has not been made from such a clinic. The senior assistants at the clinics make a very reasonable addition to their small salaries out of the fees for these reports. The admission to a clinic for this purpose is specially likely to happen where the patient has appealed against the order for sterilization. The reports in these cases are long, exhaustive and reasoned documents. For instance, I saw a report on a case of congenital syphilis and mental deficiency. The family history, personal history, physical, psychiatric, and psychological examinations were given in detail. The difficult point of whether the patient was mentally defective because of the syphilis, or because of hereditary defect and only happened concurrently to be syphilitic, was discussed in full on general grounds and in the particular circumstances of the case; and finally judgment was given, in this case that the mental deficiency was to be referred to exogenous rather than endogenous causes.

Interesting here is the fact that a certainty of congenital syphilis is not taken legally as *ipso facto* precluding a diagnosis of hereditary mental defect. The patient is assured of a full and unbiased consideration of his case in any reputable clinic. Where the doctor does not prefer to write out the report in full, special forms are provided which, if properly filled in, ensure a thoroughgoing anamnesis and examination from every point of view.

Before the introduction of the sterilization laws, Germany had no special laws for mental defectives, and practically no special institutions. Hospitalization was much less frequent than in England, and largely confined to idiots and the severer grades of defect. Mental defectives, apart from such special cases as the above, are judged principally on social grounds, to a less degree on school record and least of all on psychological tests. A special form is given for the latter, which few English or I suppose American psychologists would consider satisfactory. It consists of questions on orientation of the usual kind, on "school knowledge" of the most elementary kind (Who was Bismarck? When is Christmas?), mathematical problems (simple interest on 300 marks at 3 per cent for 3 years), general questions of an almost philosophical kind (Why do we have day and night? Why are houses built higher in towns than in the country? Why do children go to school?), differences (between "mistake" and "lie," between "Rechtsanwalt" [attorney] and "Staatsanwalt" [prosecutor]), composition of sentences (e.g., out of "soldier," "war," "father-land"), the repetition of a story, the explanation of proverbs, "general moral ideas" (Why does one learn? save money? What is truth?), memory and attention tests, and notes on the behaviour during the testing.

It is no wonder that the German does not place much reliance on such tests, considered as tests of intelligence. The requirement on which most importance is laid for a diagnosis of mental defect is a persistent failure of the person concerned to maintain any sort of a position in life for himself and his family; if this is backed by an unsatisfactory school record — e.g., twice having to stay on in the same class instead of being promoted at the end of the year, or attendance at a special school ("Hilfsschule") — the diagnosis of mental defect may be made almost regardless of the results of the "intelligence test."

One of the special problems of mental deficiency is its ascertainment. Psychiatric cases are got hold of largely through the psychiatric clinics. A few mental defectives will be discovered in the same way, if they come into the clinics in a state of excitement, or complaining of the depressive or hypochondriacal symptoms not infrequent in defectives; but these must be few. The majority are discovered in other ways. In the country the local "Bezirksarzt" is supposed to, and generally does, know every single family that lives in his district. He is accordingly able to put his hands on the local defectives, persistent low-grade misfits and failures, at any time. In the towns the matter is more difficult, and the defectives are got hold of largely accidentally, as they come to doctors or hospitals for advice on entirely unrelated subjects — e.g. for appendicitis — or as they appear as candidates for financial or social assistance at the offices of charity organizations, church missions, public assistance offices, etc. With the development of the marriage-advice centres and related scientific and social institutions, there will be still further ways of ascertainment, until this should become in the end fairly complete.

APPEALS AGAINST STERILIZATION

Appeals from the order for sterilization come before a special court. In many cases there will have been a preliminary examination and report such as has been described. However, many other points have arisen than the question of diagnosis, and a number of appeals have been reported and discussed in a paper by Bostroem.

Bostroem, in his introduction, criticizes the haphazard practice of doctors in regard to notification. There is no point in worrying the authorities with 60-year-old alcoholics and 10-year-old idiots, when the really dangerous — in regard to propagation — are not being touched. The pressing cases are the physically healthy men and women from sixteen to forty, young schizophrenics and manic-depressives in remissions, young subjects of hereditary blindness and deafness, etc. It is important to make sure of the capacity for procreation. It must not happen in future that, after months of proceedings costing a lot of money, it appears that the case should never have been brought. Further, everyone is entitled to be heard in his own defence. If not capable of taking steps himself, he must be represented. The doctor must see to this.

The following are some of the more interesting cases:

1. A man under guardianship for mental defect was held by the court to be a psychopath[1] and not sterilizable. The difference between guardianship and sterilization laws is made clear. Guardianship depends entirely on social irresponsibility. Liability to sterilization is governed by other, biological, considerations.

2. A woman at the menopause, last period some months ago, still theoretically capable of bearing children, but not likely to. Sterilization not enforced. Compelling grounds must be shown for necessity of sterilization, not merely a theoretical possibility.

3. A man, aged 50, wife at menopause. Appellant has adult children. The theoretical possibility of producing children by extramarital intercourse held not sufficient to justify sterilization. There are a number of similar decisions.

4. A man, aged 57, is in an institution, and usually allowed out only in company. He has an interest in the other sex, but only as an exhibitionist. He looks so repulsive that it is inconceivable that any woman should wish to have to do with

---

[1] Both in German psychiatry and in the sterilization law there is a sharp distinction between the psychopathic and the psychotic. Only the following conditions render their subjects liable to sterilization: inborn hereditary defect, schizophrenia, circular (manic-depressive) insanity, hereditary epilepsy, hereditary (Huntington's) chorea, hereditary blindness, hereditary deafness, severe hereditary physical abnormality, severe alcoholism. Under the term "imbecile" is understood in German a considerably wider range of mental defect than in England.

him. Sterilization was rejected on the grounds that he was under adequate supervision. His personal appearance was held to be beside the point, and no grounds for not enforcing the law.

5. A man, stupid, but a useful agricultural labourer. His brother, like himself, attended a special school. Previous history shows early death of the mother and a neglectful stepmother. He was held to lie on the boundary between normal stupidity ("landläufige Unbegabtheit") and deficiency. Sterilization not enforced. The court wished to postpone decision for a year. This is not permitted. On the other hand it is allowed to reintroduce proceedings at a later date if new facts, e.g., altered behaviour, justify it.

6. Woman of limited intelligence, husband the same. Although it was to be expected that only children of limited intelligence would be the result of this union, the limitation was not held to amount to mental defect. Sterilization rejected.

7. Three imbecile males, 14, 15, 19 years. The court allowed the appeal, because they can work on the land and show themselves useful members of society. The reduction in numbers of such people is not socially desirable. Bostroem remarks that it is all very well to be tender of "primitive personalities," but if they are imbecile they ought to be sterilized.

8. Female, aged 25. Normal school career, could never do any useful work, wanted to write stories and poems. In a girls' home was incapable even of finding her place at table, if it was changed. The court held mental defect proven on the following grounds: (a) Development uniform and continuous from childhood up. If she is mentally defective now, she was so congenitally. (b) Father is a psychopath. (c) Mother was for ten years in an asylum. Appeal dismissed.

9. Man. No proven mental defect, but he is an habitual criminal and recidivist of a bad type, guilty of crimes with violence. The court held that his abnormal behaviour justified the assumption of mental defect.

In commenting on the above cases one notes, as indeed was to be expected, a certain lack of uniformity between court and court. One sees three imbeciles, who are capable of simple work on the land, encouraged to propagate their kind, and a criminal psychopath sterilized for mental defect. One notes the admission of irrelevant evidence. It is no good evidence of hereditary mental defect to show that the parents were respectively psychopathic and insane. In fact one is inclined to doubt the diagnosis of mental defect here altogether. The child was apparently normal in schooldays, and later developed a progressive change simulating a dementia. It seems not unlikely that this was a schizophrenia of the simplex type. Of course this also justifies sterilization, but it is poor law to do the right thing on the wrong grounds.

One may note also a difference of principle between English criminal law and German sterilization law. One completed trial does not protect against a second charge for the same "offence." In the case of the three imbeciles, there may be grounds for assuming the influence on social psychiatry of the national-socialist *Weltanschauung.* Those "zuverlässige und treue Arbeitskräfte" [dependable and faithful workers] and useful members of the "Volksgemeinschaft" [community] are perhaps members of the party, and have demonstrated in that way their social desirability and suitability for procreation. This is pure supposition, but would at least be congruous. One notes that the law in its operation is tender of the merely stupid. Mental defect appears to have to be of considerable degree before becoming operative as a ground for sterilization. One remembers political speeches in which intelligence is rudely decried, and the ideal for the people is held out to be physical health and a capacity for unquestioning, uncritical obedience. For such a make-up, too high a degree of intelligence would be, if anything, a disadvantage. With this official attitude, the whole attitude towards mental defect is bound to undergo a change. Of the first importance to the German government is that every citizen should be a good national-socialist. While no hereditary constitutional tendency to national-socialism has yet been demonstrated, one may hardly blame the judges for attempting to estimate the value of the individual as a whole. One case is known to me where hospital authorities arranged that an officer in the S.A. should not be sterilized merely for a slight attack of dementia praecox.

As far as my information goes, the operation of the sterilization law is likely to prove costly. On an average it costs per woman 1,000 marks (£80) and 100-200 marks (£8-£16) each for men, inclusive of operation charges. In cases where there is an appeal, or where the patient is held in a psychiatric clinic for some weeks' observation, the cost would be considerably higher. The whole of these charges are borne by the state, which must mean, at the present rate of sterilization, a sum of about £2,000,000 a year. The patient, even if wealthy, pays nothing himself.

Certain alterations are possible in the law. Criminals are not covered by it. It is very possible that a special law will be brought into force to cover them, or certain classes of them, which will be called by a different name, be administered by different officers, have a different procedure. Criminals were purposely omitted from the present sterilization law, as far as possible to obviate the idea that sterilization is a sort of punishment. There is no foundation for the idea, sometimes found outside Germany, that the law is administered in a partial way as a punishment for political offenders.

There are other possible enlargements — e.g., to include the children of two recessive parents, and the monozygotic twin of a person already ordered to be sterilized. This could be taken as an improvement in the justice of the law. The phenotypically healthy twin is at least as dangerous eugenically as the sick twin. Further it is possible that there may be a new clause allowing voluntary sterilization to those individuals who, according to current conceptions, would be regarded as certainly heterozygotic, e.g., the children of a schizophrenic. This is hardly probable. The possibility that the law, at this date, may be converted into a law for voluntary sterilization altogether may be disregarded. It does not lie in the national-socialist philosophy to consider the possibility of getting anything done by voluntary effort.

Apart from possible changes in the law, there is a possibility of a new orientation in its application. The appeal cases show that the law is not absolutely hard and fast, but that its administrators tend to be governed by other considerations than merely the diagnosis and fertility of the person concerned. This is illustrated by the case of a musician in Frankfurt-am-Main, a man of unusual musical ability, who had an attack of mania or depression and was ordered to be sterilized. He appealed against the order, and the appeal was allowed on the grounds that unusual hereditary (here musical) talent compensated, as it were, for the manic-depressive taint. This seems to me to indicate an alteration of the official attitude, i.e., the estimation of the individual as a whole, and not merely as the bearer of one or other particular hereditary taint.

STERILIZATION AND RESEARCH

There is no doubt that the sterilization law and the whole social policy bound up with it will have a profound effect on research in Germany. Certain not entirely

287

desirable effects have shown themselves already. The fear of being notified as a suitable case for sterilization does operate as a cause of distrust and reluctance to give information among the subjects of a psychiatric research. In my own research in Munich, which was into the relatives of manic-depressives, I found an extraordinary willingness among these people to come to the institute, often at considerable personal inconvenience, for examination, and an equally great readiness to give full and sincere information about their relatives. I am sure this could not be paralleled in England. It is no doubt largely due to much greater interest in and knowledge of this subject in Germany, and the popular German conviction of its social importance. Quite a number of the relatives I saw brought family trees and documents extending back over several generations. Nevertheless there was quite a proportion of my informants who required very persistent and express reassurance that it was out of the question that the information obtained from them should be used in a way they would not like. Of the motives that influenced those persons who would not reply to any attempts to get in touch with them it is impossible to speak.

The attitude of different research workers in regard to this matter of research versus sterilization varied greatly in different research institutions. In one place I found a steadfast conviction among the more responsible workers that it was indeed undesirable that the material obtained by research should be used directly for extraneous ends, or that the public should be allowed to get the impression it could be so used. In another place I found a very curious quibbling attitude, that while certain activities of the institute were of the nature of pure research and so the data obtained thereby would not be used to provide sterilization notifications, yet other activities were not so purely research ones, and there this dispensation would not hold. For example, were subjects admitted to the institute for anthropological and medical examination, and were they at the same time to receive anything in the nature of treatment (e.g., the continuation of a diabetic diet) then a duty to notify could not be evaded. The institute in question was also intended to develop into the biological-statistical centre of its city, and into the local marriage-advice bureau, and these activities were regarded as being similarly not covered by the term research. In other words, there was a definite determination among the workers at this place to use their institute as much as possible for the extraneous purpose of providing candidates for sterilization. When one learned that the material for these anthropological and other investigations consisted practically solely of voluntary subjects who had been secured by the fair words of sisters at clinics, social workers, etc., one was left with a very disagreeable impression.

There are other important aspects of German eugenics beside the sterilization law. Eugenic qualifications are insisted on by the government for applicants for appointment to the state services — e.g., for the post office, state bank, railways, etc., as well as for the civil services proper, and for members of the S.S. and S.A. These are briefly that the applicant shall not be non-Aryan nor hereditarily tainted ("erblich belastet").

The definition of what constitutes hereditary taint has not yet been clearly laid down. Luxenburger has claimed that it should be interpreted in its more strict scientific sense, and only those persons regarded as "belastet" who according to present ideas *must* be the carriers of a pathogenic gene. These would then be only: those showing the hereditary abnormality; or the monozygotic twin of such a one; the children of parents one or both of whom have shown a recessive abnormality; the parents of a child with such a recessive abnormality; in the case of sex-linked abnormalities all children of an affected mother, the daughters of an affected father.

Luxemburger has difficulty with the siblings of schizophrenics, and suggests that only those who themselves are schizoid psychopaths should be regarded as tainted, not for instance those who are psychopaths of a non-schizoid kind. The clinical distinction would be one of some difficulty. He remarks that "In principle even the hereditarily tainted [erbkrank] families are to be encouraged, apart from those members who are to be regarded as 'belastet'." The whole family with all its members may not be regarded as "belastet"; the individual members must be considered separately, to see if they come under his rules. Luxemburger's view, however, does not seem to be the official one, at least in regard to the administration of the marriage loan.

MARRIAGE LAWS

On October 19th, 1935, entered into force the "Gesetz zum Schutze der Erbgesundheit des deutschen Volkes" [Law for the Protection of the Genetic Well-being of the German People]. This expressly forbids marriage where one of the parties suffers from an infectious disease, is under a form of guardianship, suffers from a mental disorder, or suffers from a hereditary disease in the sense of the sterilization laws. Before marriage, certificates must be obtained from the appropriate authority to the effect that no hindrance exists on any of the above grounds. Marriages which violate the law are null and void, and the parties are liable to imprisonment, as also for attempting to get around the law, for example by marrying abroad. Marriages between "Aryans" and full Jews are also forbidden. The full Jew may only marry the full Jew. Half Jews, if they accept the Jewish faith, are reckoned as full Jews. Otherwise they may only marry half Jews. Quarter Jews may not marry their like, but only "Aryans."

The certificate allowing marriage has to be obtained from the local health office ("Gesundheitsamt") These are being set up all over Germany in every district which does not yet possess one. They correspond in many ways with public health offices in England, but their activities principally consist in carrying out the new eugenic measures. At every one of the offices a special office will be set up for giving the certificates required by the above law, and for the administration of the marriage loan. At these clinics every applicant for certificate or marriage loan will receive a careful examination. For this an official form is provided, in which besides an ordinary medical examination the doctor has to note anthropological measurements, type of constitution according to Kretschmer, racial type, twinship, all details of previous illnesses with dates and notes of where treated, so that more exact particulars can be obtained if required. Further the whole family history is gone into, and details are obtained if possible of the great-grandparents, in every case of the grandparents and all their descendants, even, if possible, first cousins. Finally a summary card is drawn up, in which the above facts are summarized, and cross references to data in the possession of other social services are given, e.g., for venereal diseases, cripples, tuberculosis, obstetrics and infant welfare, insanity and psychopathy, alcoholism, school medical service. Here also the "diagnosis" is entered, e.g., non-Aryan, insane, "belastet," criminal, peculiarly gifted, etc. The special gifts, which have to be far above average to receive mention, are mental — for mathematics, languages, organization, art, music, painting, drawing and plastic art; and practical — for manual and technical occupations and sport. Similar details are noted about all members of the family.

On the basis of these findings a decision is reached as to whether the applicant is to be granted the marriage-enabling certificate, and/or the marriage loan, or as to whether he should be conditionally or unconditionally advised against marriage. The following must be disallowed the marriage loan:

I. Those who suffer or have suffered from the following hereditary abnormalities: hereditary mental defect, schizophrenia, manic-depressive psychosis, idiopathic epilepsy, Huntington's chorea, hereditary blindness, hereditary deafness, severe hereditary physical disability, severe psychopathy, severe constitutional disorder. The deaf, blind, and epileptic may only receive the loan when the disorder is clearly to be traced to exogenous causes, and where apart from this the applicant can support a family. Physical disability includes congenital dislocation of the hip, congenital clubfoot, cleft palate, split hand, spina bifida, hereditary narrowed pelvis of such a degree that it is impossible for a child to be born naturally, Friedreich's ataxia, myotonia, progressive muscular dystrophy, hereditary spastic paralysis, dwarfs less than 130 cm. in height. Constitutional disorder includes severe asthenia coupled with other abnormalities or stigmata of degeneration, juvenile diabetes, dystrophia adiposogenitalis, early and severe otosclerosis, severe lymphatism, haemophilia, myxoedema, high-grade infantilism, severe goitre — in regions with endemic goitre only those with cardiac disorder. Among the severe psychopathies are included severe cases of hysteria, homosexuality, alcoholism, drug-addiction, asocial and antisocial psychopaths (presumably includes all at least habitual criminals), and other types of psychopathy, which without being asocial or antisocial "because of its special kind and severity represents a great hindrance in the way of work and pleasure in life," where the said psychopathy shows itself as hereditary. This includes conditions with severe mood changes, depressions, anxiety states, suicidal tendencies, and compulsive symptoms.

II. Those who, without having suffered themselves from any of the above conditions, have families which show or have shown in such a severe degree the presence of hereditary illness that the children of the applicant may be regarded as materially more heavily tainted than the average population. The "Belastung" may be certain or highly probable. Apart from special consideration of the method of inheritance in a given case, it may be assumed that the applicant is "belastet" when one parent, or two siblings, or more than a third of the remaining relatives (grandparents, uncles and aunts), or one sib and two grandparents, suffer from severe and certain hereditary physical or mental abnormality. By this estimation, abnormalities of different kinds are to be reckoned together. Even lesser degree of hereditary taint is sufficient for the rejection of the application, if the proposed partner has a similar degree of tainting. Emphasis is laid on the fact that it must be ascertained that the abnormalities in question are in fact hereditable; mention is made of depressive states and psychoses of short duration, especially at advanced ages, where endocrine disturbances should be thought of as an alternative diagnosis to that of an endogenous psychosis, of symptomatic epilepsy, etc.

III. Those suffering from any infectious disorder likely to affect the health of the partner or the children. This is specially directed against venereal diseases.

IV. Where one of the partners is sterile.

V. Severe alcoholism, where it is superimposed on a basis of "hereditary inferiority," or has led to such destruction of the personality that no satisfactory family life can be expected.

At the end of the examination one of the following certificates is issued: that the applicant may marry; that he is permanently or temporarily unfit for marriage; that though the findings do not necessarily prove him unsuitable for marriage, he has been advised against the proposed union; that he is sterile and only to be recommended to marry another sterile individual or the subject of an hereditary abnormality; that he is the subject of hereditary disorder and only to be recommended to marry a sterile individual.

A number of points of great interest arise from these paragraphs. Luxenburger's definition of the scientific conception of "Belastung" goes by the board. Those are to be considered "belastet" who have a considerably greater chance than the average of carrying a pathogenic gene, not only those who theoretically must do so. Hence the government is content to prevent a number of healthy and normal people marrying and propagating, if by so doing a number of abnormal and undesirable people are also prevented. In this connection it is only rational that unlike abnormalities should be reckoned together in determining "Belastung." The heaping up of such abnormalities among the relatives obviously increases the chance of developing some sort of an abnormality, though for example, the nephew of a schizophrenic is no more likely to develop schizophrenia for having a half-brother with a cleft palate. It is possible, however, that this is not the basis of this provision, but rather a belief in a general hereditary degenerative diathesis. This view receives support from the official use of such terms as "hereditary inferiority" and such ideas as constitutional asthenia with signs of degeneration.

The policy with regard to selective breeding seems to have been settled in favour of attempting to keep abnormalities latent, rather than breeding them out. This is shown by the provision that those with a slight degree of "tainting" may marry normal persons but not those with a similar degree of tainting. They are treated in the same way, in fact, as quarter Jews.

It will be seen that the function of these "Eheberatungsstellen" [marriage-advice bureaus] is a very important one. There is first the immediate and practical one of forbidding undesirable and encouraging desirable unions. A secondary duty will no doubt be notifying cases for sterilization. Thirdly, and of increasing importance with the passage of years, will be the function of these clinics as record offices. The summary cards already referred to are kept in duplicate, one locally, the other forwarded to a central office in Berlin, and are definitely intended for statistical research. If the examinations and records are made even with only moderate care there will soon be provided a complete and fairly exhaustive family record of the whole German people. Such records thrown open to research will provide material of quite incalculable value.

The marriage loan is of the value of 600 marks (£48). It is given to those certified suitable by the marriage-advice bureaus, and no interest is demanded for the first year. The birth of a child automatically pays back 100 marks and gives another year of interest-free enjoyment of the remainder. It should be a considerable inducement to marriage and have a certain slight effect in promoting the birth of children. Much more effective in this way should be the German income-tax system. This is exceedingly complicated, but it may be roughly stated that there is a tax on single persons of about 15 per cent. Marriage reduces the amount of tax slightly, the birth of the first and subsequent children very considerably. For poor and middle-class people the possession of four children renders them almost tax-free. All reductions of income tax for children are, unlike in the English system, percentage reductions, so that better-off people get a correspondingly larger actual reduction in tax. From an eugenic point of view this is a much better system.

THE CITY AS GODPARENT

An interesting experiment has been introduced in the city of Berlin, the "Ehrenpatenschaft" [honorary sponsorship]. Families with two or three children may, if they decide to have a third or fourth, go to a city office and declare their intention. If within the term of two years the child is born, the city will stand godparent. This implies a present of 30 marks (48s.) a month until the end of the first year and 20 marks (32s.) a month subsequently until the end of the fourteenth year. If the child himself or an elder brother or sister dies, the fund ceases, but may be continued again with the birth of an additional child. Only legitimate children may receive the gift. If twins or triplets are born, all are covered. The gift is independent of the financial position of the family. It is not a form of social support, but a gift of honour. For no official purpose, e.g., for calculation of income tax, is it to be reckoned as part of the income of the family. The family and the child bear the honourable titles of "Patenfamilie" and "Patenkind der Stadt Berlin." They receive precedence in applications for flats and dwellings, for jobs and posts of whatever kind where the influence of the city authorities can make itself felt. The city even pledges itself to use its influence on their behalf in other parts of Germany, should the family move. The family has to be "of high biological value," and the conditions for this seem to be a slightly stricter form of the conditions for the marriage loan.

In considering all these eugenic measures, particularly the sterilization and marriage laws, one must not forget that their compulsory character is nothing strange to the German people. These are but two of a multitude of such laws. All the German's actions are governed and regulated. His scheme of education, what views he may express — even in the scientific world — what wireless programme he may listen to, where and what he may buy and eat and read, how he may sign his letters and say good morning to his friends, are governed by law or by a form of persuasion resting on force. The future development of the German people has been decided, on theoretical and philosophical grounds, by its leaders. The German's duty is to be moulded in the right direction. Any leadership among the people, apart from the disciplined and subordinate leadership of the type of the non-commissioned officer, is rigidly suppressed. The Führer directs with a series of ukases. With successive hammer-blows the German citizen is driven into a swastika-shaped hole. The atmosphere of compulsion pervades the whole of his life. The fact that he and his fellow men are now to be selected and bred like a herd of cattle seems to him hardly more distasteful than a hundred other interferences in his daily life. There is little doubt that these measures will have at least a partial success. If commanded with authority, the German docilely obeys. The command now is to breed.

NOTE: Sources consulted included the following: Bostroem (1935), Klein (1935), Luxenburger (1934, 1935a), Steinwallner (1935), and memoranda of the German Ministry of the Interior.

26

GENETICS, MEDICINE, AND PRACTICAL EUGENICS

TWO TYPES OF INHERITANCE

Inherited differences between human beings tend to fall sharply into two groups. First we have definite abnormalities and defects. Sometimes these are wholly determined by heredity. Sometimes there is a genetic basis, though the co-operation of other factors, often environmental, is needed if that genetic basis is to express itself as recognizable abnormality. These definite inherited departures from normality are practically always due to single genes. In the second place, however, when we turn to the hereditary differences which distinguish normal people it is rarely indeed that we find these to be due to the action of single genes. Multifactorial inheritance is the rule; that is, the effect we see is due to the combined action of many genes, each making a small contribution which is not individually distinguishable. So we get the familiar picture of continuous variation, the normal curve and certain average measures of resemblance between relatives.

The distinction between these two modes of inheritance is a radical one, but it has not always been clearly drawn. In physical characters there was from the beginning no real confusion, but this was largely the result of accidental circumstances. Physical abnormalities were investigated by medical men by the pedigree method, and were found reconcilable with a single-gene heredity. Quantitative variables, such as stature, were investigated by statistical methods by Karl Pearson and his school, and the apparently non-Mendelian type of inheritance for which they were looking was found to apply.

The inheritance of intelligence could not be adequately investigated until after the appearance of reliable quantitative tests. Up till that time it had to be judged on the basis of educational assessment or of social behaviour; thus some authorities of the early days thought in terms of qualitative distinctions between the mental defec-

---

By J. A. Fraser Roberts and Eliot Slater. Originally published in the *Eugenics Review* 40: 62–69 (1948).

tive and the normal, and of single-factor inheritance. It is only fairly recently that we have been able to estimate the relative parts played by single genes and by total genetic equipment, and to separate clinically those forms of mental deficiency or backwardness attributable to the one and to the other. We now know that the hereditary component in the determination of the majority of instances of mental deficiency is multifactorial.

When we come to the inheritance of temperamental qualities we are on less certain ground. We have no precise and reliable tests of temperament as we have of intelligence. Nevertheless, here too it seems probable that we have to look for single genes as the explanation of pathological events, and for a multiplicity of genes as the explanation of individual differences in the physiological range. Let us look first at the mental disorders of what is commonly called a "psychotic" kind, that is to say manic-depressive illnesses, schizophrenia and paranoia, involutional melancholia, and the endogenous presenile dementias. In some of them a single-factor inheritance has been demonstrated. This is so in Huntington's chorea and Pick's disease. Inheritance of the manic-depressive psychoses is compatible with a theory of a single dominant factor, with the environment too playing a considerable role, although objections can be raised to this view. The findings with schizophrenia are even more difficult to interpret. But no serious worker has wished to depart from a single-factor theory, although that single factor may be either dominant or recessive, or, most probably, schizophrenia may be not one but many diseases with different single genes responsible from case to case. Generally speaking, the evidence suggests that specific single genes are essential for the appearance of the endogenous psychoses; but that multifactorial inheritance also plays a part in determining constitutional resistance or susceptibility, just as it does in environmentally caused diseases such as tuberculosis.

Neurosis and psychopathy have probably to be looked at in quite a different way. Almost certainly they depend on qualities of temperament and personality, which are determined by multifactorial inheritance. In clinical practice we are unable to find any sharp dividing line between abnormal and normal personalities; the differences which exist must be of a graded and quantitative nature, whatever the particular temperamental trait we consider. Although our tests of temperament are nothing like as good as tests of intelligence, where they can be applied they show that the population is distributed in the normal curve. The work of Eysenck (1947) and his collaborators is particularly convincing on this point. From investigations on twins, we know that qualities of temperament and personality have a hereditary basis, and the sort of inheritance of those traits that are found running in families is readily compatible with a multifactorial theory, but very difficult to reconcile with any single-factor hypothesis.

In temperament and character, therefore, multifactorial inheritance holds, as it does in intelligence; but we must rate the importance of the environment considerably higher. Newman, Freeman and Holzinger (1937), in their classic study of uniovular twins who had been brought up apart from one another from the earliest years, showed that there were larger differences between the twins in their response to tests of temperament than to tests of intelligence. Different environments had also imposed different patterns of development, and different life stories, on personalities of the same constitutional and hereditary make-up. In his balanced study of a large series of criminal twins, Kranz (1936) concluded that the fundamental structure of the personality was largely determined by heredity, but that environment often exercised a decisive influence on behaviour. As pragmatists we are really more concerned with behaviour than with abstracted notions of the underlying person-ality; so we must make a larger allowance for environment in the problems raised by temperament, neurosis and psychopathy than we need do with those raised by intelligence and mental defect.

THEIR EUGENIC SIGNIFICANCE

From the point of view of practical eugenics, the kind of hereditary difference which is determined by multifactorial inheritance is far more important than that caused by single genes. Here are some of the reasons. First, those things determined, or partly determined, by multifactorial inheritance are more important socially. Intelligence, good physique, resistance to disease are more important to the com-munity than rare hereditary diseases, even including some of the low-grade mental deficiencies, or those diseases which though rather commoner appear to have a definite and maybe simple genetic basis. In the same way, temperamental differences are more important than the insanities. All the hereditary mental illnesses together give a risk of only about 2 per cent in the general population, whereas the disabilities caused by neurosis and psychopathy are of fateful significance to us all.

Secondly, and this is even more important, simply inherited abnormalities are individually rare or very rare. Seldom indeed does a hereditary defect attain a frequency of one in 5,000 in the population; it is usually much less than this. The sole exception is colour-blindness, but this condition should perhaps be regarded as a more or less physiological variation rather than as an abnormality. Selection then, either natural selection based on natural differing rates of reproduction, or any conscious selection that it might be decided to apply, operates on a few human beings only. With recessive genes it is only very occasionally that we can identify genetically the outwardly normal carriers, so our general conclusion is little affected. Contrast with this multifactorial inheritance, determining in part some human quality such as general intelligence. Every human being exhibits the result of the action of many genes, some good, some bad. With the birth of every single human child the balance tips a little, up or down. Selection is operating, not on one person in five thousand, or fifty thousand, or five hundred thousand, but on every child born to every couple; for upon the sum total of their good and bad genes and the relative rates at which these are increasing or diminishing depends the future of the species, whether it is advancing, whether it is holding its own or whether it is retrogressing. Here is something about which the individual can have his say. Here is something not merely about which the State can legislate effectively if it wishes, but something which is automatically affected, for better or for worse, by social and economic measures of many kinds. We cannot confine our debate to the merits of action or inaction, for the actions of individuals, of groups and of governments are already exercising a continuous influence.

There is a third reason why multifactorial inheritance is the more important practically. If the mute inglorious Milton and the village Hampden may be denied their opportunity by external circumstance, it is no less true that the potential genius, rich in good genes of many kinds, may be stultified by having the misfortune to possess just one single grossly deleterious gene. Too rigorous an attempt to eliminate such genes may prove harmful on occasion. To some extent this is so today, for it is the highly intelligent and conscientious who tend to limit the number of their children because of some harmful gene known to be present in the family group. Contrast with this the person whose unfortunate heredity is multifactorial and due to an accumulation of many bad genes. Selection in this instance is on balance practically devoid of risk.

Finally, eugenic measures are much more hopeful in qualities caused by multifactorial inheritance than they are with single genes. Even the strictest eugenic laws, such as the Draconian laws of Nazi Germany, would have remarkably little effect in reducing the incidence of recessive abnormalities below a certain level. But even a slight selective advantage will cause a growth in frequency of multifactorial genes. If we were conquered by an alien race from Mars, it would be quite a feasible project for our overlords to breed up humanity to the intellectual level of a world of first-class honours men, or down to a world of morons, and in quite a few generations. For the ease with which it lends itself to modification by almost invisible trends, multifactorial inheritance is of paramount significance in eugenics.

EUGENIC MEASURES WITH SINGLE GENES

In stressing the greater importance of multifactorial inheritance and the things with which it is concerned we are not trying to say that a consideration of inherited abnormalities is of no value, or, necessarily, that nothing can be done about them. But the field is limited and the useful application of our knowledge will often lie outside the field of eugenics. We must dismiss simple dominant and sex-linked harmful genes as of minor practical importance. In the former every possessor is marked by the abnormality and so is fully exposed to the blast of natural selection. If the effect is at all serious the rate of elimination is so high that such genes cannot be other than very rare. Recessive sex-linked genes are exposed to one-third of this exceedingly severe selective force.

Simple recessive genes present a much more intricate problem. We know that for every person we see with retinitis pigmentosa there are more than a hundred unsuspected heterozygous carriers; for every albino, two hundred and fifty; for every sufferer from alkaptonuria, two thousand outwardly normal people who carry the gene. Looking at it the other way round, while only one person in every five hundred carries the gene for such a rare condition as alkaptonuria, one person in every 70 carries the gene for albinism, and no less than one in every thirty or forty amongst us is a carrier of retinitis pigmentosa. Thus our population contains great numbers of these recessive genes; in all probability there are few of us who do not carry at least one. In this mankind corresponds to the rest of the animal and plant world, for wild populations too carry large numbers of harmful recessive genes, with little ill effect apparently on the race.

The first lesson is a negative one. There is no eugenic reason why a sufferer from a recessive abnormality, or a known carrier, should not marry and have children, though, of course, he will be wise to avoid marrying a blood relative or anyone with a family history of the same defect. It is true that harmful genes are being handed on to future generations, but we are all of us doing the same thing, the only difference being that sufferers and their relatives know it and we do not. Here we must state our disagreement with the views of Professor Ruggles Gates as expressed in his *Human Genetics* (1946) and again in *The Eugenics Review* (1947). The eugenic effect of abstinence is negligible and if everyone adopted so conscientious an attitude towards posterity no one would feel justified in raising a family.

Perhaps it is natural that in the past eugenic thought has concentrated on one particular line, namely influencing the next generation positively or negatively by increasing or decreasing the number of children of certain individuals. But the consideration of recessive defects leads us to another possibility, based on the fact that sometimes an individual can safely marry certain individuals but not others. Recessive defects crop up particularly when blood relatives marry because they tend to share the same genes in common, having received them from the same source. The incidence is greatly affected by changes even in the limited degrees of inbreeding allowed and practised in our community. The decline in the amount of inbreeding during, say, the past century must, as Haldane (1939) has shown, have greatly lowered the frequency of recessive defects. But of course mutation has been going on at its usual rate, and, as the rate of elimination has been reduced, the harmful recessive genes are slowly multiplying. Ultimately after many generations the old high incidence will once more be reached, but the proportion of carriers will be much higher. A sudden reversion to smaller, closed communities once again and relatively close inbreeding would result in a marked outbreak of recessive defects of all kinds.

In the absence of a family history of a recessive abnormality the increased absolute risk of a consanguineous marriage is small. But the relative risk, which is what matters to the whole community, is greatly increased. Would the community be wise to discourage cousin marriage? If it were prohibited the immediate effect would be to lessen appreciably the amount of recessively determined abnormality, but in the long run this would be at the price of a greater accumulation of the genes in the population. The case for interference does not seem a strong one.

Conscious control of recessive defects would be enormously easier if the heterozygous carriers could be identified. There is the promise of this in some current work. Provided that the heterozygotes could be identified with certainty the defect itself need never appear provided that marriage between the carriers were avoided. This is not merely a theoretical impossibility. It could be realized at the present time in erythroblastosis foetalis, a condition which is common compared with ordinary inherited defects, occuring say once in every 200 births. Confining ourselves to what is practically important, the abnormality need not arise if Rh negative women do not marry Rh positive men. But is it likely that 15 per cent of women will accept the proposition that they can only marry their like and that 85 per cent of the male population is barred to them? If such an attitude were, however, to become general we should see an interesting social development, for our population would split into two diverging strains, between which marriage rarely took place.

Some reference has been made to an apparently simple genetic basis, or something that looks like it, for certain not very uncommon conditions such as thyrotoxicosis, essential hypertension, or schizophrenia. But in all such instances the hereditary basis is only part of the story; the co-operation of other factors, probably environmental, is necessary if genetic potentiality is to become transformed into the disease itself. If these single genes exist they must be relatively common and widely spread. Their elimination, or even substantial reduction, is probably impossible and in schizophrenia, for example, the tendency to self-limitation is very strong. It would seem much more hopeful to concentrate on the environmental component and discover how to prevent the disease appearing in those whose genetic constitution renders them susceptible.

We are not going to claim that in all the foregoing instances there is no scope for eugenic action. The importance of such deformities and defects to the sufferers and their families may be very great. Much relief can be given by wise advice and by suitable legislation. The recent informative paper read to this *Society* by Professor Tage Kemp (1947) on fifteen years' experience in Denmark of eugenic legislation shows the importance of these humanitarian measures. But that experience also illustrates the limited scope and effect of such measures when we think of the community as a whole. In our country a few thousands of individual cases a year would be the utmost number affected, and even of those many would have, as we have seen, little eugenic significance. In those things determined by multifactorial inheritance lies the true and overwhelming importance of the application of genetics to practical eugenics.

EUGENIC ASPECTS OF PHYSIQUE AND TEMPERAMENT

There is a large genetic component in human differences in certain physical traits, for example stature. This is also true of certain mental qualities, in particular intelligence. And there is doubtless a genetic component, also multifactorial, in much that goes to determine a sound physique and also degrees of resistance to certain diseases. As we saw earlier, variation is continuous, and selection is operating over the whole range of the human population. Either the good genes are multiplying at the expense of the bad, or vice versa; or, it may be, the population in regard to some of these things is in a state more or less of equilibrium. Now we have great sympathy with those who would claim that as environmental factors are also concerned we should concentrate on these first. Let us, it might be contended, exhaust the possibilities of reducing inefficiency and disease by improvements in environment before thinking too much of the less tractable hereditary differences. And even when heredity is clearly important, the most useful practical applications may well lie not in attempting to influence relative birth-rates but in taking special precautions to safeguard those who are known to be genetically susceptible. Let us take pulmonary tuberculosis as an example. The fine twin study of Kallmann and Reisner (1943) has shown most clearly that in the present state of our community heredity is of great moment in determining whether or not a person will develop the adult form of the disease. But is the lesson of this that those with a bad family history should not marry? In our opinion, no. There are so many unfavourable things that can be inherited and this is only one. It might well be that other good qualities would more than outweigh this particular weakness. The lesson is rather to protect those likely for genetic reasons to be highly susceptible: by periodical mass-fluorography for example, by supplements to the diet, by seeing that such people do not enter the tuberculosis service, by discouraging the nursing of a tuberculosis patient by a sister.

When we turn to temperament we come up against objections of another kind. Few would deny the advantage of good build, fast and accurate neuromuscular co-ordination, strength, physical health and a high natural resistance to disease. We can surely encourage those endowed with such qualities to regard themselves as proper parents for the next generation. But in the field of temperament, our aims are much less clear. There is no such thing as a good and desirable type of temperament, and a bad and undesirable one. It takes all sorts to make a world. There is room for the quiet, the docile and the stable; but there is room also for the man of strong passions, for the natural born rebel, for the man whose moods take him from phases of elation and enhanced activity into troughs of depression. It is true, indeed, that a man like Hitler can cause much greater harm to humanity than even a million mental defectives; but we cannot say, if Hitler had had children, that they would have been any more likely to have been bad citizens than anyone else's. It is particular combinations of temperamental qualities which are productive of large effects, good or bad. Recombined in another way, the effect of the genes responsible would have been different. In fact we are too uncertain of where we want to go, and too ignorant of the foundations on which we stand, for there to be at present a practical eugenic approach to the betterment of human personality.

EUGENICS AND INTELLIGENCE

We come at last to intelligence. Even here, perhaps, the nature of our aims is not beyond *all* controversy. There are many jobs in society which do not demand a high level of intelligence; and we know that when people are set to jobs which provide no adequate outlet for their intelligence they are often unhappy and difficulties are likely to arise. But there would be general agreement that we are short of men and women of high intelligence, that the number of skilled jobs is increasing and that with the advent of mechanization unskilled jobs are becoming more and more skilled. The world in which we live is becoming more and more complex. If the average citizen is to understand it, and play his part in a democratic society, better education and better intelligence are both required. And a rise in the average level of intelligence would permit a fuller and richer mental life in the community.

The attitude of concentrating on environmental improvement and of doubting the great urgency of positive eugenic measures seems to us to be justified only if one important condition is satisfied. This is that we have no reason to suppose that those of poorer genetic endowment are reproducing appreciably faster than those who are superior. Thus we can be philosophical about heredity and pulmonary tuberculosis. Hygienic measures are proving efficacious in lessening its incidence and there is no clear evidence that those who happen to carry an excess of genes making for poor resistance are reproducing any faster than the rest of the population. In all probability we should be justified in assuming that owing to some elimination at a relatively early age the reverse is true. But suppose that we were told that those with the strongest hereditary predisposition to pulmonary tuberculosis were reproducing twice as fast as those who were most resistant, could we afford to take so detached an attitude? Surely not. And yet this is what is happening in regard to one quality — general intelligence — a quality of the highest social importance and one determined in large measure by heredity.

We do not propose to discuss the nature of what is measured by intelligence tests or to review the evidence which points to a large hereditary component. This has been done very recently by Burt (1946) with whose views we are in entire agreement. Whether we accept the estimate that three-quarters of the variance in intelligence as measured is due to heredity or whether we are ultra-cautious and simply say at least one-half, it is evident that the problem is urgent. For here is no question of speculating on the composition of a more or less stable population and debating at leisure whether some change is desirable, whether it could be made, and if so how. We are confronted with what appears to us a ruinous rate of loss of good genes and so a corresponding rate of increase of bad ones. This is the eugenic problem that far outweighs all others. We are confronted with a relatively enormous dysgenic trend, one moreover which is readily amenable to selection, should selection be attempted either directly or, better and more practicable, indirectly through those things that affect our lives and are to greater or lesser degree within our control.

There is no reason to suppose that the unfavourable differential birth-rate in regard to intelligence exists in anything like the same measure in regard to anything else. Not only is it known solely with respect to intelligence, but is only likely to exist with respect to intelligence. Nevertheless we must not forget that good quali-ties tend in general to be positively correlated and similarly for bad qualities. This means that improvement in regard to the differential birth-rate as it affects intelli-gence should automatically secure improvement in other directions also. But this in all probability would be small, important though it is to recognize that it would be in the right direction.

If the average level of intelligence of the community continues to decline, we can expect to see the effect not only on the average but much more markedly at the two extremes. The average citizen will become less fitted by natural aptitudes to understand and exercise an effective voice in the society in which he lives. But the proportion of mental defectives will rise sharply. Most critically of all, the loss of good genes will be shown in a decrease in the number of the really talented. Civiliza-tion owes disproportionally much to men of the very highest intellectual powers, to such figures as Shaw and Einstein in the present age, Pasteur and Descartes in a past one. Even a relatively small fall in average intelligence implies a catastrophic fall in the number of such men. These are the men whose intellects place them in the one-in-a-million class. With an average drop of half a dozen points on the Binet scale we can expect them to appear, not with a frequency of one in a million, but of less than one in ten million; for every ten such men today, tomorrow we should have but one.

Eugenics in the past has had too much of an aristocratic air. Perhaps the brilliant pedigree of its founder has had too much fascination. Perhaps there has been a failure to distinguish between fruitful methods of investigation and the use that can be made of them. Studies of the extremes, on men of genius on the one hand, on mental defectives on the other, are both fascinating and illuminating, but the lessons that they teach apply to the whole community. Galton himself pointed out the significance of changes in the average for changes at the extremes, just as he pointed out that among the relatives of men of outstanding ability there are a remarkable number of the outstandingly able. These are two complementary aspects of the same phenomena, but we have tended to neglect the more important one. Galton's views about distinguished families were right enough; but we need to supplement them with the observation that, all the same, the great majority of intellectual giants come from families of moderate ability as the result of an exceptionally favourable chance. Taking them by and large, the children of university professors are no doubt more intelligent than the children of clerks. But there are so many more clerks in the world than university professors that any collection of brilliant men will include more clerks' sons than professors' sons.

We need to look for a moment, not at the distribution of men of ability in the community, but at the distribution of the genes. No doubt the genes of hereditary ability are spread more thinly among those of average and slightly better than average intelligence than in the very able. But there are many more such genes in the former group than in the latter. Regarded as treasuries of potential ability, there is no comparison between the two. The principles of genetics inform us that our concern must be with the community as a whole, and not with a small and special section. The facts as we see them give rise to grave disquiet. Our task is to reverse the present trends, to change the sign of differential fertility, to encourage the more intelligent half of the community to have more, not fewer, children than the less intelligent.

SUMMARY

Inherited human differences tend to fall into two groups. First, there are definite departures from the normal, these being commonly due to the action of single genes. Secondly, there are the inherited differences that distinguish normal people, which tend strongly to show continuous variation. These are due to multifactorial inheritance. While there is some scope for eugenic action in differences of the first kind, this is small compared with the effect of even moderate degrees of selection, operating on all human beings, on differences of the second type. The outstanding eugenic problem, far outweighing all others in importance, is the present differential birth-rate with respect to intelligence, for of this human quality only do we know that the less desirable genes are multiplying rapidly at the expense of the good.

27

GALTON'S HERITAGE

Last year the world was celebrating the centenary of the publication of *The Origin of Species*. In comparison with his cousin, fame has passed Galton by. If Galton's work had less world-shaking consequences than that of Darwin, it is not because he was a man of lesser ability. In a letter of 1871 Darwin wrote:

> I have been speculating last night what makes a man a discoverer of undiscovered things; and a most perplexing problem it is. Many men who are very clever — much cleverer than the discoverers — never originate anything. As far as I can conjecture the art consists in habitually searching for the causes and meaning of everything which occurs. This implies sharp observation and requires as much knowledge as possible of the subject investigated.

Both Darwin and Galton had this compulsive curiosity.

VARIETY OF SCIENTIFIC INTERESTS

Galton's contributions were scattered over an immense field. Karl Pearson (1914-1930), and others since, have tried to find some unifying thread linking them all together. It seems to me that the only connecting thread was Galton's wayward personality. He was the scientific dilettante at his super-excellent best. Like Darwin, he never received any adequate scientific education. What he got was the first few years of a medical training and enough mathematics at Cambridge to attain a poll degree. He had no apprenticeship, no mentor, and never knew the discipline of a research laboratory. Throughout his scientific life he worked on his own, turning his hand first to one thing and then to another, as the fancy took him. It was his fortune that the fields to which he turned his attention were almost unexplored. It has been rightly said that the discoveries of fundamental importance are always made by amateurs, since in a new and untouched field there can be no experts. But the amateur who makes discoveries in new territory is usually an expert in some

Originally published in the *Eugenics Review* 52: 91–103 (1960). Figures, including three photographs of Galton, have been omitted.

more established field. Galton was an expert in nothing. Pearson says that at the age of thirty-two he knew more mathematics and physics than most biologists, more biology than mathematicians, and more pathology and physiology than either.

His scientific career began at the age of twenty-eight, when he undertook a journey of exploration in south-west Africa, to which he was attracted by the expectation of encountering big game. He was advised to put himself in touch with the Royal Geographical Society, and was briefed on how to make observations of the needed accuracy and reliability for map-making. He did his work with such efficiency as to receive the Society's Gold Medal and in due course to become a Fellow of the Royal Society. It is to the friendships and connections he made in this way that his subsequent scientific evolution must be traced. He developed an immense respect for his fellow-scientists, the reverence of the amateur for the professional. He wrote: "A collection of living magnates in various branches of intellectual achievement is always a feast to my eyes; being as they generally are such massive, vigorous, capable-looking animals" (Galton, 1908). About his own status he was modest to the point of unconsciousness. Pearson notes that Galton did not regard himself as one whose faculties gave him rank in the extreme tail of a frequency distribution: "He would have recognized such a position for half his friends, before he thought of it for himself."

Galton had a strongly mechanical bent. Even before his African expedition, in 1849 when he was twenty-seven, he had published a pamphlet on the telotype, a printing electric telegraph. This was the first of a long succession of mechanical inventions, others being an instrument for sun-signalling, a shield for the protection of riflemen, stereoscopic maps, spectacles for divers, the Galton whistle for testing the power of hearing for high notes, a wave-engine, and many others. Remarkable as the ingenuity of these contrivances must have been, one suspects that they all had the defects of lack of professionalism, since they have all suffered shipwreck on the river of time. Pearson notes that in the Galton Laboratory there was a whole series of models, "Galton's toys," the very purpose of many of them being unknown.

COMPOSITE PHOTOGRAPHY

One of Galton's devices which is of much more lasting interest and importance is his invention of composite photography. It will be remembered that, by superimposing upon one another a number of under-exposed photographs he tried to extract from them some common quality. In his way he tried to demonstrate a phthisical facies from the super-imposed photographs of tuberculous patients, and in another instance to show up the common quality in the countenances of violent criminals. He found the technique exceedingly difficult, although he tackled the mechanical problems involved with his usual untiring patience and ingenuity; and indeed the whole method was beyond solution by the technological resources of his day.

We are now beginning to enter an era in which Galton's idea may bear fruit. As an example of a modern application I may mention the work of Dr. G. D. Dawson in the Neurological Research Unit at the National Hospital. Dawson (1954) had reason to believe that in the normal subject an action potential evoked by the stimulation of a peripheral nerve could be detected by electrodes placed on the scalp over a particular part of the opposite side of the head. However the action potential would be so weak that it would be wholly obscured by adventitious electrical changes, occurring in the electrical circuits and in the scalp of the subject. In the terms of the communications engineer, the signal would be indistinguishable from the noise.

303

However, by superimposing a large number of tracings, forty or more, he obtained a thick and fuzzy band with discernible waves, whose time of onset and whose period could be roughly measured. This result led to a further great improvement in technique, by which averaging was substituted for superimposition. A rotating switch was used to sample the signal voltage at regular intervals after each stimulus. Corresponding charges were stored in capacitators and progressively summed; and the accumulated charges could be examined continuously on a cathode ray tube, from which a photographic record could be obtained. In this way the entire scatter of the observations was eliminated and a single clean line, corresponding to mean values, could be obtained, which showed even minute features of the wave-forms and allowed more accurate measurement.

It is noteworthy that Galton set himself the immensely complex task of examining the human face, while Dawson was concerned with a single wavy line. Yet Dawson needed some fifty different ordinates to describe this curve. To accomplish a corresponding task with human faces one would need something like a television scanner with storage units running in number to the order of 10,000 or so. However, simpler tasks may be found lying to hand. It has been suggested that such a problem as photography of the canals of the planet Mars, where also small regularities in appearance are swamped in adventitious light variations, could be tackled along a similar line.

There is another association between Galton and the planet Mars with an even more contemporary echo. At the end of the last century there was a near approach between Mars and the earth, which caused some discussion on the possibility of communication with an intelligent form of life on Mars, if such there was. Contrary to the generally expressed scientific opinions, in an article of 1896 Galton pointed out not only that the possibility existed but also what its method would be. The emission of dots and dashes could be used to build up first a system of numerals, then to characterize π, and from that to proceed to the communication of directions and movements, and finally of pictures. Once pictures were being sent and received, the problem would be solved. At the end of last year we learned that listening for interstellar signals is to begin at the Radio Astronomy Laboratory at Green Bank, Virginia. The Project OZMA, based on the work of R. W. Meadows, relies on the feasibility of the means of communication outlined by Galton, and on the fact that there is one particular wavelength, the radio emission line of neutral hydrogen, which would have a very high probability of being chosen for long distance communication by any advanced world.

IMAGERY

Another field, in which the stream of inspiration starting from Galton has seemed till lately to have dried up in sandy soil, is that of visual imagery. Here he was a pioneer out on his own, and he had to gather all the facts for himself. By patience and system he described an immense variety and richness of visual imagery, of spontaneous origin, which he found to be especially prominent in childhood. Number-form, for instance, which he described, is the visual form in which numbers, or numerical data such as months and days of the week, may present themselves to some people in the mind's eye. Galton describes one subject who could both imagine and mentally manipulate a slide rule, so as to be able to carry out difficult computations in his mind with speed and accuracy. Into this fascinating world Galton was not able to penetrate very far; indeed, the principal conclusion of a general and comprehensive kind which he was able to draw was that most people think of their own mental processes as being of a universal nature, to which the thinking of all others must conform. They find it almost impossible to believe that others may have ways of thinking which are to them unknown, and who may find their ways incomprehensible. The science of analysis of human communication has not progressed sufficiently to see just how far this principle will take us.

For many years no further work of any importance was done on the line pioneered by Galton. One might perhaps mention attempts made, in the first place by Golla, Hutton and Grey Walter (1943), to correlate Galton's personality types with EEG characteristics — attempts which have led to no profitable results. It is a different matter, however, when the psychologist turns to the influence of imagery on imagination and creative thinking, as has been done by Professor McKellar (1957) in a fascinating book. There are references to Galton on some thirty pages scattered throughout this work; and his ideas are the starting point for a systematic study of the appearance of imagery in normal and abnormal states of mind under experimental conditions. There is great interest in the analysis of the relations of autistic and logical thinking, and the estimation of the role played by spontaneous imagery in creativity.

McKellar draws attention to the restricting effect of imagery on abstract thought. The image that at some times supplies a fruitful model for understanding may at other times mislead, as has for instance been the case in the past with the concept of the luminiferous ether, and with the rival wave and corpuscular theories of the nature of light. Galton believed that a habit of suppressing mental imagery must characterize men who deal much with abstract ideas. But he maintained also that the visualizing faculty should be developed in education. We should be able to call up at will a clear, steady and complete image of anything recently examined; visualize it freely from any aspect; project its image on paper and draw an outline; and construct images from description.

This bringing of imagery into relation with education is of interest in connection with the educational theories of Cuisenaire and Gattegno, which are beginning to be used in schools in this country and on the Continent (Trivett, 1959). Cuisenaire, a mathematics master in a Belgian school, found that if he provided his children with ready-made number-forms, their capacity to use them to understand abstract mathematical ideas, such as the commutative law, or power and logarithms, or infinite sets, led to very rapid progress. The number forms supplied are exceedingly simple, and consist of sticks of wood, 1 cm. square in cross section, and from 1 to 10 cm. long, coloured so that each prime in succession starts a new colour sequence: the sticks 2, 4 and 8 cm. long belong to the red family, 3, 6 and 9 to the blue family, 5 and 10 are yellow and orange, and 7 is black. Such models are obviously very much more adaptable and convenient for mental manipulation than some of the eerie number-forms described by Galton, which the child develops for himself out of his untutored imagination. They indeed look like things which have been dwarfed and stunted through lack of proper nourishment. There is no knowing how much value the average man might derive from his capacity for visual and auditory imagery, if it were developed by education instead of being systematically ignored.

CORRELATION AND VARIATION

The scientific work a man does, which is fully developed and exploited by others, becomes in the course of time part of the general body of knowledge. The individual stamp is lost, so that his name may hardly be remembered, and his personal contribution is relegated to a matter of historical record. This has been the case with Galton's work on meteorology, where he has the fame of having discovered and named the anticyclone, and the great merit of having been the first to construct weather maps. So also it has been with his work on finger-prints, on twins, on anthropometry and the measurement of human variation, and in the development of the calculus of correlation. His work in any one of these fields is of an originality and a fundamental importance which would satisfy a first-class scientist for the whole of his life-work. To this there is not much one can add. The mathematical tool of correlation, which Galton developed single-handed from its beginnings, is a fantastic achievement for a man who never had the advantage of any very adequate mathematical education. However, though the calculus of correlation has become the most powerful tool available to the psychometric psychologist, and is used as a basic intrument over a great variety of scientific fields, in conceptual importance it seems to me to come second to Galton's study of quantitative variation.

When one is concerned with human attributes, the change of attitude involved in considering people as showing a characteristic to a greater or lesser degree, instead of merely having or not having it, is revolutionary. Even where the characteristic with which one is concerned is beyond the present reach of measurement, the change from the one way to the other of thinking about one's observations has the most far-reaching consequences. One may take the example of "neurosis." It used to be universal and it is still common for medical men to think of people as being either "neurotic" or "not neurotic." When one thinks in terms of more and less, "neurosis" loses its unfortunate pathological implications and comes to be seen as a mode of normal variation. A shift of this kind may be called for in the most unlikely looking places. For many scientific purposes it is more appropriate to think of maleness and femaleness as the poles of a continuous rather than a discontinuous distribution.

THE BASIS OF CREATIVITY

If we want to get an impression of Galton's personality as a creative worker, we must look, not only on the greatest of his achievements but also on his least. Galton's mind, except when he was asleep, was never still. There seem to have been but few subjects which offered a problem to a lively intelligence, and practically none where an answer might be obtained by counting and figuring, which did not claim his interest. Thus in the 247 works in Blacker's (1952) definitive bibliography, there are "Statistical Inquiries into the Efficacy of Prayer," "The Average Flush of Excitement," "Free-will, Observations and Inferences," "Measure of Fidget," "Arithmetic by Smell," "Terms of Imprisonment," "Three Generations of Lunatic Cats," "Temporary Flooring in Westminster Abbey for Ceremonial Processions," "Strawberry Cure for Gout," "Number of Strokes of the Brush in a Picture," "Cutting a Round Cake on Scientific Principles." In this bizarrely variegated collection there are some items which are wholly ephemeral and trivial, but not many; and some, like the "Inquiries into the Efficacy of Prayer" are a delight to read.

Galton's scientific work is characterized by the simplicity and lucidity of his thinking. His approach to a problem was a naive one, without preconceptions, and one is invariably impressed by the luminous intelligence with which he tackled a problem. He attained his ends mainly by ingenuity, logic and abundant patience and capacity for hard work. He also showed a naïve trustfulness and courage. Though a praeternaturally shy man, he did his own field work, applying to fellow members of learned societies for details of their private lives, and to friends and acquaintances for information about their ways of thinking and imagining. Ernest Jones (1956), in his study of genius in the person of Freud, has said that an element in the achievement of a man of scientific genius is credulity. This may well have been true of Freud, whose ideas came to him intuitively, and who had to believe passionately in their truth in order to make progress. It was not true of Galton. He, too, had his sudden flashes of intuitive insight — he names the place and time when the concept of correlation descended on him — but he relied on them relatively little. His works are characterized by self-criticism and dispassion. He was remarkably surefooted, and seldom went seriously astray. There are, however, points where he took a false path, and some of these are important. Thus he went astray on assortative mating, considering that people are attracted by their opposites up to a limiting point after which the tendency is reversed. This led to a neglect of the effect of assortative mating in the maintenance of able families. There are other instances which we shall have to notice later. Galton was secure as long as he relied on reason; it is only when he comes to the formulation of his religion and particularly eugenics conceived as a religious aim, that he steps outside the guidance of reason alone, with fateful results.

Galton's maxim was "whenever you can, count." Pearson notes that in his day the Galton Laboratory possessed no fewer than five "registrators," small mechanisms designed to be carried in the pocket, to record a count by such means as the prick of a pin on a card, without exciting the notice of the company. While Galton was having his portrait painted he was counting the strokes of the artist's brush. At a scientific meeting when he lost interest in the theme of the speaker, he would be counting the fidgety movements of the audience, and relating them to sex and age. Walking the streets of the city he recorded the percentage of attractive, indifferent and repellent-looking women he met, with the object of forming a Beauty Map of the British Isles.

A great deal of his incessant intellectual activity must be put down to the delight he must have felt in the use of his own powers. It suggests the restless playful activity of children, or the athletic young man turning handsprings at the side of a swimming-pool. Yet the psychiatrist also receives a strong impression of a compulsive quality, of a need to count for counting's sake, or for the sake of engaging a mental engine that would shake and rattle without a load.

OBSESSIONAL TRAITS

Obsessionality was a feature of Galton's family history. According to Pearson one of his father's sisters

> had a triple inkstand with three coloured inks, triple penwipers and pens; every conceivable apparatus for writing, printed envelopes for her various banks and business correspondents; printed questions for her grooms, "Has the mare had her corn?" etc.; a dozen or more cash boxes elaborately arranged to receive in separate compartments each kind of coin from each type of her property ... As many as 100 painted labels have been counted in a flower bed of hers of 12 square feet. In short, we appreciate what Francis Galton meant when he said that the desire to classify and organize which existed in his family, he felt at times as almost a danger to himself.

Galton's father was a wealthy banker of meticulously businesslike habits. He required his son to provide the most exact statements of all his expenses, and to account for the money allowed him down to the last penny. Galton says his mother was described to him as having been in her early years joyous and unconventional, but does not say that she remained so after years of marriage. It must have been from his Quaker father, and not from his mother, that he derived a weight of puritanical guilt, of whose existence one only knows from its eventual removal. The reading of *The Origin of Species* brought, he says, a real crisis in his life, and freed him from the constraint of his old superstition as if it had been a nightmare. That occurred when he was about forty, and the damage was done.

Galton was liable to nervous symptoms almost throughout his life, and twice had a breakdown. The first was at the age of twenty. In his *Memories* he writes:

> It was during my third year at Cambridge that I broke down entirely and had to lose a term and go home. I suffered from intermittent pulse and a variety of brain symptoms of an alarming kind. A mill seemed to be working inside my head; I could not banish obsessing ideas: at times I could hardly read a book, and found it painful even to look at a printed page. Fortunately I did not suffer from sleeplessness, and my digestion failed but little. Even a brief interval of complete mental rest did me good, and it seemed as if a long dose of it might wholly restore me.

Both Galton and Pearson attribute his illness to doing too much. Since this too much consisted in rather desultory reading for mathematical honours and a great deal of social life, the explanation is not very convincing. Apart from the "obsessing thoughts," there seem to have been symptoms of somatic anxiety — palpitations and dizziness are mentioned in a letter to his father of November 1842 — and some degree of depression. Early in 1843 he wrote poems, of which two begin with the lines:

> Well may we loathe this world of sin, and strain
> As an imprisoned dove to flee away;

and

> How foolish and how wicked seems the world.

Nevertheless the condition does not ring quite like a simple anxiety state, and the depressive element could not have been severe in view of the lack of interference with appetite and sleep.

His later illness, at the age of forty-four, is described as follows:

> During the whole of this interval I find from old diaries that I frequently suffered from giddiness and other maladies prejudicial to mental effort, but that I invariably became well again on completely changing my habits . . . The warning I received in 1866 was more emphatic and alarming than previously, and made a revision of my mode of life a matter of importance. Those who have not suffered from mental breakdown can hardly realize the incapacity it causes . . . After recovery seems to others to be complete, there remains for a long time an impossibility of performing certain minor actions without pain and serious mischief . . . This was a frequent experience with me respecting small problems, which successively obsessed me day and night, as I tried in vain to think them out. These affected mere twigs, so to speak, rather than large boughs of the mental processes, but for all that most painfully.

One must conclude, I think, that Galton's trouble was a liability to painful compulsive rumination.

PURITANISM

In his *Memories*, all that he has to say about his mother is confined to one short paragraph, recording nothing of her emotional relationship to him or of his feelings to her. The main feminine influence in his childhood was a much-loved sister, older by twelve years, who spent the greater part of her life lying on her back and who devoted herself to his education. Apart from her, the dominant influence on his life was certainly that of his father. Nearly all his letters as a boy and a young man are written to his father, whom he loved and who dominated him. It was his father, who pressed him on to make a career for himself; and once his father had died all plans of that kind were immediately discarded. This relationship possibly explains the extreme reserve with which Galton touches on the most personal of his experiences, though it is clear that his feelings were both warm and deep.

Pearson comments ruefully on his incomprehension of the psychology of women. When ideas came up for discussion on how women might play their part in the eugenic movement, his only notion was that they might throw open their houses for drawing-room meetings. That women might have their own ideas about the breeding of the next generation had not occurred to him. He naïvely imagined that the abler men could have the abler women for the asking, while Pearson comments that the abler men, either by choice or necessity, do not mate with the abler women, and the latter, either by choice or necessity, remain to a large extent unmarried.

Galton married in 1853, at the age of thirty-one, and enjoyed forty years of married life; yet as far as one can see, his wife had practically no influence in moulding his personality or his views. There is hardly a word about her in Pearson's biography. During their life in London she probably saw very little of him, at least alone; practically the whole of his day must have been taken up either with scientific work or with his very numerous commitments in the Royal Geographical Society, the Royal Society, the Anthropological Institute, the British Association, or the Observatory at Kew, etc. Both husband and wife came from large sibships, yet their marriage was childless. Pearson supposes that the lack of children must have been a grief to Galton, but notes also that he was alarmed by children and did not find the right words to say to them.

The couple travelled a lot abroad and were also accustomed to making visits to spas under medical direction. Not only was Galton liable to nervous symptoms, but his wife also seems to have suffered from one of those nameless forms of chronic ill-health which one finds not infrequently in the women of Victorian times. Pearson says he was wonderfully patient with her. One is compelled to wonder whether their life together was of a kind to have much chance of producing children. Galton's biographers note that the subject of sex was one which he found distressing and preferred to ignore.

Though he must have been a man of acute sensibilities, he seems to have denied himself the pleasures of the senses. His niece, Millicent Lethbridge, presumably describing his old age, wrote: "He enjoyed his food as keenly as a child, although he was a very small eater and most abstemious in every way. He delighted in after-dinner coffee, of which he allowed himself two teaspoonfuls, and that only when I, or some other coffee-drinker, was staying with him to set a bad example." She notes also that he loved the sunshine, and even on the hottest day would insist on walking on the sunny side of the street.

Nevertheless, for his London residence he chose what must have been a gloomy house, where his work-room looked out on a light-shaft. Though fond of travel, he does not seem to have been impressed by magnificent scenery. Art, whether in colour, form, or verbal expression, was no essential need for him. He was totally unmusical. He was not fond of animals, and had no comprehension and love of young things.

A FEMININE TRAIT?

To this side of his nature one gets a clue from the photographs in Pearson's *Life*. They show a lower half of the face which is ill-matched with the upper. The nose, eyes and forehead show nobility, energy and intellect. The chin is fined away and the mouth is held in a compressed and prim expression. Furthermore, as it seems to me, there is sexless or even feminine quality to the countenance, which if anything became more marked with increasing age.

He remained physically preserved into old age and there was but little sign of ageing between the fifties and the eighties. This resistance to ageing was, of course, also shown mentally. Of his old age he wrote that it was a very happy time for him, provided one accepted its numerous limitations. From his studies on Hereditary Talent he concluded that "the highest minds in the highest races seem to have been those who had the longest boyhood." In his own case he did not make a beginning with the serious business of life until he was over thirty. Pearson says he was young till his death. Even between forty and fifty he was a boy who must try his powers on all things that came his way. At the age of seventy-four he complained for the first time that his brain power was not as vigorous as formerly.

The feminine streak was also a source of strength. He was a remarkably unaggressive man. Though often taken by his work into the fringes of controversy, for instance, in the conflict between his science of finger-prints and the Bertillon system of personal identification by bodily measurement, he succeeded in not getting involved. As Blacker says, there are no polemical writings, and he seems to have made no personal enemies. In the closing years of his life there were acute disagreements between Karl Pearson, his scientific heir, and the direction of the Eugenics Education Society, who were the representatives of his faith for the future. Though he might have been torn in two by opposing loyalties, he dealt with the situation gently and without rancour, and largely held aloof.

THE HERO-WORSHIPPER

One of his most boyish and most engaging qualities was his capacity for hero-worship. His admiration for Darwin knew no limit. When he died, Galton wrote: "I feel at times quite sickened at the loss of Charles Darwin. I owed more to him than to any other man living or dead; and I never entered his presence without feeling as a man in the presence of a beloved sovereign." He was particularly impressed by intellectual eminence, but he appreciated excellence in any mode of competitive endeavour. In 1864 he was turning over ideas of breeding both dogs and men for intelligence. The trouble was that even the best were, he thought, not good enough: "The general intellectual capacity of our leaders requires to be raised, and also to be differentiated. We want abler commanders, statesmen, thinkers, inventors, and artists . . . The foremost minds of the present day seem to stagger and halt under an intellectual load too heavy for them."

Galton thought that the leaders of mankind were set apart from the rest both psychologically and biologically. Thus in his essay of 1872 on "Gregariousness in Cattle and in Men," he traced to this gregariousness "slavish aptitudes, from which the leaders of men and the heroes and prophets, are exempt." On the biological side he was of the opinion that extreme ability does not blend: "Very gifted men are usually of marked individuality, and consequently of a special type. Whenever this type is a stable one, it does not blend easily, but is transmitted almost unchanged, so that specimens of very distinguished intellectual heredity frequently occur."

On this fundamental but fallacious idea Galton's preoccupation with the "noble stirps" arose.

The role of the average man was, he thought, a very subordinate one.

> The average man is morally and intellectually an uninteresting being. The class to which he belongs is bulky and no doubt serves to help the course of social life in action. It also affords, by its inertia, a regulator that, like the fly-wheel to the steam-engine, resists sudden and irregular changes. But the average man is of no direct help towards evolution, which appears to our dim vision to be the goal of all living existence . . . Some thorough-going democrats may look with complacency on a mob of mediocrities, but to most other persons they are the reverse of attractive. The absence of heroic gifts among them [for Galton never saw the common man in times of war] would be a heavy set off against the freedom from a corresponding number of very degraded forms. The general standard of thought and morals in a mob of mediocrities must necessarily be mediocre, and, what is worse, contentedly so. The lack of living men to afford lofty examples, and to educate the virtue of reverence, leaves an irremediable blank. All men would find themselves at nearly the same dead average level, each being as meanly endowed as his neighbour.

Galton would not allow that the class of the mediocre might be leavened by men of exceptional potentialities who never showed their capacities. He did not believe in "mute inglorious Miltons": "If a man is gifted with vast intellectual ability, eagerness to work, and power of working, I cannot comprehend how such a man should be suppressed." This view shows a remarkable lack of insight into his own case. From a reading of his life story one would think that it was the sheerest accident that diverted Galton himself from a life of hunting and shooting. This was the life his brothers lived, and the life he led contentedly for some years, until an impulse took him into African exploration. Even after that he might have gone on as an explorer, had not his health been adversely affected.

Of the "lower middle classes" Galton thought still worse; they might be summed up as mentally and physically litter-scatterers. They and those still lower than them made up "the present army of ineffectives which clog progress."

Galton's excessive admiration for heroic virtues, for the leaders of men, and for the extreme deviant generally, no doubt had its emotional roots in his relation to his father, and to such later father-figures as Charles Darwin. It had, however, a rational basis. This was derived from his way of looking at normal variation.

Galton never made use of the concept of the standard deviation. He thought of people who had been measured in some characteristic as being drawn out in a long line, the man with the lowest measurement to the extreme left, and the man with the highest to the extreme right. So arranged they would show the "ogive curve," which runs almost level over the middle part of its course, but dips or rises with increasing steepness towards either extreme. This distribution was then divided conceptually into parts equal in length, quartiles, octiles or centiles—percentiles as we now call them. When looked at in this way, the man at the extreme right would exceed his neighbour to the left by a larger margin than that man would exceed his other neighbour. This led Galton to the misleading idea that there was more variation at the extremes of the distribution than about its middle. The correct view is that variability is a quality of the group as a whole, but that its effects will be more openly manifested at the extremes than near the mode.

An example which Galton chose to illustrate his idea is certainly striking. In two years of the mathematical tripos at Cambridge, out of 17,000 marks as total, the top man scored between 7,500 and 8,000. The runner-up was 2,000 marks behind, in the 5,500 to 6,000 class; while behind him, in the class 500 marks below there were no fewer than three men. Pearson says: "It was at this time that Galton first realized

311

the great principle that while between men of moderate ability there is scarcely any difference, between 'illustrious' and even 'eminent' men there are extraordinary differences." At the end of his life at the age of eighty-two he made an elegant application of this idea by calculating the proper proportions for the distribution of a sum of money between first and second prizes. Taking only 100 individuals, supposed to follow a normal distribution, the interval between the fiftieth and fifty-first is only one-tenth of the interval between the ninety-ninth and 100th. On this basis the intervals between the first and the second and between the second and the third prove to be as three to one, and it is in this ratio that the total prize money should be divided. From this Galton draws a moral:

> Differences in ability in power to create, to discover, to rule men do not go by uniform stages. We know this by experience — our Shakespeares, our Newtons, our Napoleons have no close compeers in the populations of their own generations — but we see a reason for the gulf which separates the genius from ourselves . . .

THE EXISTENCE OF AN ELITE

We must now look at Galton's ideas on the subject of an elite, since they determined the way in which he thought a eugenic policy would have to be implemented. The point I shall now maintain is that there is no class of human being which can be regarded as constituting an elite. Instead we have only individuals, who do indeed excel, but excel in a limited range of performance.

To begin with, we must distinguish between the man and his achievement. Galton does not tell us that the man, who scored 2,000 more marks than his runner-up in the mathematical Tripos, did anything very remarkable in his later career; and there is no reason to think that he did. Darwin showed more insight than Galton, when he observed that the discoverers of undiscovered things were often less clever than those who made no discoveries. There are elements of chance and will which intervene between ability on one side and achievement on the other.

Small quantitative differences in causes may lead to large or to qualitative differences in effects. This phenomenon may be met with in intelligence testing. We may pose two intelligent subjects with a problem which the one solves in three minutes and the other in thirty. If we now give them a second and more difficult problem, it may be that the first can be expected to solve it in an hour, and the second in fifty years, that is never, within the limits of a lifetime. In a walled-in courtyard full of prisoners, it may be that the one man who can jump an inch higher than his fellows will catch a glimpse of the horizon, while the others can never see more than the sky.

High achievement is the reward of the specialist, and his specialization has to be paid for by compensatory deficiencies. Take any expert off his home ground, and the mediocrity of the performance is painful. Indeed, if the subject of debate is minimally off-centre, the same can often be said. Listen to one of the BBC's "Critics" discussing a visit to a picture exhibition, or to a learned judge giving his views on juvenile delinquency, or even, let us say, to a well-known psychiatrist on the subject of human personality, and it would be pardonable to suppose that the man was clueless. To achieve his fantastic level of performance, Galton himself had to sacrifice practically everything else. Judged solely by the standards which can be attained in the arts, humanities and sciences, even the best of us are incompetents in all senses but one — mental cripples with a single hypertrophied organ. The mind of the specialist is a precision tool which can only show what it is capable of within its own limited range of application. The transcendent value to the community of the possessor of such a mind is almost entirely social and hardly at all biological.

Discussing the "Worth of Children," Galton took the view that the brains of the nation lay in what he called the W and X classes, i.e., in persons making up approximately one-third of one per cent of the population. This view is conditioned by the confusion already noted between social and biological values, or between genotype and phenotype. It is probably true that the valuable innovations, new ideas, new creations, which accrue from one generation to the next are received at the hands of one in 300 of the population or less. But the genes which provide the constitutional element in variation in intelligence are distributed throughout the entire population. There are a great many more of these valuable genes among the vast hordes of those of average intelligence, or even in the lesser hordes of those of subnormal intelligence, than there are in the chromosomes of the intellectual aristocracy. The trouble is, of course, that in the lower ranks genes of positive effect are in dilute concentration. But if we are to appraise the value of a mine, we do not take account only of the nuggets of pure gold and forget the ore.

IGNORANCE OF MENDELISM

Galton's misconceptions arose because he had to do all his work without the aid of Mendelism. Thus when he supposes that, if the W and X classes were removed from a community, it would be left with a dead level of mediocrity, he missed the fact that a single generation of random mating would restore the previous variability. The men of middle ability who make up the bulk of a population may not distinguish themselves by the creation of new social values; but, looked at biologically, they constitute the treasury of genetic variability and provide the raw material out of which the extreme deviants are made.

Finally, brief notice must be taken of Galton's disdain for the "army of ineffectives which clog progress." Of course, he was right to emphasize the way in which human progress is retarded by sheer stupidity. But the drag on progress is not the stupidity of the stupid but the stupidity of the intelligent. All the really disastrous things which have happened to mankind can be laid to the account of intelligent, indeed, frequently brilliant men. For these tragedies the intellectual proletariat are blameless.

Galton thought that eugenic policies could be furthered by encouraging the fertility of families in which eminent men had been known to occur. This was a consequence of the mode of research he had to follow in studying hereditary genius, and of the limited range of results which this approach could provide. His ignorance of Mendelism led to an important misconception of the biological nature of the family. He saw that there might be resemblances between a man and one of his grandfathers which were not shown with the intervening parent. To account for this, he derived one-quarter of the hereditary equipment of an individual from each of his two parents, one-sixteenth part from each of his grandparents, and so on, leading to a series whose sum is unity. The model is misleading. All of a man's genes come from one or other of his parents, and there is no remainder of genetic variability to be allocated elsewhere. The view that a man might base a claim for differential treatment on close relationship to an eminent man alone is quite unbiological. To take an example, we have no reason to suppose that a man of average intelligence will sire more intelligent children if he is the son of parents of superior intelligence than if his parents were as average as himself. The biological worth of an individual depends on his individual constitution, regardless of what that of other members of his family may be.

ENDS AND MEANS

This argument leads to the view that the means by which Galton proposed that eugenic ends should be attained are not the right ones. We have to abandon, I think, the whole of his ideas about diplomas of eugenic worth, the encouragement of fertility in eminent families and imposed restrictions on the fertility of the socially incompetent. They all suffer from a fatal defect, that of dividing humanity against itself. All mankind is in one boat together, and those of us who in some specified field of activity are rather less feebleminded than the average will have to do what we can for those who are rather more so.

However, if we abandon the means proposed by Galton, does it follow that we should abandon his ends? I do not think it does. To be sure, we must not blink the fact that the whole complex of ideas comprised under the heading of eugenics arouses strong opposition, not least among biologists. During his lifetime Galton had to suffer the disappointment of failing to arouse an echo among his scientific colleagues. He presented his ideas in the second Huxley lecture of the Anthropological Institute, "but the seed fell on barren soil," and the address was never published in their journal. Galton's critics pointed to the effects of the environment, as in the slums; and the resistance that any normal man would offer to interference with marriage. It was said that "at present the care for future man, the love and respect of the race, are quite beyond the pale of the morals of even the best." Karl Pearson stigmatized these ideas as unsupported by statistics, and half-baked. We are likely to rate them higher now, and the statistics are beginning to come in. Yet is it still true that even the best can take no care for the genetical future of mankind? I do not think that there is any biologist, even among those who shun this *Eugenics Society*, who would not agree that care for this aspect of our racial future should occupy us. The point on which they would insist is that social efforts, which are not supported by the weight of the evidence and by a consensus of informed opinion, should be held in reserve.

In some respects I think that our critics go too far. It is indeed true that all wild populations carry great numbers of genes of deleterious effect, and yet maintain their vitality. It is true that mankind can safely foster the infirm, and indeed permit their reproduction, without alarm for the future of the race. The variability of a race is its source of strength, and variability is the contribution of the heterozygote. But we can make a fetish of the heterozygote just as Galton made a fetish of the extreme deviant. We must have some sense of proportion. How far would the balance of heterozygote and homozygote be shifted by, say, a raising of the mean intelligence by half a standard deviation? Surely to a negligible extent; yet such a rise would transform our society. To give priority to the biological advantages of heterosis is to value reproductive vigour higher than vigour of the mind. As matters stand we are embarrassingly rich in the one and poor in the other. Stupidity is an enslavement of the spirit of man. If for biological reasons it is unsafe to contend against it, then those are risks we shall have to take. The biologists must tell us how to do it, and not that it shouldn't be done.

Perhaps it might be possible to find, entirely outside the field of genetics, principles which would have a directive influence on reproduction, which would not be dysgenic in their effect, and which might receive almost universal assent. This century is marked by increasing concern for the welfare of children. All that we might ask is that every child should be given a fair chance in life. To be an unwelcome guest in the home into which it is born does not constitute a fair start; and people who for whatever reason are unwilling to be parents should be provided with foolproof methods of avoiding conception. Furthermore if there is any accident, whether it is ill-health, or poverty, or unhappiness, which for a time would make it difficult for prospective parents to give their child the background and the upbringing it needs, they should for that time think well before they saddle a new human being with an unfair handicap. With this proviso we might safely forget criteria of eugenic worth.

28

THE INTERACTION OF SOCIAL ENVIRONMENT WITH GENOTYPE: A MODEL

It has been said that sociologists are distrustful of biogenetic explanations of human behaviour, in part because of the view that biological theories necessarily lead to predatory ethics. This has always been very surprising to me because some of our most distinguished human geneticists, such as J. B. S. Haldane and Lionel Penrose, have stood rather far to the left in social and political attitudes, and all our distinguished contemporary biologists have been contemptuous of racist theories. Familiarity with biological ways of thinking disposes us to wide tolerance. In 1946 J. B. S. Haldane gave an elegant demonstration of the ways in which genetic-environmental interactions could lead to different types of society. In the perfect society of the eugenist every genotype would be able to find the environment which suited him best, and no one genotype would consistently excel all others. In the perfect society of the environmentalist, every environment would suit some genotypes if not others, and no environment would be consistently the best for everybody. The type of society which is above all to be avoided would be one in which, wherever they went, some genotypes would always be at a disadvantage, and some environments would be universally unfavourable and avoided. The type of society which we should try to attain would be one in which genetic and environmental advantages went contrariwise. The ideal society would be one in which every existing environment would be the best for one of the existing genotypes, and every existing genotype would be able to find the environment which favoured him above all others.

I wonder whether the sociologist has been as long and as firmly persuaded of the immense importance of variety and variability as the biologist has been. In his Reith lectures some years ago Sir Peter Medawar (1960) strongly emphasized this point. He gave us, in fact, the strongest warning against genetical snobbism. All wild populations carry great numbers of genes of deleterious effect, and yet maintain their

Originally published as the vote of thanks to A. H. Halsey on the occasion of the Galton Lecture 1967 in the *Eugenics Review* 59: 149 (1967). Title added. Dr. Halsey's paper, "Sociology, Biology and Population Control," appeared in the *Eugenics Review* 59: 155–64 (1967).

vitality. The variability of a race is its source of strength, and variability is the contribution of the heterozygote. To develop Haldane's point, should we not be thinking along the same lines about societies? Perhaps it would not be the best thing for humanity if every human society has the same organization, being perhaps a copy in miniature of the United States or another of the western democracies?

In the fifty-fourth Galton Lecture Dr. Halsey has given us some splendid illustrations of the importance of sociological ideas for understanding biological processes. This is a marriage of ideas that must be fruitful. We are greatly in his debt, and all of us will wish to give him our warm and sincere thanks.

29

A BIOLOGICAL VIEW ON ANTI-SEMITISM

Where groups of human beings find themselves in conflict, it is natural for each party to blame the other. This, however, does not help at all in discovering the reasons for the conflict, or the best way of solving it. Every enlightened man must feel that outbreaks of racial or religious persecution, or of anti-Semitism, are a blot on our civilisation and a serious danger to it. Blame has been laid by the other side both on Christian education and on Jewish temperament and *mores*. If, however, we try to examine the problem dispassionately, we are led in a different direction. We see that anti-Semitism does not stand alone, but is a single, even though an important, example of a wide range of phenomena, namely class hostilities of all kinds. We find that human beings, when arranged in groups, tend only too easily to feel hostile to others not in the same group as themselves, and loyal to members of their own group. National rivalries are a case in point; but within the nation exactly the same thing is observable between smaller groups — such as between the sexes, between social classes, between political organisations, between persons who differ in accent, upbringing, education, cultural tastes, and in almost every other imaginable way.

It is likely that the tendency to react in a hostile way to others who are felt to belong to a different group is a fundamental human characteristic. It is only with great difficulty that the man of culture and insight can rid himself of such feelings. Unless he keeps a close guard on his thinking, he is only too liable to adopt emotional rather than rational thought processes. He will then be likely to confuse the individual with his class, and to allow him to possess only those faults and merits which are attributed to the class to which he belongs. The differences between the two classes are exalted at the expense of their similarities; and relative values are assigned to the one and the other. The dispassionate observer, on the other hand, notes that these judgments of value are always partial and nearly always probably

Originally published in the *Jewish Monthly* 1 (8): 22–28 (1947).

fallacious. The only observable fact is that there is a difference between the two classes. This difference in itself may be of a trivial kind, and even one that applies only to averages of the two classes taken as wholes, the individuals themselves showing a considerable overlap.

There is a growing body of evidence to show that human beings are repelled by differences and attracted by similarities. It has, for instance, been shown that husbands and wives resemble one another more closely than chance would allow, in every particular which has been made the subject of enquiry; and it seems probable that this similarity is itself a cause of the attraction which has drawn them together. Similarity in background, interests, intelligence and other qualities aid, one might well guess, that feeling of mutual understanding which is the basis of liking. Similarity of temperament, caused by a common heredity, helps to bind members of the same family together. And those human beings who show a degree of similarity not otherwise seen in nature, the so-called "similar" or uniovular twins, are known to enjoy, as a general rule, an intimacy of love and understanding but rarely found elsewhere.

If, therefore, we propose the hypothesis that anti-Semitism is not to be laid to the blame of either Jews or Christians, but is to be attributed in the first place to the relation between the two, that relation being one of difference, we have some biological justification. An examination of the facts shows that differences between Jews and Christians are of a rather wider and deeper kind than between most groupings into which a Western civilised country naturally falls. Jews are distinguished from non-Jews not only by religion, but very often also by name, cultural background, family affiliation, dietetic habits, holiday observances, and social customs of many kinds. Their occupational and economic grouping is very different from that of the population as a whole. Their favoured places of residence have a pattern of their own, so that they are not scattered broadcast through the community but mainly concentrated in certain parts. Perhaps most importantly, their average physical appearance in colouring, build and features, differs from the average of their compatriots. It does not matter that these differences are entirely irrelevant to any consideration of the worth and value of the Jews. Merely as differences, they may impede understanding and promote hostility.

The accumulation of differences is to be taken seriously; each one adds to the effect of the others. Most human groupings, at least within the structure of a society or nation, are in respect of one or only a few qualities. The Roman Catholic differs from his fellow men, so far as we know, in religion only. In a middle-class society, "Socialists" and "Tories" will be indistinguishable from one another until they start to talk politics. Societies are able to exist as unities because a cleavage of opinion, or a difference in temperament, interests, or affiliations, unites those who are divided on other issues. If one group is separated from the rest of the community in too many ways, it may come to be felt as foreign, and accordingly resented.

Other factors than mere difference are, of course, important; and among these are the degree of organisation of the groups and their relative masses. If one group is not organised at all, but consists of isolated individuals without interconnections, it will not be felt to be a group at all, and no group hostility will arise. The more closely organised it is, the more its existence as a group will be felt by others, and the more likely that those others will feel hostile towards it. Again, if one group is almost infinitesimally small in comparison with the other, the members of the larger group will only be aware of individuals, and are unlikely to become hostile. This is the present relation between coloured and white people in this country. When the smaller group becomes larger than this, hostilities begin to appear, in the first place in those parts where they are most frequent. This seems to be the present state of affairs in England with regard to the Jews; and it is noteworthy that anti-Semitism is hardly found at all in rural areas and is most virulent in those London boroughs where the density of the Jewish population is greatest.

If we accept the view that hostility between Jews and non-Jews is due to differences of physical, social, and psychological kinds, we may enquire what are the possible solutions.

The first one, which has been adopted by many generous-minded men, is the hope that by a process of liberal education we may induce members of the larger non-Jewish group to grow up mentally, as it were, abandon such primitive and emotional culture patterns, and learn to live in amity with Jews despite their differences. This has been the hope of Jews throughout the ages, and in some countries it has met with temporary encouragement. In Czarist Russia there was a recurrent danger of the pogrom; in Soviet Russia there seems to be at least no discrimination against anyone by race or creed. Nevertheless, to anyone who has seen anti-Semitic feeling appear, as if from nowhere, in otherwise tolerant people who have found themselves in competition with Jews, the hope seems a precarious one. In view of the appalling risks that can be run, it should surely not be the only recourse.

The second solution is to isolate Jews and non-Jews from one another. This is the Zionist solution, and has been gaining support rapidly. Such a solution, however, would only be a temporary one. As things are, the world is a patchwork of jarring nationalities, and one of our main hopes must be their gradual resolution. Peoples must gradually grow together, and not remain eternally divided.

The third solution would lie in the gradual dissolution of the differences themselves; and I would myself say that this solution would be a permanent and a radical one. We are not called on to contemplate the disappearance of the Jewish religion, any more than there is anything to be gained by the disappearance of, say, Quakerism. But the hope would be raised that if all those accidental and irrelevant differences which divide the Jew from the Christian were to go, mutual animosities would go with them.

It was in an effort to discover how far this process of assimilation was actually going on in this country at the present time that I made an enquiry among fifty Jewish soldier-patients of Sutton Emergency Hospital during 1944-45. These men were suffering from nervous ailments, and it is quite possible that they were not representative of British Jews as a whole. As there were no officers among them, they could only be typical of the working class and middle class non-professional Jew, such men as tailors and clerks and proprietors of small businesses. A sample taken from such a class is, however, more interesting than one taken from a more prosperous background. My results (43) may be summarised as follows:

Most of these men were not immigrants themselves, but were the sons or grandsons of immigrants. Nevertheless about 16 of the 50 surnames were English in form and not immediately recognisable as Jewish patronymics. Many names must have been changed from their original form since immigration.

First names were nearly all of a fairly typical English type, and such Jewish names as Judah and Leah were rare.

Religious upbringing had changed very much in the course of three generations. Dealing in terms of families, 46 out of 64 parental families had been brought up "strictly" or "very strictly" in the Jewish faith, in the patients' own generation 18 out of 50, in the generation of the children 19 out of 69. One only of the parents, 3 of the patients, and 30 of the families in the third generation had a lax, non-Jewish or non-religious upbringing.

In physical traits, a distinct proportion of the patients showed traits of a non-Jewish ancestry — fair skin, blue eyes, a retrousse nose, or some other similar quality.

Intermarriage with non-Jews was occurring at an increasing rate. Only one of the fathers had married a non-Jewish wife. Of the 160 marriages in the next generation, 28 were to non-Jews, i.e. about 17 per cent. Even when allowance is made for the fact that intermarriage is much more frequent in some families than in others, it seems probable that about one in every eight Jewish marriages is to someone brought up in another religion.

Insofar, then, as we are acquainted with the facts, the Jews seem to be discarding some at least of the outward characteristics that distinguish them from their fellow countrymen. Most importantly of all, it is likely that there is a substantial rate of intermarriage. This is surely a process which is on all accounts to be welcomed. There is a detestable superstition, current among Gentiles, that the Jews believe themselves to be a chosen people, and therefore inherently superior to the rest of humanity. Nothing would do so much to disabuse people of such a fanciful notion as the encouragement of religious conversion to Judaism, and of intermarriage with members of other sects.

In all the lands which they have made their homes, Jews have tended to isolate themselves from the rest of the population. In part this has been forced on them, in part they have isolated themselves in one or another respect of their own accord. Isolation has been the result of persecution, but through aiding the perpetuation of differences it has itself perpetuated hostility. It has kept the Jews together as a people, has promoted their loyalty to one another, and in the opinion of some has helped in the preservation of their faith. On the other hand it has led in country after country to restrictive practices, and even to persecutions which are a disgrace to our civilisation. On the religious side, Jewish teaching and philosophy, except as far as they are available from the Bible, have remained little known to others, and have not had the effect on world culture which a wider dissemination might have encouraged.

As parts of a reorientation of attitude, I would suggest the following points for discussion:

1. The loyalty of the Jew to his fellow-man is more fundamental than his loyalty to his fellow-Jew.

2. The largest contribution towards the dissolution of feelings of hostility would be in the dissolution of points of difference between Jews and the inhabitants of the lands in which they live.

3. As a consequence of their relative numbers, the main contribution towards mutual adaptation between Jews and non-Jews will have to be made by Jews.

4. While leaving the kernel of religious teaching intact, those modes of behaviour which have a purely symbolic or formal justification should be pruned.

5. Jewish religion and philosophy are part of the endowment of the human race, and should be shared wherever possible. An evangelical attitude towards new converts is desirable.

6. Intermarriage between Jews and non-Jews is a step in a good and friendly direction, and would be the greatest single factor in binding the two groups together.

321

30

ASSORTATIVE MATING

INTRODUCTION

The book of which this paper is a part, *Patterns of Marriage*, describes an investigation into two hundred married couples. The husbands were selected, by being married and having a home in London, from the soldiers, sailors, and airmen treated in an emergency hospital in the neighborhood of London from 1943 to 1946. Half of them had been admitted to wards for neurosis, half to medical and surgical wards. The latter group can be regarded as psychiatrically normal, and as a fairly random sample from the population of working-class Londoners. The sample was restricted by age distribution, by exclusion of persons seriously ill either mentally or physically, and by occupational distribution. The physical ailments for which the patients in the Control group had been admitted to hospital were in the nature of accidents of everyday life. There was also a selection in favour of the happily married, as those who were on bad terms with their wives tended to evade investigation. The patients admitted to the neurotic wards differed from the others only in respect of suffering from some form of nervous disorder not amounting to insanity, and largely conforming to one or other type of neurosis. The two groups can be compared in respect of all other characteristics.

PREVIOUS WORK

Since the matter was first raised in a scientific way in 1896 by Karl Pearson, there has been a great volume of work on the subject of assortative mating, nearly all of it by sociologists or psychologists in the U.S.A. Despite its importance, the subject attracted relatively little attention from psychiatrists and geneticists. Nevertheless, its great significance has been recognized.

By Eliot Slater and Moya Woodside. Originally published as Chapter 8 (pp. 127–37) in *Patterns of Marriage*. London: Cassell (1951). Part of the book's Summary added.

Dahlberg (1941) drew attention to the demographic changes in our mating habits. Mating is not at random, but is limited to those persons with whom a given individual has some chance of coming in contact. Furthermore, meetings of a certain type will be much more likely to result in a mating than meetings of another type. For instance, meetings between employer and employee are less likely to result in a marriage than are those between fellow employees. From the point of view of mating, the population can be divided up into a number of *isolates*, or groupings within which marriages are more likely to occur, than between one group and another. These isolates are of many kinds, religious, geographical, economic, social, etc. One form in which this shows itself is mating within the same family group, what is ordinarily called consanguineous marriage or inbreeding. Dahlberg has pointed out that the frequency of cousin marriage is decreasing in most countries, and in Bavaria, for instance, has dropped from .9 percent of all marriages to .2 percent in the last fifty years. He attributes this to the breaking up of isolates through the growth of communications and migration into towns. No doubt many other factors play a part, the wider tolerance shown between social classes, the lessening importance popularly attached to religious biases, and so forth. Nevertheless, although these isolates are getting larger, and overlap to a greater and greater extent, they still exist and are of great significance socially and biologically.

Dahlberg's comments draw our attention to the fact that for the most part we marry within our own kind. This may be purely an accident of opportunity; and it would be possible for such a thing to exist alongside a general human tendency to choose for a mate someone who differed from rather than resembled the chooser. This, however, has not been found. As most of the work has been done by sociologists and psychologists, it is not surprising that most of the facts at our disposal are of a social and psychological nature.

Burgess and Wallin (1943), in a recent review, give a list of fifty-one qualities in which, from their own researches, engaged couples tend to resemble one another. In four of these the degree of similarity was so small as to be statistically insignificant, but in none of them was a negative association found, i.e., in none of these qualities was there a suggestion that people engaging themselves to marriage tended to choose partners who differed from themselves. The qualities listed included family background (size of township lived in as a child, parental income and social status, church membership and attendance), education, social relations (number of friends, membership of clubs, organizations), attitudes and interests, ideas about the factors that go to make a successful marriage.

In another review of the literature, Richardson (1939) lists the reports of six workers who have tested husbands and wives for similarities in intelligence and intellectual abilities, of seven workers who have applied tests of temperament, and of another seven who have tested attitudes and interests. In all, some sixty-five different experiments have been made, and in every case there is resemblance between the partners and not its reverse. The degree of resemblance between partners is conveniently measured by the correlation coefficient (r). This is an index which can vary between 1 and -1. At the midway point, 0, it indicates that the two qualities being measured vary quite independently. An r of 0 in measurements of husbands and wives would show that they neither tended to resemble nor to differ from one another, but were apparently mating at random. An r of 1 would show that given the test result in the case of one partner one could predict the result in the case of the other with absolute certainty, and that the results were always

323

alike. An r of -1 would show that while one could still predict the test result given by one from that given by the other with complete certainty, the members of each pair varied in diametrically opposed directions, and that husbands and wives were choosing their exact opposites. In these various tests, the values of r varied very much, but they were all positive, none negative. On the whole the greatest degree of resemblance was shown in the field of attitudes and interests, where the average r was .5; in tests of intelligence the average r was .4, and in tests of temperament .1, which is very low. When these resemblances were checked against the duration of marriage, there was no sign that in marriages of longer duration husbands and wives were more alike than in those of shorter duration. In fact, we have no evidence that husbands and wives tend to grow more alike in these respects through the years. The tendency towards similarity seems to be the result of the original choice of partner.

Richardson also lists a number of investigations which have been made on pairs of friends. Once again the same thing holds, and friends, too, tend to resemble one another; there is no certainly established case where they have been found, on the whole, to differ.

In physical traits, once more, the same phenomenon has been found, although here correlations tend to assume a low value. The greatest are in measurements of height, where Smith (1941, 1946), for instance, has found a value of r of .4. He and other investigators have found resemblances between married partners in cephalic index, eye and hair colour, health, longevity, family fertility, etc.

We have to set this very impressive body of evidence against the view, frequently expressed popularly, that people are attracted by their opposites. Paradoxically, perhaps, there is no difficulty in reconciling these two views. If we assume that a general basis of similarity exists and is favourable for the occurrence of a mating, one or two features of marked contrast might then serve as an additional attraction. The swarthy husband, for instance, might find an ultra-blonde wife particularly attractive; or the man who is timid, indecisive and dependent, might feel more than usually secure with a strong, self-reliant, and protective woman. But it seems probable that such attractions can only occur frequently within a general similarity; and in massed statistics the general trend towards similarity would entirely submerge isolated and individual deviations in an opposite direction.

On common sense grounds too, one might expect that similarities over a wide field would provide the two partners with an apprehension of kinship, with the feeling that they understood one another, were in tune with one another, and might be reasonably sure of what the other would do next.

SIMILARITY AS THE BASIS OF LIKING

It is, perhaps, not without psychological significance that our words liking and likeness are etymologically related. If we look around us, in the animal as in the human world, we find that the evidences of affection and toleration are principally shown between individuals and groups which resemble one another. Different species of animals do not mix easily; and even races which, in a given spot, mix freely will frequently fail to mate with one another, however abundant the opportunities are for so doing.

In humankind we find that where two groups of individuals differ markedly from one another, a lack of understanding only too easily arises, with its consequences, perhaps, in open hostility. Differences of language, colour, nationality, religion, political organization, and social custom divide and isolate us, and provide the basis both of religious persecutions and national wars.

Similarities, on the other hand, attract us and bind us together. Men who have been educated at the same school usually continue to have a fellow feeling for one another long after their school days. The educated and intelligent man takes his pleasure in the company of others of the same degree of intelligence and education. Clubs and societies are constantly being formed to unite those of similar interests. The rich man is likely to find himself not quite at home in the society of men much poorer than himself, who cannot but have a very different attitude towards life.

The family is bound together, not only by a common history and a common cultural, social and economic background, by sharing common problems and so forth, but also by having a common blood, that is through hereditary and constitutional make-up, which is to some extent the same for all members of the family. Where this unity of blood reaches its highest point, the degree of understanding and affection also reaches its highest level. In that variety of twins called 'similar' or 'uniovular,' we observe the remarkable phenomenon of the duplication by nature of a single individual. Uniovular twins have identical hereditary equipment. Physically they often resemble one another so closely that acquaintances, friends, teachers, and even parents may have great difficulty in distinguishing one from the other; they also show, as a general rule, a very high degree of similarity in intelligence, abilities (manual, athletic, musical and artistic), in temperament and character. Their devotion to one another has been the subject of folklore and of some of the higher flights of the world's literature, and has been amply borne out by more detailed psychological and psychiatric investigation.

In fact, wherever we look in biology, sociology or psychology, we find indications that an intuitive appreciation of similarities is the basis of liking, the feeling of difference is the basis of hostility. We need not be surprised that investigations of husbands and wives in many different ways show only evidence of a trend towards similarity, and none of a trend towards difference, apart from the sex difference itself.

THE RESULTS OF OUR ENQUIRY

The findings in our sample in every way support those of other workers. We have already seen that husband and wife tend to resemble each other in the type of work on which they were engaged before marriage, but that there is no sign of a convergence of family history of physical illness on the two sides. A list of the correlation coefficients which have reached statistical significance is given in Table 30.1. Some of these are of comparatively little interest. A very high degree of similarity naturally holds in respect of the number of children born to each of the two partners, the only surprising thing about this being that the r does not approach still nearer to 1. The next highest degree of similarity is in age at marriage, where r is .5 in the Control and .7 in the Neurotic group. And there is a fair degree of correlation in the extent of pre-marital sex experience, no doubt because the behaviour of affianced pairs is necessarily much the same for both of them.

Quite a high degree of similarity is shown in intelligence, where r is .36. This is about the value obtained by other workers in the U.S.A. It means that husband and wife, on the whole, resemble each other in intelligence not much less closely than do brother and sister.

325

TABLE 30.1. SIGNIFICANT PRODUCT MOMENT CORRELATION COEFFICIENTS BETWEEN
HUSBANDS AND WIVES

	Control	Neurotic	Both
I. By Correlation of Exact Measures			
Age at marriage	.51	.72	
Stature	.27	.22	
Temperament test*			.19
II. By Grouping into Higher and Lower Halves			
Number of children	.80	.92	.86
Age at marriage	.16	.48	.32
Intelligence*	.28	.44	.36
Pre-marital sex experience	.40	.20	.30
Clinical rating of neurotic disposition	.20	.24	.22
Education	.24	.16	.20
Stature	.28	.08	.18
Good looks	.28	.00	.14
Temperament test	.08	.20	.14

All the above are positive, and statistically significant (p less than .05 at most). It is to be noted that figures under I are higher than the corresponding ones under II, and are of course to be preferred. Estimates under II are to be considered as more likely to be under than above what would be found by more rigorous investigation. These correlations are the only ones, among a larger number which were tested, which were found to be statistically significant.

*The temperament test was a 48-item questionnaire (Slater, P., 1945a). Intelligence was rated, not tested. — Editors.

After this come resemblances in height, in the clinical rating of degree of nervous predisposition, in education, in the results of the temperament test, and in degree of good looks.

Taken as a whole, the results show only positive resemblances and there are no points in which there is a sign of a systematic tendency towards difference between husband and wife.

One of the main purposes of the whole enquiry was to establish or refute this point in respect of tendencies towards neurotic illness. On this we have three pieces of evidence, two of which are independent of one another. First there is the temperament test, which had been shown by previous work to have a significant effect in distinguishing neurotic patients from comparable persons in a state of mental health. The correlation is low, but reliable (r = .19). Secondly come the results of psychiatric history taken from husbands and wives in the Neurotic and Control groups. When people are ranked by the degree to which they show nervous traits, there is a correlation in the Control group of .20, in the Neurotic group of .24. But the most significant evidence of similarity between husbands and wives is provided by the estimate we can give of the number of neurotic, psychopathic, or otherwise abnormal persons in both of the two Control groups, and among the wives of the Neurotics. As will be seen from Table 30.2, there is significantly more neurosis and psychopathy among the wives and their parents, and significantly more neurosis and neurotic traits in the wives, in the Neurotic than in the Control group.

THE SIGNIFICANCE OF ASSORTATIVE MATING
FOR PSYCHOLOGICAL MEDICINE

Previous work on assortative mating has been confined, in the realm of psychiatry, to work on the major illnesses, the insanities or psychoses. Penrose (1944), for instance, has found that in one Canadian mental hospital there were a larger number of husbands and wives admitted, at different times, than could have been expected

TABLE 30.2. PSYCHIATRIC ABNORMALITIES IN SUBJECTS AND RELATIVES

	Control						Neurotic				
	H	HF	HM	W	WF	WM	HF	HM	W	WF	WM
Normal	66	55	55	71	57	50	37	34	53	64	47
Nervous traits	23	16	28	20	25	38	28	40	20	19	39
Total: within normal limits	89	71	83	91	82	88	65	74	83	83	86
Neurotic illness	4	3	5	7	3	4	7	10	16	4	5
Psychopathic personality	4	14	3	2	5	—	17	5	1	6	4
Total: abnormal personalities	8	17	8	9	8	4	24	15	17	10	9
Mental Illness (psychosis)	2	2	—	—	3	2	—	2	—	1	—
Suicide	—	1	—	—	—	—	1	1	—	—	—
Epilepsy	1	1	—	—	1	—	1	1	—	1	—
Total: other abnormalities	3	4	—	—	4	2	2	4	—	2	—
No information	—	8	9	—	6	6	9	7	—	5	5
Total	100	100	100	100	100	100	100	100	100	100	100

H = Husband; W = Wife; F = Father; M = Mother

on the basis of chance alone; and he concluded that there was a measure of assortative mating 'with respect to traits which form part of the background of mental disease.' This background might, of course, just as easily be an environmental one (social, economic, etc.), as a background of constitutional predisposition.

The commonest, and perhaps the most terrible of the psychoses is schizophrenia. We have practically no knowledge of its causes other than that heredity plays an important part. The investigation of the hereditary basis has met with considerable difficulties, and is still an obscure problem. One of the problems was whether people with a hereditary predisposition to schizophrenia tended to marry one another. Three workers, Leistenschneider (1938), Egger (1942), and Früh (1943) have at different times investigated this in Germany. They found that the husbands and wives of schizophrenics themselves had about double the average chance of becoming schizophrenic. If there is assortative mating in this respect, it is very weak.

This, perhaps, is hardly surprising. In the mating of men and women there is no reason to postulate a metaphysical 'call of the blood'. They are, in fact, only likely to be attracted to one another by qualities of which their senses provide them with direct evidence. But the hereditary predisposition to schizophrenia as a rule remains fairly well hidden until at last it makes its appearance in obvious mental disease; and it would be risky indeed to predict, before the event, that a given individual would have an attack of schizophrenia at a later time. If those with a latent germ for schizophrenia tend to some extent to marry one another, their choice must be determined by an intuitive appreciation of rather subtle qualities of temperament, common to both of them, which are only distantly related to the tendency to mental illness.

In the field of neurotic illness, circumstances are very different. Neurotic illnesses, whether they involve symptoms of depression, anxiety, doubt, loss of memory or whatever other symptoms, are but extreme examples of what we all go through in a minor form, and regard as normal under the disappointments and hardships of our day to day life. A man becomes 'neurotic' when he has reached a breaking point, and is compelled for the time being to stop working or drop some of his usual avocations. The symptoms were there for some time before he broke down;

and an examination of his history would show that he always tended to react rather more emotionally to circumstances than does the average man. The symptoms of neurosis are, indeed, closely bound up with personality; and it is often quite possible to predict that a given man, placed in circumstances of a given type, will react with a neurotic illness in which particular symptoms will be the predominant ones.

An investigation of assortative mating has a much greater probability of reaching positive findings in the field of neurosis than in the field of the psychoses. What we have found leads us to the view that the similarities of character and temperament which appear to be a source of mutual attraction to married couples, extend also to those qualities of the mental make-up which involve a liability to nervous illness.

THE SIGNIFICANCE OF ASSORTATIVE MATING FOR EUGENICS

Any sensible programme of eugenics must base itself scientifically on what we know about population genetics. An obvious application of this arises in the problems raised by the hereditary basis of schizophrenia. As schizophrenia is so largely due to hereditary causes, it might be thought that sterilizing all schizophrenics would in time lead to the disappearance of the disease. Unfortunately, this bears little resemblance to the truth. The genetical factors which provide the predisposition to schizophrenia must be very widespread in the population, and must in the majority of cases be carried, in a possibly incomplete way, by people who remain mentally sound throughout their lives. Sterilizing the schizophrenics would remove only a very small part of the total amount of the abnormal hereditary factors circulating in the population, and even extended over many generations would reduce the incidence of schizophrenia by only a small proportion.

Our knowledge of the distribution of particular hereditary factors, or 'genes,' in the population can, in fact, warn us of the precipitate and unscientific type of compulsory eugenic measure which was enforced in Germany after 1933 by a Nazi state policy. For purposes of convenience in the complicated mathematics which the statistics of population genetics involves, it has hitherto been assumed that random mating was the rule. This is demonstrably not the case, at least in human populations; and mathematical theory will have to make some allowance for these facts. This is most clearly the case when the important subject of mental defect is being discussed. If husbands and wives are as similar in intelligence as brothers and sisters, the distribution in the population of the genes of mental defect must be a different one from that which can be calculated on the assumption of random mating. There is little reason to doubt that, in every economic class of the community, the more intelligent are, at the present time, having fewer children than the less intelligent. The correlation coefficient between intelligence and number of brothers and sisters was calculated by Fraser Roberts (1939, 1940) in a large unselected group of school children as – .22. In our sample the correlation between intelligence and number of brothers and sisters is – .23; and between intelligence and number of children – .18. The difference between these two is not significant, and there is no present reason to think that the tendency of the more intelligent to restrict their families is lessening.

Now if intelligent people have a special tendency to marry one another, and unintelligent people likewise, then when an intelligent man restricts the size of his family, he is probably also restricting the issue of an intelligent wife. The differential tendency, in fact, multiplies itself. If, on the other hand, we could introduce incentives to induce intelligent people to have rather more than a proportionate share in the procreation of the next generation, the existence of assortative mating would increase the beneficial and eugenic result.

Assortative mating has another effect. It tends to increase the variability of the population, to increase the numbers of persons showing an extreme degree of a quality, and to decrease the proportion of persons near the average. An intelligent man and woman who marry one another are more likely to have a brilliant child than if they each married persons of average intelligence. With a well-marked tendency towards assortative mating in intelligence, we have a rather larger share both of persons of high ability and of the mentally dull and backward than we should otherwise have. The tendency reinforces trends, both eugenic and dysgenic, and makes the population more genetically unstable and more responsive to carefully designed eugenic measures than it would otherwise be.

Turning now to the consequences of assortative mating in the field of personality and the predisposition to neurotic illness, the same considerations largely hold true. As a result of the existence of this tendency, we probably have a higher proportion of unusual personalities, such as, perhaps, the saintly and the philanthropic, the egotistical and the neurotic, than we would otherwise have. But in regard to tendencies to neurosis we have no present reason to believe that a differential fertility is to be found. If it exists, it is more likely to be favourable than unfavourable.[1] In the sample we have examined, the Neurotic group had on an average fewer children and a lower rate of increase of family from year to year with increasing duration of marriage, than did the Control group. The difference in fertility in the two groups is not statistically significant when duration of marriage is accounted for, but such difference as there is, is against the Neurotic.

THE SOCIAL SIGNIFICANCE OF ASSORTATIVE MATING

One important effect of the tendency of like to mate with like, is to maintain the unity of family traditions. We see this in everyday life in the tendency of families with military, political, artistic, theatrical, musical, medical, scientific, and many other interests, to marry among themselves. The tendency must be regarded as a favourable one, for it means that the seeds of culture that are handed down from generation to generation are more likely to fall on favourable ground. This is one way in which society equips itself with the multifarious specialists who are necessary to carry out the highly skilled operations on which civilization depends. There can be no doubt that a society which is well equipped with the able and highly trained, even though it is burdened with the inept and the defective, is much less likely to fail than one consisting almost wholly of mediocrities. The man-in-a-million may bring more good to a community than the harm done by a million mental defectives.

Nevertheless, we must not lose all sense of proportion in a discussion of this subject, and commit ourselves to an out-of-date aristocratic conception of society. The main treasury of hereditary human ability does not lie in the germ cells of geniuses, nor even of the exceptionally able, but lies latent in the reproductive glands of the great masses of the average and slightly above average. As Galton pointed out half a century ago, if we could raise the average ability of the community by only a small amount, we would greatly increase the number of the highly able. If the average intelligence of the community were raised by only half a stan-

---

[1] At the time of the study, 123 conceptions had so far been recorded for the Neurotic group and 155 for the Controls. — *Editors*.

dard deviation, say seven or eight points on the Binet intelligence quotient scale, the man-in-a-million would become ten such men. Probably our greatest hope of raising average intelligence would be by providing the psychological incentives for a deliberate increase in the fertility of the intelligent. If the present differential fertility could be reversed in sign, assortative mating, instead of being a danger, would become socially beneficial.

SUMMARY

Both samples show that husbands and wives tend to resemble one another in personality and temperament. There is a positive correlation of .36 in intelligence and there are lower positive correlations in the clinical rating of degree of nervous predisposition, and in the results of the temperament test. Analysis of variance in the results of this test show a correlation between husband and wife of .13; the analysis also shows that the Neurotic husbands score very significantly higher than the other groups, and that those who are happily married score significantly lower than the less happily married. It is also found that there is a significantly higher degree of homogamy in the more than in the less happily married. There was significantly more neurosis and psychopathy in the wives and their parents in the Neurotic than in the Control group. The psychological, eugenic and social significance of assortative mating is briefly discussed. A theory is proposed which postulates that the psychological basis of liking is an apprehension of similarity.

31

THE McNAUGHTON RULES AND
MODERN CONCEPTS OF RESPONSIBILITY

We are nowadays becoming increasingly aware that there is such a thing as social pathology, and that there are diseases of the body politic which are not diseases of the individuals which compose them. This awareness has come to us through the study of individual psychology, of psychosomatic disorders, and disorders of interpersonal relationships. Many of the aberrations we observe seem to have been caused by no defect or disease of the individual sufferer, but by the fact that he was caught up in unfavourable circumstances, which themselves resulted from the nature of the society in which he lives. An obvious example is juvenile delinquency: a certain amount of delinquency is traceable to disorders and defects of the individual, such as mental deficiency and epilepsy; but in the majority of cases the failure seems to be mainly caused by social inadequacies, disturbances in home life, deficiencies in training, lack of normal outlets, and factors of such kinds.

It is useless to maintain that these social evils are no concern of psychiatry and should be reserved for the economist and sociologist. Their effects are constantly to be seen by the psychiatrist in his daily work; and those of us who believe that the State exists for the welfare of the individual must also believe that, from the study of individuals and the conditions in which they thrive or break down, general directives for the planning of social organization must also be derived.

It is against such a broad background that one best approaches the peculiar problems of criminal responsibility. For many years legal and medical views on this subject have been diametrically opposed. How is it, one may ask, that two groups of professionally trained minds have found it so impossible to understand one another that they can hardly enter a discussion together without unnecessary affect? How is it, with all the growth of knowledge of the working of the human mind, that we are

Originally published in the *British Medical Journal* 2: 713–18 (1954). The spelling M'Naghten of the original paper has been changed to McNaughton. The inquest report on Sir Robert Peel's secretary, the Bethlem Hospital record of his assailant, the death certificate and the only known signature of the prisoner show the latter to be the correct spelling of his name. See Morton (1956).

still burdened with a doctrine of criminal responsibility which is more than a century out of date, while other civilized countries have progressed far beyond us? We are faced with an example of social pathology, and the history of the illness and the present status should prove interesting.

When in 1843 McNaughton shot at and killed Sir Robert Peel's secretary, believing the man to be his master, his case was not decided by the McNaughton Rules, nor was he found guilty of the act charged. These Rules and the form of the verdict in the case of insane killers were refinements introduced after his time. When it had been shown in evidence that McNaughton suffered from a number of delusions of persecution, and that the killing had been inspired by these delusions, the judge did not even leave the verdict to the consideration of the jury, but directed them to find him not guilty. At that time Broadmoor did not exist, and, though by an Act of 1800 criminal lunatics had a special legal status, arrangements for their security and care were not, perhaps, very satisfactory. The public reaction could hardly have been greater if the killer had got off scot-free. It culminated in a debate in the House of Lords, where five questions were put to the judges; and the replies of 14 of the 15 judges to the questions constitute the Rules.

THE McNAUGHTON RULES

The answer to the first question states that persons who labour under partial delusions only, and are not in other respects insane, who know, moreover, that their act is contrary to the law of the land, are nevertheless punishable for that act.

The second and third questions were answered together, and constitute the McNaughton Rules as we know them today. They state that every man is to be presumed sane, and to possess a sufficient degree of reason to be responsible for his crimes, until the contrary is proved to the satisfaction of the jury; "and that to establish a defence on the ground of insanity it must be clearly proved that, at the time of committing the act, the accused was labouring under such a defect of reason, from disease of the mind, as not to know the nature and quality of the act he was doing, or, if he did know it, that he did not know he was doing what was wrong." The answer goes on to say that the party's knowledge of right and wrong should be put to the jury with reference to the act charged, rather than generally. "If the accused was conscious that the act was one that he ought not to do, and if that act was at the same time contrary to the law of the land, he is punishable."

It is noteworthy that, since the formulation of the Rules, an element of increased rigidity has been introduced by subsequent decisions. The judges who formulated the Rules seem to have recognized the distinction between subjective right and wrong in the mind of an accused person and objective right and wrong as defined by the law of the land, and to have held the former to be the criterion. A man who believed that another was the incarnation of Satan, and that he was commanded by God to kill him, would seem to be excused by the original formulation, though not by the Rules as they are administered today. A later decision in the Appeal Court has laid it down that if a man knows his act is against the law it is enough.

The answer to the fourth question states the extent to which a delusional belief may constitute a defence, in the case of persons suffering from partial delusions only and not in other respects insane. "We think," runs the answer, "he must be considered in the same situation as to responsibility as if the facts with respect to which the delusion exists were real. For example, if under the influence of his delusion he supposes another man to be in the act of attempting to take away his life, and he kills that man, as he supposes, in self-defence, he would be exempt from punishment. If his delusion was that the deceased had inflicted a serious injury to his character and fortune, and he killed him in revenge for such supposed injury, he would be liable to punishment."

The answer to the fifth question is of no interest, as it merely defines the circumstances under which a medical witness, who has heard the evidence in court, may give evidence about the responsibility of the accused.

The judges were called on to state what the law was in 1843, and not what the law should be. The effect of their ruling was such that McNaughton himself would have been otherwise judged than he had been. The state of public opinion at the time was such as to demand a tightening up of the law, and this is a thing which lawyers are never loath to do. Nevertheless the effect of the Rules has been to stabilize the law at the time of 1843 into being the law of the country for all time. This is an event without equal in the history of English common law. For the law of murder is common law, and not statute law, and the common law is a growing organism. With the McNaughton Rules that branch of the common law which relates to the criminal responsibility of mentally abnormal persons was suddenly frozen, and all further growth and development were prevented. In the interval the world has changed almost beyond recognition; psychiatry has grown from infancy into adolescence. But the law has stayed where it was. It has learned nothing and it has forgotten nothing.

The question why this has been so is interesting. In themselves the McNaughton Rules have no authority. Even now it is only the answer to the second and third questions that has the force of law. The Rules were made in the abstract, as it were. The judges were not called on to exercise any recognizable judicial function, and were speaking merely as theoretical experts. The authority of their Rules was, in itself, no more than the authority of a textbook or treatise in the law. All the authority the Rules now have has been given to them subsequently in actual cases to which they have been applied.

DISCONTENT WITH THE RULES

Medical men have never been content with the Rules, even at the time of their formulation, and have constantly striven against them. But even lawyers have found them unsatisfactory. The most notable of these lawyers was undoubtedly Stephen, who eighty years ago had a better understanding of the nature of mental disease and the way it might affect responsibility than most of his present-day colleagues have now. The doctrine that a delusional idea should excuse only that which it would also excuse if the idea were true in fact, he exposed for the nonsense it is by pointing out that the evidential value of a delusion is that it is "in all cases the result of a disease of the brain, which interferes more or less with every function of the mind, which falsifies all the emotions, alters in an unaccountable way the natural weight of motives of conduct, weakens the will . . ." Stephen tried to introduce a way of interpreting the Rules which would bring them into conformity with clinical facts, but he was not successful. In course of time the interpretation of the Rules, in those cases in which they are specifically applied, has become stricter rather than more liberal; and their correct interpretation has now become very rigid indeed.

333

THEIR CLINICAL AND FORENSIC CONSEQUENCES

For a man to be excused, on the ground of insanity, for a criminal act of any kind he must be so mentally diseased that he either does not know the nature and quality of his act or does not know that it is wrong. "Wrong" means "against the law of England," and not against the law of God or against the moral convictions of the actor. Not knowing "the nature and quality of the act" has also been clearly defined; it means to be grossly mistaken about the physical nature of the act. In the words of Mr. Justice Cassels in the Straffen trial: "If a person was charged with having manually strangled some person, and the jury was satisfied that when he strangled that person he thought he was squeezing the juice out of an orange, that would be a failure to know the nature and quality of his act."

No one, doctor or lawyer, has disputed that, in the strict interpretation of the Rules, such as is alone sanctioned by the law, the great majority of insane people are not insane enough to come under their dispensation. From the clinical point of view only those are "McNaughton mad" (to borrow a useful phrase from Dr. Desmond Curran) who are suffering from a gross disorder of consciousness, such as is seen in a post-epileptic twilight state, an organic delirium, or the gravest degrees of dementia or mental defect. The conscience of the medical man is affronted by the suggestion that the melancholic woman who kills her child, the paranoid schizophrenic who kills his imagined persecutor, should be regarded as responsible for acts which are the immediate consequence of their illness.

This attitude is universal among medical men. Those psychiatrists who support the modern application of the McNaughton Rules do so on the ground that they work, or are made to work, so as to conform with our ideas of justice, that, in fact, they are not so strictly applied as to exclude the melancholic or the schizophrenic.

The discontent of medical men with the McNaughton Rules has not been generally shared by men of law. Nearly all of the judges and lawyers who gave evidence to the recent Royal Commission on Capital Punishment were against any modification of the Rules and wished to see them retained as they were. The lawyer's attitude to the Rules was stated pithily by Lord Bramwell in 1874, in opposing a draft Bill drawn up by Stephen. His phrase has deservedly become immortal. "I think," he said, "that, although the present law lays down such a definition of madness, that nobody is hardly ever really mad enough to be within it, yet it is a logical and good definition."

ARGUMENTS AGAINST MODIFICATION

The principal arguments which have been advanced by lawyers against any modification of the Rules can be briefly stated. Rules of some kind are necessary, it is said, because without the guidance of rules the jury would be fumbling in the dark or would become entangled in a mesh of psychiatric verbiage. If rules there must be, then these Rules are as good as any; and it is found easy to point out many and grave defects in any modification which anyone is so rash as to try to set down in precise terms. The weight which should be given to these arguments is very doubtful. There is, for instance, reason to think that when juries retire to consider the responsibility of a mentally abnormal accused person they do in fact address themselves to the question whether or not he is insane, in the ordinary lay sense of the term, and then, if they think he is, decide that he must therefore come within the Rules, whatever those Rules do in fact say.

However, the arguments advanced by lawyers in support of the Rules do not seem to be as important as the motivations which suggest them. The insane person who is legally not responsible for his criminal act and is excused thereby from suffering the consequences is a privileged person; and it is natural and proper that lawyers should feel that privilege of this kind is an anomaly, essentially highly undesirable, and that the class of those who benefit from it should be as narrowly and strictly limited as possible. From this point of view it is to some extent irrelevant that an insane criminal is not immune to the consequences of his criminal acts, but suffers consequences different in kind from those which fall to the lot of responsible people. In the case of murder, the privilege of escape from death, even though the alternative is to be immured for life, is still felt to be so very great that it offends against the idea that all persons should be equal before the law. If this country were once to abolish the death penalty, then the anomalous privilege would cease to exist; and I think the attitude of lawyers would become a very different one.

It is from their different motivations that the conflicts between medicine and the law, which are such an obnoxious feature of many criminal trials, arise. The medical man is by the nature of his profession predisposed to aid the sick man, to secure recognition for his illness and its consequences, and to defend him from the reproach that abnormalities of behaviour caused by illness are to be attributed to wickedness. The lawyer looks at matters very differently; and for him the ideals of justice and of equality between man and man before the law are paramount.

From the lawyer's point of view there are great advantages in having rules which are narrow and strict. By their means one can be almost sure of preventing any particular person from successfully claiming non-responsibility, if one so wishes, whatever the evidence may be. Sir Norwood East, a forensic psychiatrist of the greatest experience, and a warm supporter of the Rules, put it this way in his evidence to the Royal Commission: "If the judge is perfectly satisfied in his own mind that the man is insane, he is quite likely to stretch the McNaughton Rules, and does stretch them so far that they may not be used at all . . . but . . . judges were ready to apply the McNaughton Rules strictly if there was in their opinion doubt or reason to think that the person was not insane." That this was the general practice was confirmed by all other witnesses with court experience.

ADMINISTRATION OF THE RULES

This is how the matter now stands. In the majority of cases which come before the courts, the McNaughton Rules are a dead letter; in a minority of cases they are applied in their full rigour. Notorious cases, in which much public feeling was aroused, and in which they were strictly applied, are the cases of Heath, Haigh, and Straffen. The person who decides whether the Rules shall be applied strictly, loosely, or not at all is the trial judge. If he applies the Rules strictly in his summing up to the jury, and in consequence a lunatic is found to be responsible, the lunatic and his legal representatives have no redress, other than through the administrative action of the Home Secretary. No appeal to a higher court will help, as the Court of Appeal is bound by the law and its own previous decisions to support the strict application of the Rules made by the trial judge. If, however, the judge does not apply the Rules, or only applies them loosely, then if the defence of insanity succeeds there will be no appeal, no review of his summing-up, and if it fails the accused will have no reason to complain of the lenience with which the Rules were applied. This is, of course, a very satisfactory position for judges, as it amounts to a sort of "heads-I-win-tails-you-lose." In borderline cases it permits them to make reasonably sure that only those persons "get off" (as the lawyer calls it) who they think should get off. But for others, who have less confidence than the judges in the reliability of their opinions about who is and who is not insane, the position is less satisfactory.

Apart from the criticisms which can be made of the Rules themselves, grave complaint may be made of the method of their administration.

1. They are inequitable as between case and case. In the cases of some wrong-doers they are applied rigorously, in the cases of others loosely or not at all. Some mentally abnormal persons have their responsibility adjudged by different standards from those which are applied to others.

2. They are inequitable as between judge and witness. The judge is free to ignore the Rules if he so wishes, but if he so wishes he can always tie the medical witness down to them as strictly as he likes.

3. By applying or not applying the Rules in his directions to the jury the judge can exercise a large measure of control on the jury's decision. The judge, and not the jury, becomes the arbiter on what is supposedly a matter of fact.

4. The Rules are not applied candidly. If the work were to be done candidly, the judge would point out to the jury that "nobody is hardly ever really mad enough" to be covered by the Rules, and that, by that standard, the great majority of patients certified insane and permanent inmates of mental hospitals would be regarded as responsible. Once juries grasped this fact they would draw their own conclusions.

INFLUENCE ON PSYCHIATRIC EVIDENCE

The worst effect of the Rules from the medical standpoint has still to be mentioned. This is their influence, in disputed cases, on the way in which psychiatric evidence is taken and the medical witness is examined and cross-examined. As the only thing that matters is whether or not the mental abnormality of the accused passes the McNaughton test, the really important clinical aspects get passed over. No attempt is made to show in any detail in what way the accused was mentally abnormal, or what was the significance of the abnormality in the chain of cause and effect which led to the crime. The judge's summing-up in the Straffen case shows to what lengths the law goes in assigning relevance to what are, from the medical point of view, trivial, insignificant, or even wholly metaphysical and speculative aspects of the case, and to what extent the dynamics of the crime are dealt with as irrelevant. The facts in the Straffen case need only the briefest recapitulation. The killer was a feeble-minded youth who, on the occasion of a previous murder, had been found unfit to plead because of his mental deficiency. Some years later he escaped from Broadmoor, where he had been confined, and in a few hours of liberty committed another murder.

On this second occasion he was found fit to plead, and the question arose at his trial whether he was medico-legally responsible. In his address to the jury Mr. Justice Cassels said: "Ask yourselves whether you are satisfied by the defence that at the time when he did that murder he was insane within the meaning of the criminal law; not that he was feeble-minded; not that he had a lack of moral sense; not that he had no feeling for his victim or her relatives; not that he had no remorse; not that he may be weak in his judgment; not that he fails to appreciate the consequences of his act; but was he insane through a defect of reason caused by disease of the mind, so that either he did not know the nature and quality of his act, or if he did know it, he did not know that it was wrong?"

The fact that such an attitude is the one required by the law prevents the proper presentation of psychiatric evidence; it impedes scientific advance in the understanding of the relation between mental abnormality and crime; and it throws a barrier in the way of education of the public and of officers of the law in what our scientific knowledge and understanding already are. This is the lesion in social organization to which the curious concatenation of events which followed the McNaughton case has now led.

Let us see how far we have arrived with the analysis of a specimen of social pathology. In 1843 the common law was evolving by its natural slow process of development. However, knowledge of insanity was very rudimentary, and the fear of madness and the mad much greater than now. There was also then no great public assurance that a non-responsible killer was automatically rendered socially innocuous. A horrifying murder focused public attention on a largely illusory danger. The public response was, of course, emotional and irrational, and was directed against persons rather than organizational defects. What amounted to legislation, though it was not recognized as such, was completed in a hurry, without considering what was the real nature of the problem. A solution of the wrong problem having been found, it was imposed, and became a kind of permanent splint on a growing structure. Having once been imposed, vested interests grew up to keep it in place. Its effects are to mete out an unequal justice, to prevent honest and unemotional inquiry, and to prejudice the relations between medicine and the law.

OTHER COUNTRIES

An essential part in studies of pathology is played by the control case. We have seen where we have been taken in this country; how have they got on in other countries where there was no McNaughton and there have been no McNaughton Rules? The nearest country at hand is Scotland. In Scottish law, the McNaughton Rules have exerted a certain effect, in directing the way in which judges will ask juries to decide the responsibility of an accused person; but in the important group of homicides the whole position is transformed by the existence of the doctrine of diminished responsibility. This doctrine is particularly suitably applied to the borderline cases which in English law cause so much difficulty. The doctrine of diminished responsibility has arisen over the course of 100 years by a process of natural growth in the common law and depends on no statute. In answer to a charge of murder the accused may put forward a defence of diminished responsibility and will then be called on to prove that, though not insane, he yet suffered from mental weakness or abnormality bordering on insanity to such an extent that his responsibility was substantially diminished. Mental deficiency, post-traumatic personality change, even a severe neurotic state, may be adequate medical grounds to substantiate diminished responsibility.

By a recent decision psychopathic personality, by itself, has been held to be insufficient. If the jury find the responsibility of the accused was diminished in this way, then he will be found guilty not of murder but of culpable homicide, and will be sentenced to imprisonment for a period, usually several years, which is decided by the judge. In practice this law is found to be very effective and is strongly supported by all Scottish lawyers. Although there is no arbitrary system of rules,

337

such as the McNaughton Rules, to help the jury to decide whether or not responsibility is diminished, it is said that juries find no particular difficulty in deciding one way or the other.

The doctrine of diminished responsibility has also found its way into the legal systems of other lands — India and Pakistan, Western Australia, South Africa and Southern Rhodesia, and certain of the United States of America. In these countries diminished responsibility will suffice in some for a sentence of life imprisonment instead of a sentence of death, or for the recording instead of the pronouncing of a sentence of death, or for a recommendation for mercy from the jury, or for reduction of the degree of murder from first to second degree.

In no other European countries than our own is any legal definition of the degree of insanity which shall exclude responsibility found necessary; and the decision whether the mental abnormality of the accused was sufficient to relieve him of the liability to punishment is in effect left to the jury to decide on medical and other evidence.

In the Scandinavian countries forensic psychiatry presents an altogether different picture from that in the English-speaking world. In Sweden, for instance, evidence on the psychiatric aspects of a crime is given almost exclusively by specialists in the service of the State. Psychiatrists act as counsellors in the courts — that is, as subsidiary judges and aids to the trial judge himself. The courts may ask for a psychiatric examination of the accused, not only if it is suspected that the crime was committed in a mentally abnormal state, but also if medical evidence is needed to help decide what penal treatment would be the most appropriate. No legal definition of psychiatric non-responsibility is used as a yardstick, and, quite simply, the perpetrator of a crime is excused from punishment if the crime was committed under the influence of psychosis, or mental deficiency, or another mental abnormality of such a fundamental nature that it must be considered to be on a par with psychosis.

Thus the severer sequelae of brain injuries, encephalitis, etc., and very severe forms of psychopathy will be so considered, especially if they have already in the past interfered with a normal social life; for instance, by causing repeated admission to a mental hospital. The very concept of non-responsibility is hardly taken into account, the real grounds for excusing a man from punishment being that, in his case, punishment is an irrational method of treating him, his proper treatment, whether therapeutic or solely custodial, being best left in medical hands. The administrative method of dealing with such cases is not different from that employed for other patients who are a social danger but have not committed crimes, and admission to an ordinary and not a special criminal psychiatric hospital is the mode of disposal.

What is true of Sweden is also largely true of Denmark and Norway. Capital punishment does not exist in these lands, which means that conflicts between legal and medical viewpoints in an acute form and with maximum publicity do not occur. Medical opinion almost always prevails in the courts, but its effect is often to add to any sentence of punishment, which may itself be reduced on psychiatric grounds or wholly omitted, a further period of subjection to safety measures. The effect of this is greatly to diminish the enthusiasm with which the defence will be inclined to seek for psychiatric examination. The psychotic subject is not sentenced to any form of punishment, but will be sent to a hospital. Psychopaths tend to be regarded as responsible for their acts, but may be subjected to safety measures in lieu of or in addition to any punishment.

THE MEANING OF "RESPONSIBILITY"

In Scandinavia, therefore, we arrive at the opposite pole from that at which we are placed in this country. The pragmatic solution of the question, "What are we to do with this man?" is regarded as the important task, rather than the theoretical solution of the question, "How are we to adjudge this crime?" This brings us to the important problem of what it is we mean when we talk about "responsibility."

For the English lawyer the meaning of the word is clear. For the lawyer "responsible" means only "liable by the law of England to be convicted and punished for a criminal act." This meaning is, for our present purposes, entirely useless, as it is entirely arbitrary. What we have to do is to decide whether any scientific meaning can be given to the word "responsible." As the ordinary man uses the word, an ethical judgment is implicit, and what he really means is that a "responsible" man is one whom one can properly hold responsible, whom one can call to account for his acts.

To the mind of the ordinary man, the lunatic is certainly non-responsible, and the average healthy citizen is as certainly responsible. Doubts and difficulties arise, however, when the mentally abnormal but not grossly insane individual is considered. Furthermore, we may usefully ask whether the insane patient is to be regarded as non-responsible for all his acts. Is he non-responsible when he cleans his teeth in the morning instead of at night before he goes to bed? Is he to be regarded as responsible if he resolutely refuses to have his brain damaged by leucotomy? And is the normal man always to be regarded as responsible? As a case in point, when he cowers whimpering at the bottom of a trench when he has received the order to advance under fire? Is it in conformity with our principles of justice to sentence such a man to imprisonment for cowardice?

If medical men are to be required to give evidence about diminished responsibility it would be possible to use the concept of causation to help the ends of justice. If it seemed that illness or defect or disease had entered as a material element into the causation of the crime, there would be so much reason to regard responsibility as diminished. Even then there would be difficulties. In the case of Raven, who butchered his parents-in-law, there were strong reasons for regarding him as epileptic, but the crime could be interpreted as a cold-blooded one, motivated on the desire for material gain. Unless we are to take the stand that the whole personality is involved in every crime and that any existing abnormality is inevitably involved in its causation, we are liable to land in difficulties, and be called on to make decisions which are bound in some degree to be arbitrary.

Finally, how are we to regard the psychopath? If defects of intelligence are to be allowed weight, are we justified in excluding defects of personality? Is there any satisfactory distinction to be made between the psychopathic criminal and the criminal of bad character? When giving evidence before the Royal Commission the prison medical officers were asked to say what was the difference between a "thug" and a psychopath; and the answer came, "A thug is a thug because he wants to be a thug; a psychopath cannot help it." I confess myself that I cannot see either the force or the practical usefulness of this distinction. Can the thug help wanting to be a thug? And is the man who does a deed of shame to be regarded as abnormal if he subsequently regrets it, but to be regarded as normal and a criminal if he subsequently glories in it or views it with indifference?

AN UNSCIENTIFIC APPROACH

These considerations lead one to the view that attempts to measure the responsibility of others are essentially unscientific. There is nothing objective about the idea which could possibly provide a standard of measurement. Even as a value judgment, responsibility offers extraordinary difficulties. I suspect that when we give opinions about the responsibility of others we are really reporting on our own states of mind. Perhaps we are doing little more than identifying ourselves with the criminal and asking ourselves whether or not we could have been guilty of his crime. If we then feel that we could have done it only after going mad, we may give one sort of answer; if we feel that we could have done it, but only by suppressing the whole of our better nature, then we shall give another sort of answer. Responsibility, it is worth noting, does have some meaning subjectively, in our judgments on our own actions. It is only when we apply the concept to the actions of others that it breaks down.

No theory of mental medicine could develop without the working hypothesis of determinism. When a man acts in a given way at a certain time under a particular set of circumstances we must assume, if we are going to understand his conduct at all, that it was determined by such things as his own make-up, his physical and mental state at the time, and the circumstances and his appreciation of them. The "free will," on which both law and religion are based, proves a heuristically sterile idea. If we attempt to inject it into our analysis of causation it only introduces an element of the unknowable. If we are to inquire at all we must assume that the processes of inquiry will eventually enable us to answer the questions we put; and we are precluded from supposing that there are decisive causes, producing observable effects, which are for ever beyond the reach of inquiry.

Now if every act which a man performs is determined by his own nature on the one side and circumstances on the other, then no other way of acting was open to him. The application of such concepts as responsibility, innocence, and guilt becomes nonsensical. In psychiatry we do very well without them. It may be important to discover whether a patient feels guilty, but we find no need to say, ourselves, he is guilty. If we refrain from making use of such judgments of value, not only is it easier to understand our patient's behaviour, and to predict what that behaviour will be in future circumstances, but our personal rapport with the patient is easier too.

This is the point at which the Scandinavian system has arrived. The whole idea of responsibility, even the idea of diminished responsibility, is there gradually dropping out of use as being unnecessary for practical purposes. The question is asked instead, will the criminal be benefited by punishment?

PUNISHMENT

This brings us to the questions what is punishment, and how is it justified. Punishment, I take it, consists in making special arrangements to secure that certain modes of behaviour shall be succeeded by disagreeable consequences. Its corollary is the provision of rewards for desired behaviour. The two together are merely a way of conditioning stimuli, a procedure which is valuable, even necessary, in the training of animals and children as well as of adults. The aims of punishment are often said

340

to be deterrent, reformatory, and retributive. The first two of these three are clearly connected with training, and justify as pragmatically useful the application of punishment to non-responsible as well as responsible beings. Something quite different is involved in retribution.

Retribution seems to involve the idea of making a payment. Its justification is purely emotional, and has a basis in the group psychology of the society which requires the payment and the individual psychology of the offender who has to make it. There seems to be an emotional need for it on both sides, and an equally emotional feeling that, once punishment has been undergone, the ill deed has been wiped off the slate as it were, and can be forgotten. The retributive element in punishment is very often condemned by rationalists; but it must not be forgotten that it is the element which balances offences with appropriate punishments, and will not permit an excessive punishment for a minor misdeed. It is in regard to our feeling that the non-responsible person should be excused retribution, that responsibility becomes important for justice.

How, then, are we to reconcile these antagonists, the line of thought that teaches us that responsibility is almost meaningless from an objective viewpoint, and the thought that shows that some people are to be dealt with differently from others? A compromise might be made along the following lines.

ABNORMALITY OF CRIME

Statistically, crime is abnormal in the sense of being unusual. For it to occur there must have been something unusual either in the criminal or in the circumstances which motivated the crime. If a man finds half a crown on the floor of his office, picks it up, and keeps it, what is statistically unusual is the combination of circumstances. The man himself is not particularly likely to be unusual; in fact, it is the man who would make some effort to find the loser who would be the unusual one. The great majority of minor offences — trying to smuggle some trifle through the customs, riding a bicycle after dark without a light, and so on — are of this kind. It would be highly uneconomic, in the application of deterrent measures, to bother oneself about the possible abnormalities in the wrongdoer. He may be adjudged as average, and subjected to the procedure appropriate to the average case. If, however, we find that X is now being tried for his thirtieth offence of indecently exposing himself, the evidence is overwhelming that it is not the circumstances which are unusual but the man. We might then very properly apply the Scandinavian system of trying to say what is the best way of handling the man, and abandon methods of treating him which would be appropriate only to the average case.

What is so obviously true of the recidivist criminal may also be very often true of the single very abnormal crime. Murder, in the statistical sense, is highly abnormal; in England and Wales there are only about 150 murders a year. Murder is also in a majority of cases the act of a man who is mentally ill. In this country, over the course of fifty years, in 22% of murders known to the police the suspect committed suicide. Of murderers brought to trial at Assizes, 14% were found unfit to plead. Of those found guilty of the act charged 39% were found guilty but insane. Of those sentenced to death 4% were respited to Broadmoor, and a further 42% had their sentences commuted to penal servitude, in a proportion of cases on psychiatric grounds. It is then hardly surprising that no one has been able to produce any convincing evidence that capital punishment acts as a deterrent for such a pathological event.

CONCLUSION

At the present stage in the development of criminal law, we are half-way between the irreconcilable aims of fitting the punishment to the crime and fitting the punishment to the criminal. It would not seem possible to abandon either aim entirely and replace it by the other. But it should not be beyond the reach of inquiry to find the principles of classification which would provide the basis of a just and efficient penology, to find the means of distinguishing the crimes in which the element of personal deviation is large from those in which it is small, to classify the kinds of deviation and measure their degree, and to work out the means of treatment of the causes, both in individuals and in societies, which lead to crime.

32

THE JUDICIAL PROCESS AND THE ASCERTAINMENT OF FACT

The psychiatrist is a not infrequent visitor in courts of criminal justice, and of course observes the scene from his own particular point of view. As a witness, he is naturally under close examination by judge and counsel; and these gentlemen come to conclusions about psychiatric habits of mind which are frequently expressed with great robustness, both in and out of court. In the same way the psychiatrist, whose professional habit it is to inquire into the ways of behaviour and the motives of his fellow-men, watches the performance put up by those with whom he is engaged, and forms conclusions of his own. The opportunity of expressing them, however, comes all too rarely; and this is why I am grateful to be given such a chance today.

The judicial process does not seem to be designed primarily for the ascertainment of fact; and if it is not so designed, it is hardly surprising that it is not very successful. It is true that an effort is made to elicit facts of a certain kind; but these are facts in a legal and not in a scientific or even in a popular sense. A Lord Chief Justice once told a company of which I was a member, that facts were what was found by a jury. For instance, if a jury found that the accused was not insane, then it was a fact that he was not insane, no matter what any number of medical men might say. Fact of this kind is of an altogether lower order than scientific (or verifiable) fact. But lawyers have had to put up with Brummagem goods for so long, that I do not think they always recognise the better article when they are given it.

However, ascertainment of fact, even in this limited sense, is not the primary purpose of the judicial process. This purpose is, I believe, something quite different, namely, to display the might and majesty of the law. Why else do we observe, with an astonishment only mitigated by ennui, the elaborate ritual, the Oyez, the calling on the Almighty, the may-it-please-your-lordships, the fancy dress, the hordes of police kept waiting in attendance? These measures were designed centuries ago to amaze the peasantry and to strike fear even into the arrogant feudal baron. They

Originally published in the *Modern Law Review* 24: 721–24 (1961).

were, perhaps, appropriate to an age of simplicity, when respect would only be given when claimed by pomp and show. Surely this time is past. The judge earns respect by the fairness and the ability with which he does his task, and these are not increased by the wearing of a wig. A wig, in fact, by the effort it discloses to evoke respect by the trickery of simple suggestion, in the mind of the thoughtful man excites only derision.

Pomp and spectacle do of course play a part in the graces of life. There is no section of the community which does not make use of ceremony, on ceremonial occasions. But most professions put aside the frippery, the chains, the hoods, the wands of office, when they get down to daily tasks; and the way the legal profession clings to this sort of nonsense is anachronistic. It has a number of bad effects. By overawing the simple and inexperienced witness, it saps his confidence and increases his tendency to confusion. It has been found impossible to conduct children's courts in this way. The other victim is the judge himself, who is seldom able to resist the suggestion, daily reinforced over the years, that he in his proper person is something above the common run of humanity.

There is a motivation, even more basic, which has its ill effects on the ascertainment of fact. To the ordinary citizen, the primary aim of administering the criminal law is to protect the public against wrongdoing. This is, of course, not a lawyer's idea; but I think the lawyers should explain this to the public in words of one or two syllables. Punishment of wrongdoing, restricted to the doing of illegal acts, has, so it is held, a retributive and a deterrent aspect. For these purposes it has to be awarded in due form, conspicuously, so that justice may be seen to be done. Any failure to maintain the due form negates the whole process. Higher courts do not hesitate to quash a sentence, and let loose a known enemy of society, if there has been even a minor lapse in the formalities. Punishments tend to be so severe, at the upper end running into deprivation of life and imprisonment for forty years, that the officers of the law, as humane men, become reluctant to inflict them, without requiring unrealistic standards of proof. We are constantly being reminded that the police know very well who is the author of such and such a crime, but that they are unable to take action because their knowledge is based on facts, cogent enough for moral certainty, but lacking possibility of proof by legal standards. Now it is one of the best established tenets of criminology that people are stopped from prohibited actions by the degree of certainty and not by the degree of severity of punishment. What the public needs from the legal profession is not more emphasis in stigmatising the evildoer who has been caught out, but the arrest of a higher proportion of the badly behaved from their antisocial courses.

Mr. Du Cann, in his book *Miscarriages of Justice* (1960), criticises British justice on a number of counts. The procedure of a criminal trial is not inquisitorial but accusatory. It is loaded with a hidebound traditionalism and theatricalism. Get rid, he says, of the useless formulae; get rid of the dock; provide desks and writing facilities for the accused, the jurymen, and others. Use all up-to-date business methods. Get rid of the oaths and substitute affirmations. Perjury is rife; bring the perjurors to book. The single judge system is at fault; judges are too often deaf, ill, or senile. Oral advocacy by professional pleaders can, and often does, deflect the straight course of justice. The laws themselves are chaotic, obsolete statutes cluttered by case-law. Substitute a criminal code.

Of these many points I should like to emphasise but two. However much they are persuaded of the opposite, judges are made of the common stuff of humanity. If a man's powers begin to fail, it is not possible for him to have full insight into the change. The man whose memory is getting weaker, whose judgment is impaired, whose sympathies are withering, seldom realises what is happening, and always thinks much better of his powers than does the outside observer. One may be glad that it has at last been recognised that judges, like professors and doctors, suffer from our common lot, and that a retiring age has been fixed. But when one considers the fatefulness of the decisions that lie in a judge's hands, it would seem well to have available for them the same possibilities of medical supervision, and if necessary compulsory retirement on medical grounds, as exist elsewhere in the civil services. A further point emerges. The aphorism that power corrupts is as true of judges as of other men. Long exercise of the magisterial function has a deleterious effect on the personality. The danger would be less if the duties of convicting and of passing sentence were in different hands. Certainly the considerations which should be borne in mind on the two occasions are of a very different kind. Information of a kind not available to judges, for instance about the effect of punishments on criminals of different kinds and the ways in which their subsequent careers are affected by them, should be constantly brought up to date and be made available to the sentencing authority.

The weightiest of Mr. Du Cann's criticisms is his point that the procedure of the courts is accusatory and not inquisitorial. A struggle is staged in which each team tries to pull the balance as hard as possible over to the one side or the other. Hence the violent oscillations, as prosecution or defence win a temporary advantage, hence the drama of the scene, hence the intrusion of powerful but irrelevant motive forces, such as the skill of the pleader. When the whole course of the trial is designed to interfere with any cold-blooded appraisal by the jury, it is a miracle that their common sense prevails as often as it does. But the battle is relentless. Neither side will concede a point which can possibly be maintained, even in the face of a total lack of evidential support. The medical witness finds himself in a peculiarly invidious position. The tradition of having all witnesses called by one side or the other casts the shadow of partiality over all he says. Counsel on his own side tries to push him just as far as he can be made to go, and it is rare for him to retire from the box without being trapped into expressing an opinion with greater confidence or emphasis than in a cool moment he would think justified. Lawyers complain bitterly about the way in which experts can be brought to disagree with fellow experts; but it is they who have forced this situation. I know any number of senior colleagues who refuse to be called in this capacity, because they know they will not be allowed to stand squarely between prosecution and defence, leaning neither to one side nor the other. The courts never see these men. The expert witnesses they get have been shopped for, by an agent who hires not the most balanced opinion but the warmest protagonist. I see no solution for this absurd state of affairs, except that witnesses should be called by the court. On appearance, they should be examined by the judge or the judge's assessor, and cross-examined by both of the opposing counsel. No good scientific witness would object even to the most gruelling examination provided it were carried out with respect for his good faith instead of with the implicit suggestion that he is, himself, out to make a case.

Finally, we must not forget the fantastic cost in public money of these unseemly battles. If at an early stage the two sides could agree on what matters were so well established as to be acceptable without debate, and the matters which would have to be thrashed out, much time would be saved and things would be much easier for the jury. The oscillations of the scales would be less violent, and one could have a firmer hope that the instrument, more delicately held, would find an end-point nearer the true equipoise. Quicker trials in a less fervid atmosphere would speed justice and save much human distress.

I am told that the problem of delinquency and crime is graver now than it has ever been. Everyone is blamed for this, parents, teachers, doctors, psychologists, public welfare officials, everyone but the men whose proud claim it is to be the peculiar guardians of all that is law-abiding. We accept this claim; but we ask them to consider how far their antiquated methods have contributed to the present situation.

Note by Editor of "Modern Law Review". This subject [The Judicial Process and the Ascertainment of Fact] was discussed at a meeting of lawyers and sociologists held at the Institute of Advanced Legal Studies. Certain short papers, including this, were read at the opening of the discussion. It was felt by the lawyers present that the impressions of a psychologist [*sic*] would be of general interest to the profession and accordingly Dr. Slater was asked to permit publication in this *Review*.

33

CONTRIBUTIONS TO A PATHOGRAPHY OF THE MUSICIANS: 1. ROBERT SCHUMANN

INTRODUCTION

In his monumental study of human genius, Lange-Eichbaum (1956) has pointed out how much there is of the subjective in the very concept itself. "Genius" is a matter of public reputation, and is not measured solely in terms of achievement or ability. The geniuses of one age may not be so regarded in the next; and there is a rise and fall in fame which has little to do with objective appraisal. Lange-Eichbaum has also pointed out the extent to which any mental abnormality shown by the candidate for the title of genius affects the subjective factor in judgment. For if it is present, it provides hints of the mysterious, the strange, and the awesome which, playing on the personality like a light from beyond this world, inevitably impress the beholder.

It is a fact that, when we come to consider the personality of some Great Man, we are likely to lose some of our capacity for a cool judgment. We always try to understand other human beings with the aid of introspection; to some degree we identify ourselves with them, and compare their characters and way of behaving with our own. Doing this with one of the great, we have the feeling of being dwarfed. If we feel drawn to the man and his work, we are likely to take him for a hero and to shut our eyes to blemishes. If, however, we find his personality strange or difficult to understand, then we may only be able to bear the comparison by trying to cut down the man or his work to our own scale. We can do this more easily if at some point we are able to look down on him from above, from a superior level of sanity, or social competence, or moral integrity.

Nevertheless, an impartial study of such people is a matter of great importance. We should know whether great achievements arise only from a disharmony or a

By Eliot Slater and Alfred Meyer. Originally published in *Confinia Psychiatrica* 2: 65–94 (1959). The extracts from the Schumanns' letters and diaries and other passages which appeared in German in the original have been translated by the Editors. Portraits of Schumann have been omitted.

pathological fault, or whether they do not always require some element of more than normal health and vitality in a personality however otherwise diseased. We should know what are the conditions necessary for talent to develop and for it to show in achievement; what are the ills to which the man of gifts is liable; what is the effect upon him of encouragement and frustration, of strain or illness, of tragedy, of success. For in this of all ages the reminder may be permitted that, for any life or progress in our society, we depend on those who have some more than average talent, great or small; from unleavened mediocrity there can come nothing but spiritual stagnation.

For the answering of such questions as these there is little value in the conventional type of study, in which the author has made his own selection of great men; it is not possible to guard against a personal bias in this method. A fundamental advance on such work is provided by Adele Juda's book *Höchstbegabung* (1953). This is the first venture into a systematic pathography in this field, and provides material on which reliable conclusions could be based. Juda took as her subjects 113 artists and 181 men of science, and investigated their lives and their medical histories, as well as those of their relatives, ancestors and descendants. The probands were chosen for her by experts in the fields of achievement in which the probands had themselves worked; thus her composers were chosen for her by musicologists, her chemists and her mathematicians were chosen by chemists and mathematicians. These experts were required only to supply the names of persons, speaking the German tongue, who had been the ablest and most creative in their field, of all born since the year 1650. Choice was based on achievement only, regardless of whether the proband was normal or abnormal, whether or not he merited the title of genius.[1]

The results of Juda's very thorough investigation, which she did not live to see published, are presented in the form of statistical expectations. These run: in the artists, schizophrenia 2.8%, manic-depressive 0, unclear endogenous psychoses 2.0%, psychopathic personality 27.3%; in the scientists, schizophrenia 0, manic-depressive 4.0%, unclear endogenous psychoses 0, psychopathic personality 19.4%. Psychopaths were rarely "erregbar" (excitable) or "haltlos" (unstable), comparatively frequently "Sonderlinge" (eccentric) or "Thymopathe". There was then a little, but only a little, more psychosis in both groups than could have been expected if they had been members of the general population. But in both groups there was about double the normal expectation of psychopaths. This is a decisive counter-demonstration to the vulgar belief that men of genius are by and large mad or half-mad, and it shows that not only is normality of personality compatible with the highest achievement but also that the majority of men of the greatest achievement are normal. It still leaves open, however, as a problem requiring the closest study, the relationship of "genius" with abnormality of personality.

In the course of her work Juda collected a large amount of valuable biographical material, sorted psychiatrically, and supplemented by her own appreciation. This material, in so far as it relates to the probands, has been most kindly placed at our disposal by the late Professor Bruno Schulz, of the Genealogical Department of the Deutsche Forschungsanstalt für Psychiatrie in Munich. Furthermore, we have been absolved from the usual requirement that the names of probands should not be published or divulged. This is both necessary and permissible for a number of

---

[1] However, it should be noted that none of the representatives of the modern twelve-note school composers were included.

reasons. It is necessary because we propose to go into biographical details, and it is essential that our statements should be open to criticism and correction if needed; it is permissible because the probands are all historical figures who have already been the subjects of biographical and pathographic publications. For our work the data which were obtained by Juda have been supplemented mainly from a variety of sources in the English language, which will appear in the bibliography.[2]

Juda's material of German-speaking composers consists of the persons named in Table 33.1, together with one other who has been omitted, as he is still alive. Of

TABLE 33.1. JUDA'S PROBANDS IN ORDER OF DATE OF BIRTH

Composer	Born	Died
*Handel, George Frederick	23. 2.1685	14. 4.1759
*Bach, Johann Sebastian	21. 3.1685	28. 7.1750
Bach, Wilhelm Friedemann	22.11.1710	1. 7.1784
*Gluck, Christoph Willibald	2. 7.1714	15.11.1787
Stamitz, Johann Wenzl Anton	19. 6.1717	27. 3.1757
*Haydn, Josef	1. 4.1732	31. 5.1809
*Mozart, Wolfgang Amadeus	27. 1.1756	5.12.1791
*Beethoven, Ludwig van	16.12.1770	26. 3.1827
*Weber, Karl Maria von	18.12.1786	5. 6.1826
Marschner, Heinrich	16. 8.1795	14.12.1861
Loewe, Carl Johann Gottfried	30.11.1796	20. 4.1869
*Schubert, Franz Seraph Peter	31. 1.1797	19.11.1828
Lortzing, Albert Gustav	23.10.1801	21. 1.1851
*Mendelssohn-Bartholdy, Felix	3. 2.1809	4.11.1847
*Schumann, Robert	8. 6.1810	29. 7.1856
Liszt, Franz	22.10.1811	27. 7.1886
*Wagner, Richard	22. 5.1813	13. 2.1883
Franz, Robert	28. 6.1815	24.10.1892
*Bruckner, Anton	4. 9.1824	11.10.1896
Cornelius, Carl August Peter	24.12.1824	26.10.1874
Strauss, Johann	25.10.1825	3. 6.1899
*Brahms, Johannes	7. 5.1833	3. 4.1897
Wolf, Hugo	13. 3.1860	22. 2.1903
Mahler, Gustav	7. 7.1860	18. 5.1911
Strauss, Richard	11. 6.1864	8. 9.1949
Pfitzner, Hans	5. 5.1869	22. 5.1949
*Reger, Max	19. 3.1873	10. 5.1916

these people, some had their names proposed by all of Juda's assessors, and are marked with an asterisk in the list, some only by a majority. Out of the entire list of 27 persons, Juda considered that 10 were psychiatrically abnormal. Those whom she classed as psychopaths of one or another kind were: Friedemann Bach, Gluck, Liszt, Mahler, Pfitzner, Schubert, Johann Strauss the younger, and Wagner; those whom she classified as psychotic were Gluck, Schumann and Wolf. In addition to these three, we consider that two others, Handel and Mozart, should be taken into consideration, as the possibility of a psychotic illness does arise. The diagnostic problem of the nature of the psychosis, if any, is not of any difficulty in the cases of Gluck, Mozart and Wolf; but with Handel and Schumann there are difficulties which will have to be resolved before the general problem of an enhanced tendency to psychosis in the composers can be considered. In the paper which follows the case of Schumann is particularly discussed. In a second paper (89) we propose to consider

[2] Following our usual procedure, the Schumann bibliography has been integrated with the consolidated list of references. Sources not specifically cited in the text are Alley and Alley (1956), Basch (1931), Braun (1940), and Brion (1956). — Editors.

the evidence of psychosis or neurological disease in Gluck, Handel, Mozart and Wolf; and in a third paper we hope to take up the central problems of the relationship of creativity to abnormality of personality.

THE PROBLEM

Robert Schumann was born on the 8th June, 1810. On the 27th February, 1854, he threw himself into the Rhine, but was rescued. On the following 3rd March he went of his own free will into the mental hospital at Endenich; and he ended his days there on the 29th June, 1856.

The Superintendent of the asylum at Endenich, Dr. Richarz, called Schumann's illness "partial paralysis", and from the context of his report it is clear that by that term he meant general paresis. The first suggestion that a diagnostic problem was involved was made by Möbius in 1906. After considering the evidence, he concluded that Schumann had suffered from a succession of schizophrenic illnesses from youth on; he rejected the diagnosis of any final organic illness. This view was countered by Gruhle (1906), who argued that the facts adduced by Möbius led, instead, to a different conclusion, i.e., that during the earlier part of his life Schumann was cyclothymic, but that his last illness was an organic disease of the brain, most probably general paresis. Since then many other writers have taken up the problem. In the review of the literature provided by Lange-Eichbaum, the writers quoted are almost equally divided between three views, that of Möbius, that of Gruhle, and an intermediate one which sees the psychosis as an organic one arising on the basis of a psychopathic personality. The personal opinion of Lange-Eichbaum, which is sustained by Kurth, the editor of the last edition of his work, is in conformity with the last of these three. Juda herself did not go further than to classify the case as one of endogenous psychosis of unclear nature, with a final organic psychosis not to be excluded.

Of recent work, that of Garrison (1934), Wörner (1949) and of Reinhard (1956) should be mentioned. Garrison concerns himself principally with the family history, but states that Schumann was schizophrenic. Wörner argues that an earlier schizophrenic state was followed by a final organic psychosis. Reinhard believes that a final general paresis can be confidently excluded, and the psychosis was an endogenous one, nature not clear.

Our own view is approximately that of Gruhle; but in view of the discrepancies of opinion, we propose to reexamine the relevant evidence in order to establish it on a firm foundation.

It was not possible for us to consult all the contributions quoted by Lange-Eichbaum in the original; but it is hoped that no major point has escaped our attention.

THE EVIDENCE

Family Background and Personality

Robert Schumann was the youngest of six children, of whom four brothers and one sister survived childhood. There was mental illness in the family. In his biography of Schumann, Young (1957) says that his father August had a nervous breakdown from which he never entirely recovered. He is said to have had attacks of giddiness, and to have had a melancholic tendency; but there is no evidence known to us that he had a mental illness. Juda classified him as normal. He was a publisher and successful in business, but also a writer on his own account and with an interest in romantic literature though no talent for music. He died when Robert was sixteen, so that Robert was for a number of years under the guardianship of his mother. She was a dominant personality, who resisted his attraction to music as a profession, but was psychiatrically normal. The eldest child, Robert's sister Emilie, became mentally ill at the age of 17 and drowned herself at 29. She was regarded as a case of dementia praecox by Möbius, and this diagnosis was accepted by Juda, although it is by no means certain. Robert's three brothers, who all died before him, of brain fever, cancer, and tuberculosis, were all mentally normal.

Robert and Clara Schumann had eight children, one of whom, Ludwig, began to show signs of mental illness by the age of 20, and two years later was regarded as incurable. He died in a mental hospital at the age of 51. Juda considers that this case, too, was most probably one of schizophrenia. All of the other children were mentally normal, though one son took morphine in the course of a chronic physical ailment. From the family history alone, therefore, a suggestion of schizophrenia in Robert's case arises.

Schumann seems to have changed in personality during the course of his life-time. As a young man he was sociable, fond of a gay life, interested in girls, cham-pagne, cigars, and billiards, and he had a number of minor love affairs. He was somewhat irresponsible and unsteady in his intentions and even after giving up the law for music, he varied from time to time in the application he brought to his studies.

With all this, however, and underneath his romanticism, his idealism, his vague optimism, his unpractical ways, he had a fundamental seriousness. He pursued Clara through all difficulties until he won her; and the devotion of the two to one another only increased with the years.

Wasielewski (1906) gives a portrait of Robert in middle life as a man of more than average height, with slow and deliberate gait. His expression was mild and kindly, but with a good deal of reserve. He had little conversation, none on ordinary matters; but in an intimate circle would become quite eloquent on subjects which moved him. In the course of time he became more and more taciturn, and even to questions would not reply, or would answer in a murmur, in fragments of sentences, as if he were thinking the answer out for himself. Apart from his eyes, the most attractive feature was his mouth, finely cut, with lips thrust a little forward as if to whistle. Möbius says that this was a mannerism, and did not appear till after 1833. He was very fond of his children, but somewhat distant and passive as a father; he was a most tender and loving husband. The life he preferred to lead was an exceedingly quiet one; and one of great regularity, the same routine being followed every day. Throughout his life he had strong interests in romantic literature and poetry. He edited the *Neue Zeitschrift für Musik*, and, in the numerous essays and reviews which he wrote for this journal, he showed amply his remarkable generosity of spirit, full of warm appreciation of the merits of younger composers, without envy or reserve. The same warmth and natural feeling ("Innigkeit") pervade his composi-tions, particularly his short piano pieces and songs. Perhaps the natural expression of his personality in his music is not quite as direct as, for instance, that of Schubert. This may have been due, partly as Abraham (1954) suggests to strong literary interests which somewhat deflected his musical inspiration, partly to the strong influence of the phantastic romanticism of Jean Paul and others.

351

In a self-description, made by choice of adjectives, which Möbius quotes, Schumann chose as appropriate: quiet, shy, hypochondriacal, good-humoured, genial, sociable, highminded, sensitive, emotional, enthusiastic, tenderhearted. One might add that he himself characterised the main contrasts of his personality by the pseudonyms of Florestan, the gay, energetic iconoclast, and Eusebius, the gentle, pious and melancholy.

Schumann was, socially, never very competent. In Dresden the Schumanns found themselves in a provincial society entirely dominated by a philistine Court. It is not surprising that they shut themselves away in a circle of their own. When they came to Düsseldorf, though they were received with the greatest friendliness and enthusiasm, they never fitted in with the gay light-hearted Rhinelanders. The collapse of Robert's career there must be partly attributed to mutual lack of understanding. Young (1957) says that he appeared at committee meetings as seldom as possible, and never stayed more than a few minutes; he generally delivered his instructions to the choral society in writing, through a committee member.

However, one cannot speak of a pathological withdrawal. Throughout his life he continued to make intimate and devoted friends, such as Mendelssohn, Jenny Lind, Hiller, Joachim, Brahms. He first met Brahms when he was a very sick man, and on the point of his final breakdown.

Schumann was something of a hypochondriac, and throughout his life was afraid of death and of madness. He was extremely shocked and upset by all the deaths of near and dear ones, of his sister-in-law Rosalie, his brothers, and of Mendelssohn. After Mendelssohn's death he feared that he would die in the same way, i.e., after a succession of strokes. More than once in his life he expressed the fear that he would lose his reason; and at other times he had a fear of heights and of metal objects.

On the sexual side, we must regard him as normal in every way. A normal sexual life with his wife must have continued throughout their time together. She bore him eight children, in 1841, 1843, 1845, 1847, 1848, 1849, 1850, and 1854, and in 1852 she had a miscarriage.

Schumann's Illness: First Stage

From early on in his life, Schumann was troubled by variations of mood, which cannot be adequately accounted for by circumstances. Nussbaum (1923) showed that while outwardly taciturn he could be eloquent in his letters. The following calendar can be drawn up.

1828: Predominant mood melancholic. "Often I am utterly tortured by this petty life with its pitiful people." "I do not feel well in the company of people who don't understand me and for whom I cannot care."

1829: One and a half years of almost continuous happiness, with humorous letters, demands for money from home, much in society, complete forgetfulness of law studies. Occasional interruptions by short depressive moods. "The wooden Prussian soldiers, — tedious company at meals — my imagination dulled — Moselle wine without sparkle — heavy food — myself extraordinarily heavy spirited" [all described as *ledern*, i.e. leathery, in German].

1830: In October, recurrence of melancholy; compaints of indecisiveness. "My heart is dead and desolate like the future."

1831: Persistence of melancholy; in May it takes him three weeks to complete a letter. Very few letters during the summer. In September an agitated mood; for some weeks a fear of cholera and fear of death; this succeeded by an apathetic mood. On the 31st December sudden recovery of mood.

1832: Mood elevated; plans for going to America as a virtuoso; in June "Head and heart full of divine happiness." August: "I also sense a power and a marvellous feeling of tenseness in my whole body."

1833: In June: "Full of the happiest and gayest imaginings, in which indeed pain itself often turns to beauty." A severe feeling of illness in the autumn, when the deaths of his brother Julius and his sister-in-law Rosalie occurred. In a letter to Clara of 11th February 1832 he described this time: "Already back in 1833 a feeling of dejection began to set in . . . I received little recognition: on top of this came the loss of my right hand for playing . . . . This was in the summer of 1833. Yet I seldom felt happy; something was missing; the melancholy which ruled me still more after the death of my dear brother increased still further. And that is how I felt when I heard of Rosalie's death. — On this only a few words, — in the night of the 17th–18th October 1833, all at once I was seized by the most terrifying thought that a man can ever have — the most terrifying that heaven can inflict on us — that of losing one's reason — and this possessed me with such an intensity that it silenced all consolation, all prayers, as so much scorn and mockery."

It is noteworthy that Schumann injured the third (ring) finger of his right hand, in a contraption he had invented for the practising of finger movements, between the end of May and the beginning of June. The effects of this accident were such as to close for him the career of a piano virtuoso. But the depression did not occur then, but in October. Wasielewski states that he had heard that on the night Schumann describes, he had wanted to throw himself out of the window, but adds that the report is unconfirmed. Möbius states that Schumann's fear of heights and upper storeys dated from this night.

1834: The depression, which had persisted since October, began to yield in January. In May almost well. In August an elated mood.

1836: In the summer: "However I still spend many splendid hours at the piano, in the exchange of ideas with first-rate people, knowing that one is working in a worthy environment, and hoping for still more and better achievements. It is this exalted mood which often ends up in a spirit of overconfidence, in which I want to take the entire world by storm. Exhaustion follows hard on its heels, and then I have to raise my spirits by spurious means." In June: "The melancholy weather and increasing suffering, of which I can tell no one, had devastated me." December: "in a deadly anguish of heart."

1837: September: "Comfort me, please God, and let me not be destroyed by despair. I am assailed at the very roots of my existence." On 28th November, to Clara: "And now too, since you set so little store by my ring — since yesterday I no longer care for yours, and no longer wear it. I dreamed I passed by a deep stream, when I suddenly had the idea and threw the ring in — then I was overcome by the desire to throw myself in after it."

1838: February, Clara writes: ". . . I have never known you so gay." March shows a hysterical note: "I woke up and could not get to sleep again — then, as my thoughts penetrated more and more deeply into you and the life of your mind and dreams, I suddenly cried out with greatest intensity: 'Clara, I am calling you.' — And then I heard quite strongly, as though close to me, 'Robert, I am here with you'." April: "And then how well I am feeling physically, so that I am in full possession of my strength and youth." In June and July, again melancholic. In August: "These past days I have been so terribly sad, sick, and exhausted, that I thought my end was near." Towards autumn, better.

1839: February, an anxiety attack. April, ruminations about death. July: "Only I am often very ill now, so singularly weak in my whole body, particularly in my head. . . . Everything affects me so frightfully." "For days on end I am silent — without thoughts and only muttering to myself." "Once the first excitement is over, I am overcome by such a strong vital urge, a desire for activity, that I turn my hand to any kind of work."

This account is extracted principally from *Der junge Schumann* (Schumann, A., 1917), and from Nussbaum's (1923) extensive quotations from Schumann's letters. From the time of his marriage in 1840, the material available in letters is less and the principal source of information is the joint diary kept by Robert and Clara, later kept by Clara alone. The best source for Schumann's life and later illness is the biography by Litzmann (1918).

The Second Stage

With his marriage, there came no end to Schumann's mood changes, although he was extremely happy with Clara and devoted to her. It seems clear that she was the dominant partner in their relationship, and that though she maintained an attitude of wifely submission, in fact he fell more and more under her influence. His life took on an unvarying daily routine, with hours set aside for composition, for a long walk, and for society of a small and intimate kind. It was probably under her influence, too, that he tried to rise superior to his romantic, half-literary and lyrical nature, and to model himself on the classics and attempt larger forms.

. The first years of his marriage were very good years for Robert, and a large part of his best work was done then; 1840 was one of his peak years. However, at the end of 1842 and at the beginning of 1843 he was suffering from nervous weakness, and had to give up composing for some months. This was succeeded in March 1843 by a period of elevation of mood; and Clara records that he was then working on the *Peri* with such enthusiasm that it made her anxious.

In the autumn of 1843 Robert was very indecisive about the Russian journey, which was then being arranged; and in February 1844 he was in a low state which is anxiously recorded by Clara. In April, however, the couple set forth for St. Petersburg and Moscow. Robert broke down on the way, and had to interrupt the journey at Dorpat, where he spent six days in bed. A deep melancholy was accompanied by anxiety symptoms and physical complaints such as giddy attacks. He was incapable at this time of any work of composition; but he wrote five melancholic poems which show, according to Litzmann, remarkable helplessness both in form and content. If this is right, it must be put down to psychic inhibition, since Robert was a professional writer of articles on music, and an enthusiastic reader of poetry.

In May 1844, back home again, he began to feel better; but it was only a short and incomplete intermission. In August he was suffering again from a total nervous collapse, making work impossible. In September he was still worse, and unable to leave his room. In October they went to Dresden to stay with the Wiecks. Clara writes: "There were now eight terrible days. Robert did not sleep a single night, seeing in his imagination the most dreadful pictures; early in the morning I would find him drenched in tears; he gave himself up for lost."

It was at this time that he first made contact with a homoeopathic doctor, Dr. Helbig, who remained his physician for a number of years. In a report quoted by

Möbius, Helbig describes numerous phobias, fear of death, of heights, of metal objects, etc., and physical symptoms such as tiredness, tremor, cold feet. Highly significant symptoms he mentions are insomnia and a diurnal rhythm, the patient feeling his worst in the morning hours. Helbig also makes the first mention of auditory symptoms ("Gehörstäuschungen") as occurring at this time.

In November and December there was gradual improvement. But again the following year, in May 1845, he had more of his trouble and there were again attacks of giddiness. The symptoms persisted into August, so that a proposed journey to Bonn had to be cancelled.

In May 1846, as well as more giddy attacks, there was the first definite mention of tinnitus. This was a constant singing and roaring in the ears, and a distressing effect by which noises became musical tones. He was deeply hypochondriacal, weighed down with physical fatigue, full of melancholy ideas. He could not bear the sight of the asylum from his window.

However, from July 1846 he made steady improvement, indeed an apparently complete remission, which lasted for over a year. In September 1847 there was a slight return of the hypochondriacal mood; but he was in good health over Christmas 1847 and full of joy in work. Then in January 1848 there was a sudden relapse, improving somewhat during February, but leaving him in only moderate health and spirits over the summer. By the winter he had dropped again into a low state, which lasted into January 1849, when the death of his brother Karl had a shattering effect on him.

Once again there was a complete remission; and 1849 proved to be the high point in productivity of his career, with invention and versatility at their height. His mood was so much better, that there is a suggestion of more than normal elation: unlike his wont, he ordered in large quantities of expensive wine.

In 1850, during preparations for the performance of *Genoveva* in Leipzig, symptoms recurred, including the fear of heights. He had to exchange an upper-floor bedroom in the hotel for one on the ground floor. Otherwise, in the earlier part of the year, his health was fairly good. On the first of September the family moved to Düsseldorf. They were at first disappointed in their new home. Clara wrote that Robert was in a highly nervous, irritated, excited mood. From early on, Schumann's official duties as musical director in Düsseldorf did not go well, his principal fault being that he was incapable of maintaining discipline. He and Clara were equally blind to his deficiencies. An article in the Düsseldorf paper in May 1851, criticising the concert direction, was felt by the Schumanns as an insult. Nevertheless his mood did not suffer. In May 1851, after a successful concert, Clara wrote that Robert was unusually happy. By September, Clara's complaints in the diary of the Düsseldorfer have become bitter and persistent; in a single year, Robert's relations with the local musical society, which had begun in a mood of great friendliness, had been entirely spoilt.

In 1852, symptoms showed which we must take as ominous: a certain apathy and dreaminess, an occasional clumsiness of speech. By the summer he had reached the point where the preparation and conducting of the first two concerts of the season had to be taken by Julius Tausch as his deputy. He took over the direction again in December, but was ill received by the public. Three of the Committee of the *Gesangverein* approached with a request that he should resign as unfit. Efforts by others at a compromise were regarded by Clara as an infamous intrigue. Another year had to go by before, on the 9th November 1853, Schumann decided to conduct no more.

In April 1852 there were more physical symptoms, thought to be rheumatic, and insomnia and a depressive mood. In May he was better, but worse again in June. In July he had "ein nervöser Krampfanfall" (a convulsive attack?), while out walking; and after it there were hypochondriacal ideas. After this he was a good deal better for a number of months, apart from more giddiness in October.

In 1853 melancholic and anxiety states were remarkably few, despite the fact that his official difficulties were now reaching a head. In the spring of the year he took a great interest in table-rapping seances, to the surprise and misgiving of his friends. On his birthday, the 8th June, he was well and happy. A little later, on the 30th July, he had a sudden attack of what the doctor called lumbago, which Nussbaum thinks was a cerebral vascular stroke. Nussbaum says that the physician, Dr. Kalt, actually remarked "Der ist ein verlorener Mann, hat ein unheilbares Gehirnleiden (Gehirnerweichung)."[3] [He is a lost man, has an incurable brain disease (softening of the brain).] On the 30th August speech disturbances were noted. The physical symptoms did not impair Schumann's mood. On the 10th September he was outstandingly gay. Again there is a suggestion of elevation of mood above the normal. On their fourteenth wedding anniversary, Robert gave Clara a piano, which certainly delighted her, but also caused her great concern on account of the expense. The 30th September is a day of moment, as it was the day on which Brahms paid his first visit, to become a firm friend of both of them and a devoted admirer, indeed lover in all but the physical sense, of Clara. Robert immediately conceived the greatest admiration for Brahms' genius, and gave it expression in the renowned article "Neue Bahnen" [New Paths].

In November the Schumanns went off on a triumphal tour of Holland, Robert in gay, almost elevated mood, which was not in the least impaired by the fact that he had just had to resign his post. While on this tour, he had a temporary return of auditory symptoms; and from this time all creative activity ceased. Instead, he developed for a time a preoccupation with making an anthology of the sayings of famous authors on the subject of music.

On the night of the 10th February, 1854, he had a sudden attack of tinnitus, the same note sounding in his head all night. On Saturday the 11th he was better during the day, but bad again all night and all through the Sunday, apart from an intermission of two hours. Again sounds came to him as musical tones. Later, a hallucinatory element entered in, for the tinnitus progressed to the point where he was hearing entire pieces, as from a full orchestra, from beginning to end.

On the night of Friday 17th February, he was up in the night to write down a theme which he said the angels had sung to him. When he had finished he lay down, rapt in phantasy for the rest of the night, always with open eyes lifted to heaven. He believed that angels hovered over him and gave him glorious revelations, all in wonderful music. However, the next morning there was a dreadful change, and the angel voices changed to the voices of devils. They told him he was a sinner and they would throw him into Hell. He saw them about him in the shapes of tigers and hyaenas. Later in the day he quietened down to the point where he could get up and set himself to the correction of musical manuscript. On the next day, Sunday 19th, there was a return of hallucinations, in a state of consciousness at least partially preserved. He was firmly convinced that he was surrounded by spirits, but recognized the presence of his wife and spoke to her.

[3] In common German parlance, synonymous with general paresis.

On Monday 20th, he was listening to the angel voices all day, his face full of happiness, and he tried to write down some of the music he heard. From the next day, Tuesday, the hallucinatory voices were more in words than music. He spent the time writing variations on an angelic theme, and he also wrote two business letters. He gave directions on what was to be done when he was dead, and he said farewell.

On Sunday 26th he was rather better. He received a visitor and played to him a sonata by a young composer who interested him, ending in a state of joyful exaltation. At the evening meal, he ate a lot and in fearful haste. He suddenly stood up and said he must go to the asylum, and went and laid out all the things he would wish to take with him. The following morning he was deeply melancholic and told Clara that he was not worthy of her love. He set himself to write a fair copy of his variations, but suddenly broke off and left the room. Without the others realising it, he went out of the house into stormy rain without boots or other protection. An hour later he was brought home again, having thrown himself into the Rhine, but seen to do so and immediately rescued. He must have taken off his wedding ring and thrown it into the river first; for it was never recovered, and at a later time a note was found: "Dear Clara, I will throw my wedding ring into the Rhine, you do the same, both rings will then unite." So he carried out in fact his dream of November 1837.

Clara was not allowed to see him again after this, before he was taken to hospital. He left a week later, on Saturday 4th March. She wrote: "Robert dressed in a great hurry, climbed with Hasenclever and his two male nurses into the carriage, and did not ask after me, nor after his children." Robert settled happily into the asylum, and took an immediate liking to his personal nurse. In succeeding weeks he spent part of the time quietly in bed, or taking a walk, or talking to the doctors; but he also had spells of agitation in which he would walk up and down his room or kneel and wring his hands. On the 31st March Clara recorded with sorrow that Robert asked for flowers, but never for news of her. When he did receive a bouquet from her, he smiled in a pleased way, nodded his head, but said nothing. At the end of April he was worse again, with auditory hallucinations and confused talk, with never a mention of Clara. At the end of May he was unusually cheerful, and on the 21st July Clara received flowers Robert had sent her.

For the knowledge of Robert's state in the asylum, we are principally dependent on letters to Clara from friends, especially Brahms. Very little is available in medical reports. The report by Richarz, given in 1873, quoted by Wasielewski, says that spells of hallucination were repeated again and again, but that they tended to change in type from auditory hallucinations to hallucinations of taste and smell. Gradual and progressive impairment of his intellectual powers was very slow, and never reached an extreme degree. At the latter end of his illness he frequently refused food, and he eventually became extremely emaciated. The hospital notes themselves are not available; when Möbius enquired after them, they could not be found, and Möbius thought that they had been removed from the hospital records at Endenich by Richarz himself. We have to rely therefore on technically less competent sources.

On the 13th August, 1854, Brahms wrote a letter to Clara describing a visit to Endenich. He saw and heard Robert from a place where he was himself concealed. Robert was telling his doctor of a walk to the cemetery; his talk was clear and sensible, not confused. Brahms records that during the entire conversation, Robert held a white pocket handkerchief to his mouth. He was looking well and strong, and had put on some weight. Dr. Peters told Brahms that he was very changeable, and periods of clarity and confusion followed in quick succession. The day before, while drinking his wine, he had suddenly stopped, said there was poison in it, and had thrown the rest on the floor. He wrote much, but illegibly; once, "Robert Schumann, Ehrenmitglied des Himmels [Honorary Member of Heaven]". The doctor also commented on his weakness of memory, and his incapacity to remember what he had done an hour ago.

On the 15th September, 1854, Robert wrote Clara a letter. Superficially, it contains nothing grossly abnormal. Yet Litzmann is right when he comments on it, that it is like a voice from the grave, from someone who does not know that he is dead; touching, childishly tender, but wholly concerned with the past. He asks Clara whether she plays as well as ever, where the album is, whether she still has his letters written from Vienna to Paris. In fact, trivialities, thrown together in an indiscriminate way, with never a word about the vital and tragic issues that faced them both.

There appears to have been no consistent change during the winter of 1854-55; musical hallucinations continued to occur. On the 23rd February, 1855, Brahms wrote Clara a letter describing a second visit to Robert. He says:

> Robert Schumann received me with the same warmth and gaiety as on the first occasion. . . . He immediately showed me your latest letter and told me what a delightful surprise it had been. . . . I showed him your portrait — you should have seen the depth of his emotion. . . . He asked for news of the children. He complained that writing paper was not given to him to write to his wife. When he got writing paper, he sat down at his table with a charming expression on his face and started several times to write to you. Finally he gave up, saying that he was too agitated. He mentioned several times that his publisher should not wait for his corrections and I told him that he had already received them long ago. He insisted with violence that it was impossible for the publisher to have received them. We discussed the matter for some time and I was unable to convince him.

Brahms goes on to describe how Robert wanted to play a duet with him, and that it was not very successful.

The things which will interest the psychiatrist in this letter are the clear signs of defects of memory, and the lack of recognition by the patient of their existence. When he is corrected he is first pathologically obstinate, and then has a catastrophic reaction, showing a pathological increase in emotional lability. It is also important to note that general emotional responsiveness is maintained and natural.

On the 5th May 1855 Robert wrote his last letter to Clara, after which he descends into a perpetual silence. This is:

> Dear Clara,
>   On the 1st May I sent you a spring greeting; but the following days were very restless; you will learn more from my letter, which you will receive by the day after tomorrow. A shadow blows through it; but the rest of its contents, my dearest, will gladden you.
>   I did not know when our dear one's birthday was; therefore I must put on wings, so that the despatch arrives with the score tomorrow.
>   I am enclosing the drawing of Felix Mendelssohn, for you to put (it) in the album. A priceless memento.
>   Farewell, dear love.
>   Your Robert.

The psychiatrist notes that, while a normal affect is still preserved, this letter is completely fragmentary and incoherent.

Brahms made another visit in April 1856. Schumann received him with signs of pleasure, but could only express himself in single inarticulate words. At another visit on the 8th June, Brahms found that Schumann scarcely noticed him, but spent the time poring over an atlas and picking words out from it. That month Schumann was losing strength fast, and was mostly confined to bed with swollen feet. On the 27th July Clara went to see him. He smiled at her, and tried to put an arm around her, with great difficulty as he could not control his limbs. His expression was clouded but mild. His speech was practically unintelligible: he said, looking at her, "Liebe . . . ich kenne . . ." ["Dear . . . I know . . ."] and Clara concluded that he wished to say, "Liebe Clara, ich kenne dich" ["Dear Clara, I know you"]. On the 28th his limbs were in almost continuous convulsion, and on the 29th he died.

The results of the autopsy were published in 1873 by Richarz, the Superintendent of the asylum at Endenich; they are quoted by Wasielewski. The abnormalities in the cranial cavity consisted of: (1) growth of bone at the base of the skull, forming exostoses which in some places penetrated the dura mater; (2) thickening of the leptomeninges and adherence of the pia mater with the cerebral cortex in several places; (3) considerable atrophy of the brain; its weight was below that which would have corresponded with his age; (4) hyperaemia, especially at the base. Part of these findings have been modified by Schaafhausen's re-examination of Schumann's skull, quoted by Möbius. Schaafhausen did not find any appreciable new growth of bone and, judging the intracranial capacity, he arrived at the conclusion that the atrophy of the brain was not as considerable as assumed by Richarz.

PREVIOUS SOLUTIONS OF THE DIAGNOSTIC PROBLEM

The postmortem findings are, measured against modern standards, incomplete and vague, and do not permit of definite conclusions, though the findings are compatible with dementia paralytica. In view of Schaafhausen's negative findings the diagnosis of a disease of the cranial bones (as maintained, for instance, by Stanford and Forsyth [1917]) seems to be without foundation. Richarz himself, more on clinical than postmortem grounds, was definitely in favour of an organic disease against one of the hereditary dementias, which were, in the terminology of the time, the equivalent of dementia praecox (schizophrenia). His description of Schumann's illness as one which combines the signs of speech disturbances with elation leading to dementia, certainly alludes to dementia paralytica, as it was then defined. Richarz called the disease in Schumann's case "incomplete paralysis", probably referring to Bayle's "la paralysie générale incomplète". He thought that, with Schumann, elation was replaced by melancholia; but he disregards the marked and sustained phase of elation which had preceded the attempt at suicide.

Möbius, in his book on Schumann's illness, gives a fairly full but still incomplete account of it, and he discusses the differential diagnosis in detail. However, he only considers the alternatives of general paresis and dementia praecox, and not that of manic-depressive illness. Correctly pointing out that Schumann was liable to nervous illness from youth on, he takes the view that this must have been schizophrenic. Once this is accepted, then he thinks there is insufficient evidence to call for a superadded organic illness during the last years.

Without going back to the original data, but accepting those provided by Möbius, Gruhle pointed out the alternative which Möbius had missed. The very facts which led Möbius to a diagnosis of schizophrenia lead Gruhle to a diagnosis of cyclothymia. The personality traits, looked at in detail, are all those of the cyclothymic personality. Then the many recurrent illnesses, if they had been schizophrenic, must have damaged Schumann's creativity. One might find a patient, who had an early attack of catatonia, and thereafter recovering worked well through many years of health. But Schumann had hardly a single complete year when he was fully healthy; and yet he was always able to recover his productivity when health improved again after a spell of illness. Gruhle thinks nothing of the diagnostic value of the *moue* as for whistling; the taciturnity was psychomotor inhibition; the irritability was cyclothymic; hypomanic signs were the ordering of expensive wine and the sudden overthrow of firmly made decisions. Gruhle says that the outspoken psychic inhibition shown during phases of illness, accompanied by an intense subjective feeling of illness, point with certainty to the manic-depressive syndrome. He quotes a number of examples from Schumann's self-descriptions, giving vivid expression of his feeling of illness and incapacity. This phenomenological evaluation has a very modern ring.

Gruhle admits that the last illness, which he takes as beginning about 1850, cannot be manic-depressive. There is much that speaks for general paralysis: the speech disturbance, the impaired judgment, the rapid dilapidation interrupted by short improvements, the eventual deterioration to death. Yet there can be no certainty about this. The illness might have been not general paresis but some other severe organic psychosis, perhaps of a luetic kind.

According to Feis (1910), Dupré in 1907 supported the view that Schumann was subject to manic-depressive phases. A rather different opinion was expressed by Pascal (1908), in a noteworthy article in which the biographical data and the arguments of Möbius are subjected to analysis and criticism from the clinical standpoint. In her view, Schumann had ten major depressive attacks, but in the interim periods between them was left with some persisting symptoms, especially in the nature of obsessive fears, scruples and doubts. She cannot see that he ever had symptoms of a hypomanic kind, and regards the depressive states as reactive to psychic traumata, particularly overwork. She criticises Möbius' arguments for a diagnosis of dementia praecox with severity and in detail, and has no doubt that the last illness, coming on after 1850, was a general paresis. Before that he had been, not a manic-depressive, but a constitutional psychasthenic, in English parlance an obsessional personality.

Gruhle's view, that dementia praecox can be definitely excluded, is still not universally agreed. An important document is Nussbaum's unpublished thesis. After an extensive exposition of the mood changes in Schumann's earlier life, Nussbaum considers that they have to be taken as manic-depressive, showing no schizophrenic feature. Yet he feels that later changes were schizophrenic in nature, and that the final illness was either general paresis or else a continuation of the schizophrenia "which probably is often of organic origin". This failure to consider the differentiation of schizophrenic from organic states robs this part of Nussbaum's thesis of much of its value.

The most recent work which sustains the view that Schumann's illness was schizophrenic is that of Wörner. He supports this in the main on the change in personality which occurred between about 1840 and 1849. Furthermore, since Schumann's later work is not as highly regarded as his earlier work, taking lessened achievement with change in personality a case is made for (schizophrenic) deterioration.

This view appears to be unjustified, since it receives no support from the musicologist. Thus Abraham in *Grove's Dictionary* (1954) explains the fall in level, at least at dates earlier than the last two years, along normal psychological lines. Abraham points out that in his youth, 1828-40, Schumann was the composer of small forms. He was at his best with simple and clear melodic ideas which he gave in a rich, diffused romantic light. The turning point was in 1841 when, partly under the influence of his wife, he turned to larger forms. His inability to cover a larger canvas is painfully apparent in his first symphony in B-flat as well as in his sonatas. Only genuine dramatic talent reveals itself in *Manfred* and *Faust*, as well as in his only opera, *Genoveva*. Some of the manifestations that have been taken for symptoms of mental decay — melodic and thematic angularity, increased harmonic complication — betoken nothing more than a normal development of musical style, influenced partly by the Zeitgeist and partly by intensive study of J. S. Bach. A more profound failure is recognisable in the last two years of his life. A certain element of heavy, sometimes bombastic, banality may have already appeared earlier. But such fairly late works as the Rhenish symphony (1850), the D minor violin sonata (1851) and the song *Der Gärtner*, Op. 107 (1851-52), show that the general decline must not be dated too early.

Joan Chissell, in her biography (1948), takes a similar view. She points out that in such an early work as the F sharp minor sonata of 1835, Schumann was having difficulty in filling out time, and using sequence, decoration and mere repetition, in a thick matted texture, in the endeavour to do so. On the other hand the Rhenish symphony of 1850 and the two violin sonatas of 1851 are masterpieces; and only after that year is his spontaneous imagination smothered and destroyed.

DISCUSSION

If we are to come to any final opinion about the nature of Schumann's illness, we must first try to decide what it was that killed him. There can, we think, be no reasonable doubt that when Schumann was in Endenich he was suffering from organic disease of the brain. When, twelve days after the onset of acute psychotic symptoms, he voluntarily went to the asylum, he was in a fatuously euphoric state, entirely forgetful of his wife and family. From the letters of Brahms we get a clear picture of Schumann in hospital retaining his emotional responsiveness, even when intellectual failure had become profound. Gross failure of memory was reported by the doctor as present a few months after his admission to hospital. In course of time intellectual failure reached the point of not being able to speak or write coherently, and it was succeeded by increasing physical weakness and emaciation, decubitus, incapacity to carry out ordinary voluntary movements, and death in convulsions. During the earlier part of his stay there were hallucinatory episodes and short-lived delusional ideas, a prominent feature of these states is their transitory nature, and they have every appearance of being organically determined phenomena. The existence of some form of organic disease of the brain seems to be beyond dispute.

Going back into the past, we find the first mention of symptoms characteristic of an affection of the nervous system not earlier than 1844. In that year there is the first mention of attacks of giddiness, and Dr. Helbig reports "Gehörstäuschungen." We do not know exactly what was meant by this word, but it seems improbable that it meant auditory hallucinations. It is much more probable that some form of tinnitus was intended, since that is the auditory symptom which is more precisely described later. Giddiness recurred in 1845, and tinnitus in 1846. It is then described in unmistakable terms as a constant singing and roaring in the ears, and an effect by which noises became musical tones.

From this time until 1852 there is a gap, and no symptoms of a characteristically organic kind are recorded. In 1852, however, they reappeared in more ominous form, first as a dreamy apathy and disturbance of speech, then the occurrence of a "convulsive" attack. From that time deterioration was steady. There were more speech difficulties and more auditory symptoms in 1853; and in February 1854 there came the sudden outbreak of a florid psychosis. In the course of a week Schumann was reduced from normal mentality to a state of raving.

Of this state the first sign was an intense tinnitus, which was soon translated into a continuous and vivid auditory hallucinosis. It is interesting that the hallucinations took at first a musical form, only later to become voices. One might suppose that stimulation of the auditory centres by pathological stimuli caused this reaction in his case because so much of his normal mental activity was musical rather than verbal. In this delirium-like psychosis, it is not easy to say how large a part was played by clouding of consciousness. At times at least it was not wholly clouded over, since he could recognise his wife at his side; but there is a suggestion of a twilight state with a varying degree of clouding. The hallucinosis, also, was variable in degree, and at times passed off. We hear of his getting quieter, getting up and setting about the correction of manuscript, of writing business letters, and still later receiving and entertaining a visitor. Other symptoms were fleeting delusional ideas and sudden impulsive actions. The total picture is a very familiar one, that of a delirious state, an exogenous organic reaction.

We agree with Gruhle that dementia paralytica is by far the most probable diagnosis, and accounts for the entire course of the illness from 1852 onwards. There are other possibilities, such as presenile and arteriosclerotic dementia, hypertensive encephalopathy, vitamin deficiency (pellagra, aneurin deficiency or related deficiencies which are known to occur in depressives or after chronic alcoholism), a deep-seated new growth, etc. MacMaster (1928) thought of (obviously atypical) tuberculous meningitis. But on careful consideration none of these alternatives fits all the facts as well as syphilitic disease.

Relating this hypothesis with his productivity, we can say that an organic psychosis, such as dementia paralytica, would explain the failure of Schumann's musical powers in 1852 and later. Furthermore, the type of failure is consonant with organic changes. Schumann was quite productive in 1852 and 1853. All critics are agreed that these later works are without merit, the last occasions when he reached his old mastery being the violin sonatas of 1851. Of the work of 1853, Chissell notes that mental tiredness and emotional apathy were accompanied by an unhesitating flow. It seems very probable that organic psychotic changes were making their effects felt in 1852, and unlikely that their onset was any earlier than 1851. We have, then, to account for the tinnitus and giddy attacks which appeared much earlier, i.e., in 1845. Consistently with the diagnosis of dementia paralytica, these may be attributed to a luetic infection. A combination of cerebrospinal syphilis and dementia paralytica, though rare, is well known to occur; and, following Lange-Eichbaum, there seems to have been a similar sequence in the illness of Nietzsche. An exceedingly far-fetched suggestion is also, perhaps, just worth mentioning, that of a lesion such as a tumour of the temporal lobe. The later appearance of gustatory and olfactory hallucinations might be thought to fit in with this, but otherwise there is nothing to support it. Ménière's disease, as a cause for tinnitus and giddiness, can be excluded, since there is no evidence that Schumann ever became deaf.

Having reached this point, we now have to consider the nature of the depressive and anxiety states which afflicted Schumann from the age of eighteen onwards. We believe that any impartial examination of the self-descriptions, such as those we have quoted, leads irresistibly to the conclusion that these were cyclothymic in nature. Let us, however, first consider the alternative hypothesis, which is so constantly repeated, that Schumann was schizophrenic.

The whole basis for a diagnosis of schizophrenia depends on a schizophrenic interpretation of the final psychosis of 1854-56, and a determination to regard earlier symptoms as caused in the same way. This was the position taken by Möbius, who said, in a paragraph which has often been quoted:

"Angst und Verstimmung, wunderliche Manieren, Neigung zur Stummheit, Misstrauen, Gehörstäuschungen, schwere Sprache, allmähliches Abnehmen der Geisteskräfte, alles schubweise hervortretend und langsam, aber unaufhaltsam zunehmend, das ist die Krankheit, die jetzt Dementia praecox genannt wird."[4]

In the light of the description which has been provided, this clinical summary can be seen to be inaccurate. There were numerous phases of illness from youth on, always with complete recovery and no indication of progression until the 1850's. The speech difficulties and mental impairment are confined to the last years, and are organic in nature. The auditory symptoms are peripheral in nature, until the delirious state of February 1854 brings genuine hallucinations. The only "hallucinatory" experience before that time is the hypnagogic hallucination of February 1838. Evidence for mistrust or a paranoid reaction at any time in life is very scanty: at Düsseldorf Clara was more mistrustful than Robert. The states of anxiety and depression are, surely, characteristic of cyclothymia and not of schizophrenia.

The "Neigung zur Stummheit," which Nussbaum also calls "Mutismus," is worth a little more discussion. There can be no doubt that in the course of his married life Schumann became very taciturn; yet evidence is lacking that his taciturnity was pathological. At times, especially in an intimate circle, he would be very talkative, when the subject discussed was one which interested or moved him. Nussbaum's "Schnauzkrampf" and Möbius' "wunderliche Manieren" appear both to be overstatements of a position of the lips at rest suggestive of whistling, and of a habit Schumann had of walking up and down in his room on tiptoe. Both of these would appear to fall well within the range of normal mannerisms.

The family history is a point which counts in favour of schizophrenia. The mental illnesses of both his sister and his son have been diagnosed as schizophrenic; this diagnosis seems very probable in the case of the son, less so in the case of his sister Emilie. However this is a point which cannot carry great weight. We have to diagnose schizophrenia by the clinical features shown by the patient himself, and to do so with any justification we have to show the presence of at least one or two incontestably schizophrenic symptoms. We can find no evidence of any schizophrenic symptoms in the illness itself; and the most that can be safely asserted is that Schumann's basic personality, which of course lent an individual colouring to the features of the illness, was not of an exclusively cyclothymic kind. His unrealistic idealism, his dreaminess and romanticism are certainly character traits which are not typical of the cyclothymic extravert, and could perhaps, together with his mannerisms, be regarded as schizoid. In such qualities as these one might justifiably trace the influence of the familial predisposition. The fact remains that Schumann never showed any overt symptom, and that the whole course of his illness is of a totally different kind.

[4] [Anxiety and depression, strange mannerisms, tendency to muteness, mistrust, auditory hallucinations, difficult speech, gradual reduction of mental powers, all progressing in stages and increasing slowly but continuously, this is the disease which we now call dementia praecox.]

The portraits of Schumann show a markedly pyknic habitus, with soft, rounded, almost feminine features. His personality also had qualities which might be called soft or feminine. In youth he was extremely extraverted, gay, active, and sociable, without a sign of schizoid sensitivity or withdrawal. In his married life he changed much, in a way which can be accounted for by the increasing predominance of depressive moods, and by the domesticating influence of Clara. Schumann was, of course, a complex personality, to which his classification as cyclothymic does not do full justice.

However, the course of the mood changes is characteristically cyclothymic. There were depressive phases in 1828, 1830, 1831, 1833, 1836, 1838, 1839, 1842, several such in 1844 taking up nearly the whole of the year, 1847, 1848. In 1829, 1832, 1833, 1836, 1838, 1843, 1849 and 1851 there were phases of marked elevation of mood, sometimes of a rather extreme degree. On two or three occasions, Schumann recorded in self-descriptions emotional states of a mixed kind ("tot und selig zugleich," [lifeless and blissful at the same time] "so arm und reich, so matt und kräftig, so abgelebt und so lebenslustig" [so poor and rich, so exhausted and vigorous, so worn out and so high spirited]). There is a suggestion of correlation of mood changes with the seasons. Many of the down-swings took place in the autumn, with a number of others in the spring; the principal up-swings also occurred in the months February to June. However there was no consistent regularity; the main mood changes in 1836, 1842 and 1848 were in December.

If one examines a chart of Schumann's production against the years, the inhibitory effect of his depressive phases and the excitatory effect of the elevated phases are made strikingly obvious (Table 33.2). 1840 and 1849 were his peak years, and in both of them he was in a consistently elevated mood throughout the year. In most of the other years he had some weeks or months of depression, not enough to distinguish one year from another on the chart; but the year 1844 was remarkable for low spirits practically throughout the entire year. It is also noteworthy that, regardless of quality, his production was consistently high in the four years 1850-53. Despite the onset of symptoms of an organic type, he was unusually free from depressive and hypochondriacal moods during these years, apart from a phase of depression in April and May 1852. The fact that the organic symptoms themselves had no inhibitory effect on his productivity is confirmatory evidence that the earlier and the later psychiatric illnesses were different in nature.

Gruhle laid stress on two signs which he regarded as pathognomonic of endogenous depression, both shown by Schumann to a conspicuous degree; the inhibitory effect of the depression on mental life, and the subjective experience of intense physical malaise. There are other points which we may add. In his depressions Schumann suffered from an intractable insomnia, which Dr. Helbig said had resisted all previous medicines; from Clara's account of finding her husband in the morning awake and drowned in tears, it would seem that the insomnia was of that type, with early morning waking, which is most characteristic of endogenous depression. Helbig also observed a marked diurnal rhythm, with the morning hours being the worst, a feature which is again typical of the endogenous depression. Psychogenic precipitation for the depressive phases is not easily to be found, and in general these moods do not appear to be of the reactive type. They could not be alleviated by distractions, and, until they spontaneously remitted, Schumann was hypochondriacal, oppressed by irrational fears and bodily malaise, dependent and self-reproachful. The evidence of a manic-depressive constitution could hardly be more complete.

TABLE 33.2. SCHUMANN'S WORKS BY YEAR AND OPUS NUMBER

1829	'30	'31	'32	'33	'34	'35	'36	'37	'38	'39	'40	'41	'42	'43	'44	'45	'46	'47	'48	'49	'50	'51	'52	'53
																				146				
																				145				
																				141				
											142									138				
											127									137				
											077									108				
											057									106				
											053									102				
											051									101				
											049									098				
											048									095				
											045									094		136		
											043									093		128		
											042									092		121		
											040									091		119		
											039									086		117		
											036									085	144	116		
											035									082	130	113		
											034									079	129	112		143
											033									078	125	111		134
											031									076	097	110		133
											030	120								075	096	109	148	132
									032		029	064				072		084	115	074	090	107	147	131
			124						021	028	027	054				060		080	081	073	089	105	140	126
			004			022	017		018	023	026	052	047			058		065	071	070	088	104	139	123
			003	010		011	014	012	016	020	025	038	044	050		056	061	063	068	069	087	103	135	118
007	001	008	002	005	099	009	013	006	015	019	024	037	041	046		055	059	062	066	067	083	100	122	114

SUMMARY

The controversy about Robert Schumann's mental illness has never been satisfactorily resolved. Möbius' diagnosis of dementia praecox has been severely criticised by Gruhle, who regarded Schumann as a manic-depressive succumbing finally to an organic brain disease, probably dementia paralytica. Subsequent reviewers have more or less adopted either the one or the other of these diagnoses, schizophrenia finding more favour recently.

The present authors have re-examined the available evidence and consider the interpretation of Gruhle to be preferred. The terminal psychosis presents unambiguous organic features, and may well have been a dementia paralytica, with atypical prodromata, but typical course and outcome. When that is eliminated from the picture, no signs or symptoms of schizophrenia remain to be accounted for. The earlier illnesses, both depressive and hypomanic, are essentially affective in symptomatology and all ended in complete recovery.

RETROSPECT

Perhaps it was in part the working of an instinctive internal direction-finder, and not merely good fortune, which led me in the end to combine genetics with psychiatry. I believed what my teachers told me, that work along genetical lines might help one to understand these illnesses, abnormal states that showed themselves in such subtle ways that most medical men preferred to have nothing to do with them — and so left them to the trick cyclist. What a challenge, then, to be sent out into a largely uncharted, a mysterious, dark and rather uncanny world, and to go provided with the lamp which the basic life sciences had lit!

Both self-esteem and humility were encouraged by the double apprenticeship. One cannot really dive any deeper or climb any higher — or further out along a limb — than one is put in the way of doing with these two disciplines. On the one hand I was admitted, as a kind of lay brother, to the great halls of science. On the other hand I became a member of a kind of international Diners' Club, with the possibility of entry as a temporary guest to a number of professional coteries, such as law and the humanities. The psychiatrist is given permission to interest himself in a great variety of human affairs, and is sometimes even listened to, when he thinks he has something to say. This is a privilege greatly enjoyed by all. Who among us has not fallen a victim to the charms of "Psychiatry Unlimited"?

It is probably a good thing for psychiatrists to tell the world about its awful ways; and maybe we have something useful to contribute in discussing, say, the breakdown of marriages, the range of human sexuality, the nature of the stresses that society imposes, and why people break the law. No harm is done as long as the audience takes the psychiatrist in along with other expert witnesses, and treats his information and his ideas on their merits. It is bad for both sides when, as sometimes, we are regarded as speaking with authority. Results then may be disastrous (*viz.* the effects of psychiatric dogma on child management), until a new generation has automatically dethroned the "authorities" of the last.

This "Retrospect" has been specially written for *Man, Mind, and Heredity* in winter 1969–70.

THE PSYCHIATRIST AND THE LAW

These excursions meant a lot to me. Most of them were written under a certain amount of emotional pressure. The accumulated affect that pushed out the essay on the McNaughton Rules (p. 331), was built up during the sessions of the Royal Commission on Capital Punishment, which sat from 1949 to 1953. It was a revelation to see the ways in which the minds of lawyers worked. The witness who made the deepest impression on me was the Lord Chief Justice of the day, who was built like a heavy-weight boxer, and radiated dominance and "strength of personality."

After our Chairman, Sir Ernest Gowers[1] had had his go at putting questions to the succession of witnesses who appeared before us (and a very notable group of public figures they were, not only in England and Scotland, but also in the U.S.A. and in Scandinavia, Belgium, and the Netherlands), it was "Buggins's turn" for the individual members of the Commission. So it was that, on the 5th January 1950, I found myself in a position, perhaps unique for living psychiatrists, to submit the Lord Chief Justice of my country to cross-examination, like the canary that ate the cat. The animal proved indigestible.

On the subject of the McNaughton Rules, it seemed that the L.C.J. had no difficulty in combining the opinions (a) that these Rules were satisfactory and did not need modification, (b) that juries would at times go further than the directions of the trial judge allowed, and expand the Rules to cover cases in which their sympathies were aroused, and (c) that it was quite proper for juries to do this. This is what we call English pragmatism and common sense, and it has got us where we are today.

Stranger still was the attitude exposed in the following exchange:

Q. Take the interesting case of Ley, whom you mentioned. You had no doubt he was insane?
L.C.J. No, I thought he was insane from the way he gave his evidence, that there was something wrong with him, because he did not even attempt to set up a defence, or his defence was: "I did not do it, every word that is said in this case is a lie." "Of course," you said, "this man cannot be normal because at any rate he would try to set up some defence, if he was." But that he knew what he had done, that he knew it was wicked, that he intended to destroy that boy and would have destroyed another man if he had been able to get hold of him, there was no doubt.
Q. And he would hardly be covered by the McNaughton Rules?
L.C.J. He was not covered by the McNaughton Rules, at least, I thought he was not, because he knew what he was doing, and he knew that what he was doing was wicked and wrong. Of course, he did not set up a defence of insanity. He was reprieved on the ground that he was a paranoiac, and he died within six weeks.

*　　*　　*

Q. To revert to the case of Ley, I suppose you would not have wished that man to hang? You would not think it proper that he should hang?
L.C.J. I should have thought it was very proper that he should have been hanged.
Q. Even though he was insane, and presumably, from the ecclesiastical point of view, not in a fit state to make his peace with God?
L.C.J. He could make his peace with God, I think, quite well. I do not know what his religion was, but the only reason he committed the murder was because he mistakenly believed that the man had committed adultery with his mistress. What excuse did he have? Supposing it was true that the boy had committed adultery with his mistress, it was no excuse for kidnapping him, and then brutally murdering him in the basement of a house in South Kensington.

[1] A son of the renowned neurologist William Gowers, and himself a very distinguished ex-civil servant, the Chairman of several important Royal Commissions.

Q. I think the medical point of view would be that the disease had altered his personality so as to make such wickedness possible.

L.C.J. If that is the medical point of view, I am afraid, frankly, that it does not appeal to me at all. If that was the case, I think it is one of the reasons why he should be put out of the way.

The effect of these answers on me was stunning; I could hardly believe I had heard aright.[2] At lunch, after the morning hearing, the eminent judge entertained us with stories both comic and grim. With his immense vitality and gusto he dominated our table, and we put up no resistance but gave him his head. For me, he loomed enormous across the white cloth, a shape of darkness, from whose penetrating eyes shone a ferocious energy and a powerful (and malign) intelligence. I looked at him like a being from another world, as indeed he was — a world in which psychiatric insights are unheard of, or if heard of are not attended to, or if attended to are not understood, or if understood are discounted as irrelevant, or mistaken, or mischievous, or valueless.[3]

I wonder whether lawyers understand either the nature of the information which the psychiatrist can obtain for them, or how it should be applied. They seem to believe that the world of psychiatry, like the world of law, is a human artefact. But what the psychiatrist can find out and can report about the past history, the mental make-up, and the motivations of an accused man is evidence about a real world in which events occur. The real world has primacy and, in the last resort, legal concepts and legal fictions must conform to it. One gets the impression of but little desire to understand this real world. Psychiatric evidence, and indeed evidence of all kinds, has to be stretched and strained to fit the legal concepts, which are jealously preserved. For the legal mind it is more important for the game to be played according to the rules, than for sensible decisions to be made.

I was once invited to give an open lecture in the University of Oxford; and when it was over, I was taken by my host to dine with the dons at the high table at Magdalen College. After a dinner, excellent at a number of levels of experience, which continued for some time after the undergraduates had left the body of the hall, a select party of us were conducted in the light of a summer evening through the courts to a Combination Room looking over the deer-park. We seated ourselves round the table on which there were bowls of dessert, carafes of wine, and costly silver, porcelain and crystal. Two of our number were formally dressed for the evening; and it appeared that one of them was some kind of an appendage and the other was the Assize Judge on circuit. This urbane gentleman was graciously pleased to learn that I was a psychiatrist, and informed me that he had had a psychiatrist before him that very day. The man had been called to give evidence in a case of homicide, and had been able to persuade him, the judge, that the case was one of diminished responsibility, and the accused was a psychopath. In consequence the

[2] Such opinions, so uncompromisingly expressed, caused the Lord Chief Justice a good deal of embarrassment later, when they were exploited by both journalists and counsel. See Abel-Smith and Stevens (1968), p. 182, footnote.

[3] It is not unknown for judges publicly to question the honesty of psychiatric witnesses, men of high standing and irreproachable character, who have done no worse than give evidence that displeased them. To quote again from Abel-Smith and Stevens (1968), p. 184, footnote: "Lord Justice Harman said of a psychiatrist acting as an expert witness: 'A doctor is a paid advocate who speaks for the person who pays the fee'." If it is true that psychiatrists and other medical men prostitute themselves, then it follows that officers of justice are procurers and courts are brothels.

judge had felt able to sentence the accused to a considerably shorter number of years of imprisonment, for manslaughter, than would otherwise have been possible. Provoked by the benign smile, and the confident expectation of good opinion which such clemency deserved, I felt it incumbent on me to tell his Honour that he had got it all wrong. A man whose responsibility for his acts was impaired was a greater danger to the community than a man whose responsibility was intact; and the appropriate measure would be to remove him from society for a longer rather than a shorter term.

The result was not altogether happy. In England the Assize Judge travels from county town to county town as a representative of the sovereign. He is met on arrival by the civic authorities and conducted in state to the Judge's Lodgings, where he is installed with his own staff of domestics which he has brought along with him. He is isolated from the world in which he moves as a superior being, and he is accustomed to having his *obiter dicta* treated with little if any less respect than his judicial pronouncements. It was unfitting on my part to treat him — as I saw him — as just another professional man. One does well, in England, when addressing a functionary, or any important or self-important personage, to give him the degree of deference which one can see he expects. When I was young I used to rebel against this. Now I am wiser, and Konrad Lorenz has convinced me that the social hierarchy fulfils a vital function, and works most satisfactorily for all when the established ritual gestures are punctiliously performed.

"THE CRIME OF PUNISHMENT"

Re-reading what I wrote those years ago in Papers 31 and 32, I find little I wish to withdraw, or even change very much, though I am sorry not to have put the argument against "free will" more cogently. My feeling now is to go further. Having just finished reading Karl Menninger's (1966) splendid crusading work *The Crime of Punishment*, I am tempted to formulate my own ideas.

The most serious of the very many problems we face seems to me to be the heavy and increasing toll taken by the highly intelligent and skilfully organised professional criminals. Perhaps this is only ten percent or so of the total wastage caused by crime, but it is these men who, by defying the social order, constitute its most dangerous threat. It is the success and the immunity of these criminals that erode our values. Why is it that such crime flourishes? Surely, in part at least, as Menninger points out, because we refuse to take it seriously. The professional criminal is at all stages treated as if he were a member of our society and a member in good standing, when in fact he has opted out, at least for the time being, and is its determined and ruthless enemy. How can we deal with the challenge he offers, and still maintain decent standards of behaviour? If our efforts to cope with him are ineffective, are they any more successful with the amateur and the occasional offender? Are the principles we use to guide us conceived on the right lines? I would submit that they are not, and in their place offer what follows, drawn up in an order of precedence, so that later clauses operate only in the conditions defined in the earlier ones:

I. At all stages and at all times suspects and offenders, even the worst, must be treated with decency and humanity.

II. We recognise that all processes of ascertainment of fact are liable to error. The conclusion that the person X did the criminal act A is to be based not on an attempted certainty, but on a substantial balance of probabilities. Not infrequently it will prove to be an incorrect conclusion, and then the processes by which the official decision is reversed and amends are made is to run smoothly and efficiently.

III. We recognise that in penology the "justice" of an award cannot be defined and cannot be validated. In taking administrative action on the finding that X did A, the first and over-riding consideration is to be the safety of the community. From II it follows that nothing is to be done to the individual against his consent which cannot be subsequently reversed or adequately recompensed.

IV. Before such administrative action is taken, offenders are to be classified according to guidelines derived from our knowledge of psychiatry. Persons of good character and normal personality are to be dealt with by standard processes (rebuke, penalty, punishment, probation, etc.), with broad adherence to a "tariff" system. It is recognised that punishment will not be required, or be deserved, or be the effective method of treatment, in a substantial minority of offenders, e.g.:

a. those of good character whose social controls have broken down under exceptional or massive stresses;

b. the psychiatrically ill, the psychotic, the neurotic, the psychopathic, who will need treatment along psychiatric lines, either while they continue to live in the community under safeguards, or while living in adequately equipped enclaves;

c. the professional criminal, whose way of life is to prey upon the community. He is to be recognised as an enemy of society and being in effect the national of a foreign hostile state. Now that he has been taken prisoner of war, he is not to be allowed back into the community until his antisocial allegiance has ended.

V. Since deterrence rests much more on the probability of detection and punishment than on its severity, all processes should be favoured which lead to the conviction of offenders, while at the same time their punishments are made milder. In the processes involved in detection and conviction, the police are the first line of defence against crime. They must be given the public recognition and the esteem which their work deserves. They should be an elite force, no less so than the armed forces of national defence, with the highest standards of conduct and *esprit de corps*, well rewarded and honoured. Their position as guardians of public safety should get for them the friendly cooperation of all good citizens. Consonant with their standing and their standards, they should be freed from much of the present bureaucratic and legalistic controls on how they go about to apprehend the criminal; but lapses from high professional standards of conduct should be strictly dealt with.

VI. The adversary system in trials is to be abandoned, and an inquisitorial, or investigatory process substituted. The aim of the hearings will be to find out what happened and why. The past record and personality of an accused, being highly relevant information, are to be available from the start. Other rules of evidence are to be modernised and made efficient.

VII. The processes gone through to conclude that X did A are to be held distinct from those gone through to decide the appropriate administrative action, and both processes are to involve a different set of agents of decision. Both organisations are to be backed by efficient research services, criminological, penological, sociological, psychological, psychiatric, medical, etc.

INTENSITY AND EXTENSITY

Alas 'tis true I have gone here and there,
And made myself a motley to the view.

William Shakespeare, *Sonnet* CX

Over a lifetime, my aim in choosing problems for investigation has not been a single-minded one. Men of great scientific achievement have nearly always concentrated their efforts. Out of a welter of problems accessible to their expertise, they choose a key one. They are not to be deterred by difficulties, but they require a reasonable possibility of success. As Popper has pointed out, the method of work always involves playing hunches. Once a key solution is obtained, once a piece is fitted into a focal place in the jigsaw, then other pieces, single or articulated, fall naturally into place. More of the total picture emerges; and new problems then show themselves, whose very existence till that time had not been guessed.

The danger of the single-minded approach is that the hunch may fail; it may lead into a blind-alley, in which a lifetime of work can be spent in achieving nothing. That was not a risk I ran. The concentration and the heroism of the true professional scientist have not been within my powers. Cyclothymia, neurosis, schizophrenia, hysteria were taken up and dropped in turn when I did not know what was the next step to take. If now, casting an eye over the whole, one can see any unifying design, that does not come from any deliberate planning. If a restless curiosity led to probing attacks at any point where the defences of the unknown might offer a soft spot, that could be regarded as a pragmatic policy. It had also its romantic side. It was probably more important for me to enjoy the work I was doing than to be secure in the knowledge that, if it succeeded, something of fundamental importance would be learned. Many of the professional jobs done have been of trivial significance; and in my leisure time uncounted hours have been spent on labours which one can only call piffling.[4]

I have worried myself over a number of questions for which I had to find an answer, valid for myself if not for others. Once I had the answer, right for me, and had got it off my chest, it nagged me no longer; and the chances were that I would never return to it again. Is there such a thing as extra-sensory perception? If there is, then surely the what and the how of it are more important and more fundamental problems than any others to be dreamed of in our philosophy. I gave a lot of reading time, and quite a lot of thought, to this question at two periods, separated by many years. After the first, I came to the conclusion that the workers in this field were not serious, i.e., they did not attempt to set up rigorous conditions; perhaps there was something in it, perhaps there was not. This was most unsatisfactory. A second period of questioning led me to a conclusion, a negative one.[5] As far as I am concerned, the matter is finished; and I can't even be bothered to read of the latest work. Let other sceptics spend time looking into it; it is not for me.

---

[4] For instance, I spent a lot of time analyzing the results obtained in international chess tournaments to see whether there was such a thing as a best chess opening, as according to games theory there ought to be.

[5] See the review on ESP (126) that occasioned lively rejoinders in the correspondence columns of the *British Journal of Psychiatry*. – Editors.

GROUP INTOLERANCE

An obvious example of work done to settle my own disquiet is the small set of papers written around the "Jewish question". My own family life was completely free of any antisemitic feeling or indeed racialist tendencies of any kind. But I did meet such prejudices in school and university life. Prejudices of this generic kind have a fatal attraction for the young and immature in spirit. By classifying human-kind into two groups, a majority (minority) to which you and I belong, and a minority (majority) of others, inferior and excluded, we unite with one another in a cosy and protective world which claims our loyalty and promises us support. It is the same tribal togetherness which I learned in my first year at boarding school, when a whole classful of fifteen-year-olds, I among them, turned on an unfortunate prefect sent to keep order, and drove him from the room with sadistically directed riot and disorder.

Antisemitism in England was the feeblest flicker here and there until Hitler and his disciple Mosley appeared on the scene. When I arrived at the Maudsley in 1931, some of the senior psychiatrists were Jews who distinguished themselves as a group from the rest of us mainly by absenting themselves from duty on Jewish festivals and by refraining from certain articles at the midday lunch table. While we all liked and respected these colleagues, I think we would have had to be angelic not to be the slightest irked by the self-sought differentiation. It would seem as if, incompre-hensibly, *we* and our ways were rejected by *them*. That one should have such feelings at all was degrading. Where did they come from? Why should we, the non-Jewish, have the guilt of feeling antisemitic?[6] Were the Jews right, that it was entirely our fault and nothing to do with them? Or were they too to be blamed?

When I arrived in Nazi Germany the need to come to terms with myself over this issue became a matter of urgency. I solved the problem for the time being by a strong repudiation of all Nazi racist ideas, indeed rejoicing when I was able to proclaim my repudiation in my marriage.

But the to and fro did not entirely cease then. Even during the war, waged on our side against the Nazi ideology, our minds showed symptoms of the infection from time to time. Somehow one should attempt to discover whether there was any truth in the group differences that were maintained and again denied. Was there any truth in the belief that while the Jews were more intelligent on average than we, they were more neurotic? A little bit of head-counting I conducted suggested that among enlisted men Jews were several times more likely than non-Jews to be ad-mitted to our psychiatric centre, and to be discharged from the Army on psychiatric grounds. Then how was this difference to be accounted for? And how was it to be combined with the tenet which I held as an article of faith that group differences are no basis for value judgments? I could not allow that the Jewish race, if it was a "race," could be either chosen or rejected; it was an integral part of humanity, like all other such groups.

I would not change anything I wrote in Paper 29, though the same basic problem now shows a different face. In England antisemitism has diminished to vanishing point, and we are bedevilled by a greater bogy. Important group differences based

[6] Perhaps "we" is quite wrong; perhaps I was the only one. We never discussed it, that I can remember.

on cultural patterns and language are made conspicuous by having a coloured label attached to them. We cannot deal with the practical problems this causes by pretending that the differences don't matter, and that the silly mob is being upset by labels. The real differences are the main problem. They have their worth and value, and they must not be played down, even though we are determined that all groups are to be allowed the same status in human dignity. If a harmonious society can be built on heterogeneous communities living alongside one another, it is so much the richer, provided there are the transcultural communications which enable us to enrich our experience and our awareness from this diversity. Communication there must be, and sexual and reproductive exchange must be a part of it.

But with this added richness, there are added dangers. Group differences divide loyalties and provide a culture medium for hostilities. If these are serious, it may only be possible to deal with them either by separating the groups and reducing contacts or by dissolving group boundaries and mixing all in an inextricably compounded mishmash of individuals. The final aim of the assimilative process would be to reduce intra-pair ties to being no stronger within groups than across groups. This is probably impossible, and very doubtfully desirable. It is unrealistic, however, to suppose that all that is necessary is to pass laws against racial discrimination, and by educative processes to prolong the universal acceptancies of childhood into adult life. Children in infant schools do not form themselves into gangs, coteries, clubs, and mutually exclusive clusters; but let them only grow old enough, and they will do so, however they have been indoctrinated.

It is probably true that the greater the genetic and cultural homogeneity of a society, the easier it is to allow room for individual extravagances and eccentricities. The greater the genetic and cultural heterogeneity, the greater must be the social pressure for conformism in any highly developed community, especially with a high population density. Extremely intricately involved factors must be interacting with one another in producing concord or discord; and we seem to know practically nothing about them.

MODELS FOR TREATMENT AND MODELS FOR RESEARCH

As one of my editors put it, "the idea may get around that a genetic and organically minded neo-Kraepelinian has little time for social and personal factors as they affect the illnesses of his patients." Do I wish to defend myself against this? Altogether, I must have spent a good deal longer in looking after patients entrusted to my care than in researching the conditions from which they were suffering. In treating a patient one has to try to be all-wise, and it is not unusual to suppose that one is. One must take account of everything that might be helping to make him ill, or that might be used to try to get him better. It is best to keep a certain distance from the patient, with a view to seeing his problems objectively; but even so, one must be warmly engaged on his behalf. One must be prepared, for instance, to spend time and trouble defending his interests vis-à-vis employers, community services, and relatives. One can't do this without taking personal and social factors very much into account, both when trying to understand the patient and when trying to help him.

Where genetics comes in is in helping to settle the diagnosis, a vitally necessary task and one in which knowledge of the social and personal background does not often give much help. I do not believe you can do your best for a schizophrenic patient without first deciding that his trouble is schizophrenia. But it makes no difference to treatment if one knows he has a family history positive for this disorder, or knows that he has not.

374

In the therapeutic situation, the medical model has proved to be the most consistently successful one; I think it is a necessity and that it is irreplaceable. Most of our patients are ill, and we cannot afford to try out other "models" until we can be sure that there is no illness and that the medical approach is inappropriate and best replaced by a wholly different way of looking at the situation.

In requiring a "diagnosis," this strategy makes one try to conceive of this man — this patient one is talking to, with all his individual qualities — in relation with predecessors, the other patients one has studied oneself, and the abstractions of the text-books. It matters very little whether one calls the condition a "disease" or a "syndrome" or a "reaction type"; at least, these are not counters which do a lot of work for me. One matches this patient with the others, in respects which the accumulated experience of generations of psychiatrists has shown to be important. The extent and the ways in which this patient resembles those others provide the main indications for treatment, and the main guides for predicting an outcome.

With new and more powerful methods of classification, our present diagnostic systems may become obsolete, replaced perhaps by statistical taxonomy. But the basic logic and the rationale for prognosis and treatment will be the same. When the individual patient, despite his uniqueness, has been identified with a point in a multidimensional universe, whose many parameters are tracked by many millions of observations, it will still be the relationships between that point and all the others, whether considered in clusters or not, which will tell the working doctor what to do.

When we leave the therapeutic, i.e., medical, situation, we are not compelled to take the medical model along with us. If we are dealing with large groups of patients or with populations, or with administration, welfare, or research, we can use quite different instruments. Trained as a doctor, I am of course stuck with the medical model; I don't think that doctors who have abandoned it have done very well. Necessarily, I took the model with me into the planning of research and the consideration of its results. It proved very useful, rigorous enough and adaptable enough, and I never felt it had let me down. So I *believe* that it corresponds with the realities we are trying to grasp.

Of course, what was necessary for me has not been a necessity for others who can and do enter research with models of a very different kind. I may or may not be able to understand the way they think; if science is a common language shared by us, I should be able to understand their conclusions, perhaps apply them, perhaps be in the position to check them. But they must forgive him, if the neo-Kraepelinian sticks to his own pathway.

What I have tried to be as a doctor and what I have tried to do as a journal editor are another matter, but it is true that in research I have had relatively little time for examining the role of social and personal factors in contributing to psychiatric illness. I might have found more time, if the results of environmental research had lent themselves to being checked with more precision, in the type of studies in which I became involved.

RESEARCH AS A DISCIPLINE

When one takes up research as a professional activity one dedicates oneself, for the time being and while in that field, to the pursuit of truth. To be sure, however one tries, one is myopic or astigmatic by constitution, blinkered by past indoctrinations, perhaps even suffering from some form of hysterical amblyopia. But one can refrain from putting on the distorting spectacles on offer or try the effect of taking off the pair one normally wears and has grown used to. In sciences concerned with soft data and subjectively toned observations, blind techniques are helpful but are not enough. It is necessary to aim at being unbiased, to lean against rather than towards the motivations by which one is impelled. A conscious effort of mind and a lasting self-discipline are called for. Those who are not prepared to try are a danger, and they would be better placed in fields in which uncritical enthusiasm brings the rewards. In his spare time the research worker should feel free to campaign and to crusade. When he turns to his professional task, figuratively or in fact, he should put on his white coat. While he wears that coat, he must accept the findings his work brings him, regardless of his preconceptions. Given a chance, he should put those preconceptions on trial by setting up the experiment or starting the enquiry which would seem to have the best chance of disproving them. Genuine observations, which bear the various hall-marks of authenticity, must be received dispassionately and handled with respect, whether they come from his own work or from that of others, whether they tend to support or to rebut the working hypotheses which he uses as his tools. Above all, he must not identify himself with the results of his work or with the hypotheses to which they give rise. His loyalty to his brain-children must be of a strictly limited kind, and go no further than seeing that they are given the chance of a fair fight when they come in conflict with others.

I have tried to live up to these standards, when I remembered; I have tried to abandon the disproved hypothesis with a good grace, when it became untenable. When our Unit went out to get the results of a follow-up of twin subjects of "hysteria," I confidently expected that positive concordances would emerge, higher in the MZ than in the DZ pairs. When quite different results came in, I imagine I was disappointed and I can remember feeling very perplexed. New ideas had to be taken into account; and I had to think the thing through from the ground up, to the point where I doubted the very existence of a hysterical syndrome (or reaction type, or personality type). It was painful. It meant I had to go back on ideas I had published, and had, for instance, to re-write a section on "hysteria" in the textbook of psychiatry of which I was part author. It was a *volte face* as uncomfortable and as invigorating as when a growing acquaintance with German phenomenological teaching drove me out of the comfortable school of Adolf Meyer.

Not to be willing to give up old ideas when the evidence is produced which shows they have to be modified, is the sin against the light, not only for research workers though for them above all. Soon after the Tienari (1963) results came out, showing a zero concordance rate in the MZ co-twins of schizophrenics, a colleague with a background in the social aspects of psychiatry remarked, "You know, all of us at the X Hospital, when we saw those results, just whooped for joy!"

Perhaps it is not waste of time to consider the implications of this remark. The speaker had presumably adopted a sociogenic or psychogenic or at least environmental theory of the causation of schizophrenia and for a number of years had been aware of but had refused to accept the results of family and twin research in schizophrenia. These results had obviously not been considered on their merits but had been reacted to emotionally and had been felt as in some way hostile to the accepted environmental theory. This could only have been because the genetical results were not understood, since, if understood, they would have been felt to be complementary rather than contradictory. One can also conclude that the environmental theory had been accepted as some kind of a credo, accepted with passion, identified with high aims and ideals, and given an unquestioning loyalty. This could only have been because the environmental hypothesis itself had never been looked at with understanding, since all theories of causation are ethically indifferent. The mental set that resulted meant that no evidence could be considered on its merits, but valued only in so far as it tended to confirm already accepted ideas. When Tienari came along with a piece of evidence which confirmed those ideas, the conclusion was at once drawn that all the genetical work that had gone before was now disproved. A warm surge of certainties confirmed flooded the system, and the soul sang for joy.

Tienari's results compelled others, including myself, to reconsider our positions; but I think we were able to do so without any very extravagant emotional reaction. This is the nub of the matter. It is a pity to be blinded by emotion; but it is the wilful self-blinding which causes so much of the avoidable difficulties against which workers in such fields as psychiatry and behavioural genetics have to pit themselves. It is indeed necessary to take up a position, for argument's sake, or to have a point of departure for further work. But such positions are necessities of convenience and should claim no loyalty. We must not weep when we are forcibly moved on, or compelled to retreat.

A primary requirement for good clinical work with patients is the working hypothesis that one knows the answers. Until one has convinced oneself of that, one can hardly make a beginning with treatment, or with settling any number of other practical issues. Over the years the good clinician, becoming more and more experienced and skilful, gets more and more sure of himself, so that in the end he can look around his arena with sublime wisdom and certainty. For research work, the requisite working hypothesis is that one doesn't know the answers, but that, if one can only succeed in putting the right questions, some answer may emerge. Over the years one comes to learn a certain humility; if one begins to doubt some of the clinician's certainties, it is not because one is at all sure that one has anything more certainly true to put in their place.

Speaking for myself, I like a monogenic theory for schizophrenia. It provides me with the kind of tool I like to handle. Wherever you start digging with it, it turns up questions, in family psychiatry, social psychiatry, epidemiology, just as much as, say, in chemical pathology. Burch's (1964) plurigenic theory does not appeal to me at all. I cannot use it heuristically, and I don't see how anyone else can. Perhaps one day a team of immunologists will come along with a demonstration of auto-immune processes actually going on in schizophrenics; and then the theory will be on another footing. I guess that the polygenic theory of schizophrenia, favoured by my editors (Gottesman and Shields, 1967), appeals particularly to them because it fits in naturally with established ways of thinking, and is not merely a remarkably successful explanatory hypothesis, but also a good working tool. I would think that it must be preferred by psychologists and social scientists, while a monogenic theory would have more appeal for doctors, pathologists, chemists, and straight geneticists. This is small comfort for me, as doctors, pathologists, etc., usually run as hard as they can when schizophrenia looms over the horizon.

It seems to me that genetical theories have an essential part to play in the understanding of schizophrenia. Even if one is mainly interested in, say, family dynamics, problems become easier to handle if one is prepared to allow some importance to the genotype. Nearly all the socially and psychodynamically interested schizophrenia workers (notably Alanen 1966, Kringlen 1967, Tienari 1963) have convinced themselves that there is a genetical aspect to causation, even if that is not the aspect to which they wish to devote their own endeavours.

377

I have written this as if I thought that the working hypothesis one adopts is determined solely by one's past learning and one's temperament. This is, of course, only half true. As new facts emerge, one does get driven from hypothesis to hypothesis. It is my belief that the genetical facts, in their multiplicity and their systematic order, are now too powerful to be resisted by an open-minded psychiatrist; the strongholds of the pan-psychic and purely environmental theories are no longer defensible.

If we turn now to manic-depression, the situation is rather different, and has not advanced so far. Monogenic theories are beginning to look increasingly improbable (though they cannot be excluded for a part of the range of affective psychoses); it is polygenic theories that would seem to be the best bet. But they have to be complicated by making a much larger allowance for heterogeneity of the clinical material than is necessary in the case of schizophrenia. Maybe there are affective disorders, say the "neurotic" or "reactive depressions," in which genetical variance contributes very little to causation, or symptomatology, or course, or treatment susceptibilities. But we can be reasonably sure that over the greater part of the range of the affective disorders, genetical factors play a significant role.

HYPOTHESES AND BELIEFS

If then we are to give no faith, but only a provisional credence, to any scientific hypothesis, should we — can we — inflict on ourselves the austerity of no beliefs? Each of us has his own world of values, in which all tenets are in the nature of articles of a creed and cannot claim to be logically necessary consequences drawn from the public domain of observable reality. However, it should be possible to build a bridge between the two, given a single axiom of universal acceptability. The discourse of values would still be without logical foundation in the discourse of fact, but it could proceed logically thereafter, by building on that bridge. This was the method used by the Greek geometricians, and got us so far that in a later era the systematic overthrow of their axioms could be undertaken without pulling the whole structure down about our ears. What kind of axiom should we be looking for? Does nature, or the evolutionary process, or the mind of man offer us in any dimension a contrast of observable states to which we would all agree in assigning a plus or minus sign in the scale of values? On this issue I should like to return to a point of view developed during the war years (Slater and Woodside, 57).

When we examine human behaviour we find that the individual man is faced at many moments of the day with alternative courses of conduct. He has to make a choice, and he formulates this for himself by trying to decide which of two modes of procedure is the "better." The primary datum is the contrast between "better" and "worse," and "right" and "wrong," "good" and "evil" are secondary constructions from this. With the idea of an absolute goodness we have now come to associate the idea of God; and from the idea of God we reach such insoluble dilemmas as, how could a perfectly good and omnipotent God make a world in which evil abounds? Such questions are seen to be meaningless when we return to the more fundamental contrast between the comparatives "better" and "worse" and see them as merely alternative directions in which one may move, as in fact a necessary dimension of any world in which there is self-consciousness and in which development is occurring. If we can take this step, the study of ethics becomes an experimental science. We are faced with the work of finding out what things are preferred by human beings and of extracting from a multiplicity of observations general principles of universal validity.

Seen in this perspective, human beings appear as individuals each of whom is endowed with a polarity, leading him to orientate himself in a particular way towards the environment and to turn his steps in a given direction. In the same way, the free-swimming animalcule in a bath of water moves away from regions of excessive salinity, or towards a food particle. The direction chosen by human beings is away from circumstances which on the whole are disliked towards those which are felt to be preferable. As all human beings share much that is common in their mental and physical make-up, humanity as a whole seems to be striving towards a vaguely apprehended goal. It would be the task of experimental ethics to discover, by the analysis of processes of choice, what is universally felt to be desirable.

From this point the argument went on to consider some of the snags that would be met; for instance, what people imagine they desire may not be what their behaviour shows they do desire. Pending the solution by exhaustive experiment, it was proposed, in the best medical tradition, that good health might have sufficient universality of appeal, and be sufficiently precisely definable, to provide an ethical yard-stick for measuring social changes, or behaviour, etc.

Is it possible to jump the gap from what we know to what we value by assumptions which few would be willing to deny, such as that health is better than sickness, that a rich world would be a better place than an impoverished one, that the vigorous use of one's capacities is better than letting them rust, that diversity is better than uniformity, that it is a wise policy to keep one's options open? If it were possible to assume these values, guide-lines for the management of community affairs could be drawn.

One of our recent acquisitions of knowledge is an understanding of the uniqueness of the human individual. Though we have only begun to explore the range of genetic variability in man, we already know enough, say about protein and enzyme systems, to be able to calculate that each single individual is an extremely improbable event — perhaps so improbable as not likely to be duplicated (except rather roughly in a monozygotic twin partner) either elsewhere on the face of the globe, or potentially for all time. A fact so fundamental should be part of the foundations of all the life sciences, and, by extension, of the social sciences. We do not begin life as a *tabula rasa,* a clean slate of uniform manufacture, differing from one another afterwards only by what has been written on us. We are not stamped out of one common metal, but are made of different alloys. We vary in refractoriness to all the moulding processes through which we are forced, and we take the imprinting to which we are subjected with very different degrees of fidelity.

We know that when a species loses its genetic variability it is in danger of extinction. The genetic variability of man is certainly no less than that of most other species; but in spite of — perhaps because of — our immense numbers, we face a variety of threats. Should we aim at conserving this variability? Does the uniqueness, the irreplaceability of the individual lend anything to the dignity or the moral stature with which we should think him endowed? We shall never have another Mozart, not if the world goes on for another billion years. We did not treat him very well when he was with us, and he died very young. Was that a fault of the generation in which he lived? And how are we doing today?

The story of evolution makes it plain that all living things are of one kin. Is this something that we should feel, that should be part of our *Weltanschauung?* Is the ruthless exploitation of, say, our cousins the mammals in any way an ethical issue? The biology of the pollutants has brought it home to us that we and all our kin are in one universal life-cycle. We cannot poison our pests without poisoning more friendly relatives and in the end poisoning ourselves. Empty the stuff into the rivers, and a little later it will be found in the fish we trawl from Arctic fisheries. This is a brute fact. Does it carry any moral overtones?

While we occupy the world, we are its masters. We can beautify it very little; we can conserve it only with difficulty; we can smash it, or destroy it by negligence, with ease and nonchalance. There is no logical reason why we shouldn't. We are here on a very short tenancy, and it will be later generations which will have to try to pick up the bits. Realists will agree that that will be their problem, and it is not ours. So let us casually eliminate our wild life, species by species. Let us turn our towns into confluent conurbations, and cover our countryside with motorways. Let us watch Venice sink under the sea. We shall not be here when they start to blame us.

PUBLICATIONS OF ELIOT SLATER[1]

1935

1. Slater, E. The incidence of mental disorder. *Ann. Eugen.* 6: 172-86.
2. Curran, D., and Slater, E. Mental disorder in general practice: a plea for clinical psychiatry. *Lancet* 1: 69-71.

1936

3.* Slater, E. German eugenics in practice. *Eugen. Rev.* 27: 285-95. [25]
4.* Slater, E. The inheritance of manic-depressive insanity. *Proc. Roy. Soc. Med.* 29: 981-90 (Section of Psychiatry pp. 39-48). [4]
5. Slater, E. The inheritance of manic-depressive insanity and its relation to mental defect. *J. Ment. Sci.* 82: 626-34.
6. Slater, E. The inheritance of mental disorder. *Eugen. Rev.* 28: 277-84. (Reprinted in *Mental Hygiene*, 1937, 3: 28-37.)

1937

7. Slater, E. Mental disorder and the social problem group. In *A Social Problem Group?* ed. O.P. Blacker, pp. 37-49. London: Oxford University Press.

1938

8. Slater, E. Mental diseases, heredity. In *British Encyclopaedia of Medical Practice*, ed. H. Rolleston, vol. 8, pp. 552-63. London: Butterworth.
9. Slater, E. Zur Periodik des manisch-depressiven Irreseins [On the periodicity of manic-depressive insanity]. *Z. Ges. Neurol. Psychiat.* 162: 794-801.
10.* Slater, E. Zur Erbpathologie des manisch-depressiven Irreseins. Die Eltern und Kinder von Manisch-Depressiven [On the inheritance of manic-depressive insanity: the parents and children of manic-depressives]. *Z. Ges. Neurol. Psychiat.* 163: 1-47. [5]
11. Slater, E. A critical review: Twin research in psychiatry. *J. Neurol. Psychiat.* 1: 239-58.
12. Mayer-Gross, W., and Slater, E. Psychoses. 1. Affective psychoses. In *British Encyclopaedia of Medical Practice*, ed. H. Rolleston, vol. 10, pp. 267-91. London: Butterworth.

---

[1] The list is selective as regards book reviews, etc. Publications reprinted in this book, in whole or in part, are marked with an asterisk; the numbers in square brackets identify the Papers in the volume.

1939

13. Slater, E. Über Begriff und Anwendbarkeit der Manifestationswahrscheinlichkeit [On the concept and applicability of the probability of manifestation]. *Allg. Z. Psychiat.* 112: 148-52.
14. Guttmann, E., Mayer-Gross, W., and Slater, E. Short-distance prognosis of schizophrenia. *J. Neurol. Psychiat.* 2 (New Series): 25-34.
15. Shrimpton, E.A.G., and Slater E. Die Berechnung des Standardfehlers für die Weinbergsche Morbiditätstafel [The calculation of the standard error for the Weinberg morbidity table]. *Z. Ges. Neurol. Psychiat.* 166: 715-18.

1940

16. Slater, E. Professor Edward Mapother. *Character and Personality* 9: 1-5.
17. Sargant, W., and Slater, E. Acute war neuroses. *Lancet* 2: 1-2.

1941

18. Slater, E. The inheritance of twinning. *Proc. 7th Internat. Genet. Congress 1939*, ed. R.C. Punnett, p. 266 (abstract). Cambridge: Cambridge Univ. Press.
19. Slater, E. War neuroses — General symptomatology and constitutional factors. *Med. Press and Circular* 205: 133-35.
20. Debenham, G.R., Hill, D., Sargant, W., and Slater, E. Treatment of war neurosis. *Lancet* 1: 107-109.
21.* Sargant, W., and Slater, E. Amnesic syndromes in war. *Proc. Roy. Soc. Med.* 34: 757-64. [15]

1942

22. Slater, E. Psychosis associated with vitamin B. deficiency. *Brit. Med. J.* 1: 257-58.
23. Lewis, A., and Slater, E. Neurosis in soldiers. *Lancet* 1: 496-98.

1943

24.* Slater, E. The neurotic constitution. A statistical study of two thousand neurotic soldiers. *J. Neurol. Psychiat.* 6: 1-16. [16]

1944

25. Slater, E. A demographic study of a psychopathic population. *Ann. Eugen.* 12: 121-37.
26. Slater, E. Genetics in psychiatry. *J. Ment. Sci.* 90: 17-35.
27. Slater, E. The war-time development of British psychiatry. *Nevro-patologia i Psikhiatria* 13: 59-63 (in Russian).
28.* Slater, E., and Slater, P. A heuristic theory of neurosis. *J. Neurol. Psychiat.* 7: 49-55. [17]
29.* Sargant, W., and Slater, E. *An Introduction to Physical Methods of Treatment in Psychiatry.* 2nd ed. 1948; 3rd ed. 1954; 4th ed. 1963, Edinburgh: Livingstone; and Baltimore: Williams and Wilkins. [2]

1945

30. Slater, E. Psychological aspects of family life. In *Rebuilding Family Life in the Post-War World*, ed. J. Marchant, pp. 92-106. London: Odhams.
31. Slater, E. Psychological factors in cutaneous affections. *Brit. Med. Bull.* 3: 185-86.
32. Slater E. Modern tendencies in eugenics. *Health Education J.* 3: 182-85.
33.* Slater, E. Neurosis and sexuality. *J. Neurol. Neurosurg. Psychiat.* 8: 12-14. [18]
34.* Craike, W.H., and Slater, E., (with the assistance of George Burden). Folie à deux in uniovular twins reared apart. *Brain* 68: 213-21. [6]
35. Heppenstall, M.E., Hill, D., and Slater, E. The EEG in the prognosis of war neurosis. *Brain* 68: 17-22.
36. Garai, O., (with a statistical note by Eliot Slater). Immersion as a factor in the development of hypertension. *Brit. Heart J.* 7: 200-206.

1946

37. Slater, E. An investigation into assortative mating. *Eugen. Rev.* 38: 27-28.
38. Slater, E. The modern family. *Plain View* 9: 224-30.
39. Carse, J., and Slater, E. Lymphocytosis after electrical convulsion. *J. Neurol. Neurosurg. Psychiat.* 9: 1-4.
40. Gainsborough, H., and Slater, E. A study of peptic ulcer. *Brit. Med. J.* 2: 253-58.

1947

41. Slater, E. A note on Jewish-Christian intermarriage. *Eugen. Rev.* 39: 17-21.
42.* Slater, E. A biological view on anti-Semitism. *Jewish Monthly* 1 (8): 22-28. [29]
43. Slater, E. Neurosis and religious affiliation. *J. Ment. Sci.* 93: 392-96.
44.* Slater, E. Genetical causes of schizophrenic symptoms. *Mschr. Psychiat.* 113: 50-58. [7]
45. Slater, E., and Slater, P. A study in the assessment of homosexual traits. *Brit. J. Med. Psychol.* 21: 61-74.
46. Mannheim, M.J., and Slater, E. The psychopathology of a correspondence column. *Brit. J. Med. Psychol.* 21: 50-60.

1948

47. Slater, E. Psychopathic personality as a genetical concept. *J. Ment. Sci.* 94: 277-82.
48.* Roberts, J.A.F., and Slater, E. Genetics, medicine and practical eugenics. *Eugen. Rev.* 40: 62-69. [26]

1949

49. Slater, E. The basic principles of psychiatry. *Nursing Times* 45: ii, 682-83.
50. Slater, E. The inheritance of twinning. *Hereditas* (Proceedings, 8th International Congress on Genetics, Stockholm, 1948), pp. 665-66 (abstract).

1950

51. Slater, E. Consciousness. In *The Physical Basis of Mind,* ed. P. Laslett, pp. 36-45. Oxford: Blackwell.
52. Slater, E. Perspectives in psychiatric genetics. In *Perspectives in Neuropsychiatry*, ed. D. Richter, pp. 173-82. London: H.K. Lewis.
53. Slater, E. Psychiatric genetics. In *Recent Progress in Psychiatry*, ed. G.W.T.H. Fleming, vol. 2, pp. 1-25. London: Churchill.
54. Slater, E. Kriegserfahrungen und Psychopathiebegriff [The experiences of wartime and the concept of psychopathy]. *Mschr. Psychiat.* 119: 207-26.
55. Slater, E. The genetical aspects of personality and neurosis. *Congrès international de Psychiatrie, Rapports VI,* pp. 119-54. Paris: Hermann.
56. Sargant, W., and Slater, E. The influence of the 1939-45 war on British psychiatry. *Congrès international de Psychiatrie, Comptes Rendus VI,* pp. 180-96. Paris: Hermann.

1951

57.* Slater, E., and Woodside, M. *Patterns of Marriage.* London: Cassell. [30]
58. Slater, E. Evaluation of electric convulsion therapy as compared with conservative methods of treatment in depressive states. *J. Ment. Sci.* 97: 567-69.
59. Hallpike, C.S., Harrison, M.S., and Slater, E. Abnormalities of the caloric test results in certain varieties of mental disorder. *Acta Otolaryng.* 39: 151-59.

1952

60. Lewis, A., and Slater, E. Psychiatry in the Emergency Medical Service. In *History of the Second World War: Medicine and Pathology,* ed. V.Z. Cope, pp. 390-407. London: Her Majesty's Stationery Office.
61. Slater, E. El estudio de los gemelos en psiquiatria [Twin study in psychiatry]. *Actas Luso-Esp. Neurol. Psiquiat.* 7: 122-34.

1953

62. Slater, E. Statistics for the chess computer and the factor of mobility. *Transactions of the Institute of Radio Engineers Professional Group on Information Theory*, pp. 150-52, 198-200. London: Ministry of Supply.
63.* Slater, E., (with the assistance of Shields, J.). Psychotic and Neurotic Illnesses in Twins. *Med. Res. Coun. Spec. Rep. Ser., No. 278.* London: Her Majesty's Stationery Office. [9]
64.* Slater, E. Psychiatry. In *Clinical Genetics*, ed. A. Sorsby, pp. 332-49. London: Butterworth. [8]
65. Slater, E. Mental diseases, heredity. In *British Encyclopaedia of Medical Practice*, 2nd ed., vol. 8, pp. 543-55. London: Butterworth.
66. Slater, E. Genetic investigations in twins. *J. Ment. Sci.* 99: 44-52.
67. Slater, E. Sex-linked recessives in mental illness? *Acta Genet. (Basel)* 4: 273-80.

1954

68. Mayer-Gross, W., Slater, E., and Roth, M. *Clinical Psychiatry*. London: Cassell. (2nd ed. 1960; for 3rd ed., extensively rewritten, see 137.)
69.* Slater, E. The M'Naghten Rules and modern concepts of responsibility. *Brit. Med. J.* 2: 713-18. [31]
70. Polonio, P., and Slater, E. A prognostic study of insulin treatment in schizophrenia. *J. Ment. Sci.* 100: 442-50.
71. Sargant, W., and Slater, E. Physical methods of treatment in psychiatry. In *Refresher Course for General Practitioners*, ed. H. Clegg, pp. 177-88. London: British Medical Association.

1955

72. Slater, E. La psychiatrie en Grande-Bretagne [Psychiatry in Great Britain]. In *Encyclopédie Medico-Chirurgicale*. Paris.
73. Slater, E., and Shields, J. Twins in psychological medicine. Paper read to the British Association, reported in *Nature (Lond.)* 176: 532-33.
74. Alexander, C.H.O'D., and Slater, E. The relative strengths of the openings. *Brit. Chess Mag.* 75: 177-80.

1956

75. Elithorn, A., and Slater, E. Prefrontal leucotomy. Views of patients and their relatives. *Brit. Med. J.* 2: 739-42.
76. Shields, J. and Slater, E. An investigation into the children of cousins. *Acta Genet. (Basel)* 6: 60-79.

1957

77.* Slater, E. Areas of interdoctrinal acceptance: An organicist speaks. In *Integrating the Approaches to Mental Disease*, ed. H.D. Kruse, pp. 41-43. New York: Hoeber-Harper. [1]
78. Slater, E. The twin-study method in wider perspective: Discussion. First International Conference on Human Genetics, Copenhagen, 1957. *Acta Genet. (Basel)* 7: 20.
79. Nixon, W.L.B., and Slater, E. A second investigation into the children of cousins. *Acta Genet. (Basel)* 7: 513-32.

1958

80. Slater, E. The sibs and children of homosexuals. In *Symposium on Nuclear Sex*, eds. D.R. Smith and W.M. Davidson, pp. 79-83. London: Heinemann.
81. Slater, E. The biologist and the fear of death. *Plain View* 12: 29-42. (Republished with minor revisions in 1969, as "Death: the biological aspect" in *Euthanasia and the Right to Death*, ed. A. B. Downing, pp. 49-60. London: Peter Owen.)
82.* Slater, E. The monogenic theory of schizophrenia. *Acta Genet. (Basel)* 8: 50-56. [10]

83. Elithorn, A., Glithero, E., and Slater, E. Leucotomy for pain. *J. Neurol. Neurosurg. Psychiat.* 21: 249-61.

1959

84. Cowie, V., and Slater, E. Psychiatric genetics. In *Recent Progress in Psychiatry*, ed. G.W.T.H. Fleming, vol. III, pp.1-53. London: Churchill.
85.* Slater, E., and Meyer, A. Contributions to a pathography of the musicians: 1. Robert Schumann. *Confin. Psychiat.* 2: 65-94. [33]

1960

86.* Slater, E. Galton's heritage. *Eugen. Rev.* 52, 91-103. [27]
87. Slater, E. Mapother memorial. VI: The psychiatrist. *Bethlem-Maudsley Hospital Gazette* 4 (1): 7-10.
88. Shields, J., and Slater, E. Heredity and psychological abnormality. In *Handbook of Abnormal Psychology*, ed. H.J. Eysenck, pp. 298-343. London: Pitman Medical. (Issued by Basic Books, New Yor, 1961).
89. Slater, E., and Meyer, A. Contributions to a pathography of the musicians: 2. Organic and psychotic disorders. *Confin. Psychiat.* 3: 129-45.

1961

90. Slater, E. Some considerations on mental health and genetic disease. In *Biological Problems Arising from the Control of Pests and Diseases*, ed. R.K.S. Wood, pp. 81-88. London: Institute of Biology.
91. Slater, E. Heredity of mental diseases. In *Clinical Aspects of Genetics* (The Proceedings of a Conference held in London at the R.C.P., 17-18 March, 1961), ed. F. Avery Jones, pp. 23-29. London: Pitman Medical.
92. Slater, E. Colère et irritabilité sont-ils des caractères essentiels de la personnalité des compositeurs allemands? [Are temper and irritability essential characteristics of the German composers?] *Vie Méd.* 42: S$_3$, 59-60.
93.* Slater, E. The judicial process and the ascertainment of fact. *Mod. Law Rev.* 24: 721-24. [32]
94.* Slater, E. The thirty-fifth Maudsley lecture: 'Hysteria 311'. *J. Ment. Sci.* 107: 359-81. [19]
95.* Slater, E., and Zilkha, K. A case of Turner mosaic with myopathy and schizophrenia. *Proc. Roy. Soc. Med.* 54: 674-75. [11]

1962

96. Slater, E. Trends in psychiatric genetics in England. In *Expanding Goals of Genetics in Psychiatry*, ed. F.J. Kallmann, pp. 219-27. New York: Grune & Stratton.
97. Slater, E. Psychological aspects. In *Modern views on "Stroke" illness* (Symposium held at the RSM, London, 23 January 1962), pp. 41-48. London: The Chest and Heart Association.
98.* Slater, E. Birth order and maternal age of homosexuals. *Lancet* 1: 69-71. [22]
99. Beard, A.W., and Slater, E. The schizophrenic-like psychoses of epilepsy. *Proc. Roy. Soc. Med.* 55: 311-16. Section of Psychiatry, pp. 1-6, (abridged).

1963

100.* Slater, E. Diagnosis of zygosity by finger prints. *Acta Psychiat. Scand.* 39: 78-84. [23]
101. Slater, E. Genetical factors in neurosis. *Proc. 2nd. Internat. Congr. Hum. Genet., (Rome, 1961)*, pp. 1686–91. Rome: Istituto G. Mendel.
102. Slater, E. The colour imagery of poets. *Schweiz. Arch. Neurol. Neurochir. Psychiat.* 91: 303-8.
103. Cowie, V., and Slater, E. Maternal age and miscarriage in the mothers of mongols. *Acta Genet. (Basel)* 13: 77-83.
104.* Slater, E., Beard, A.W., and Glithero, E. The schizophrenia-like psychoses of epilepsy. *Brit. J. Psychiat.* 109: 95-150. [12]

1964

105. Slater, E. Genetical factors in neurosis. *Brit. J. Psychol.* 55: 265-69.
106.* Slater, E. Review of *Psychogenic Psychoses* by P.M. Faergeman and *Die schizophrenie-ähnlichen Emotionspsychosen* by F. Labhardt. *Brit. J. Psychiat.* 110: 114-18. [13]
107. Slater, P., Shields, J., and Slater, E. A quadratic discriminant of zygosity from fingerprints. *J. Med. Genet.* 1: 42-46.

1965

108. Slater, E. Clinical aspects of genetic mental disorders. In *Biochemical Aspects of Neurological Disorders* (2nd series), ed. J.N. Cumings and M. Kremer, pp. 271-85. Oxford: Blackwell.
109. Slater, E. Diagnosis of "Hysteria". *Brit. Med. J.* 1: 1395-99.
110. Slater, E. Discussion of paper by M. Bleuler, "Conception of schizophrenia within the last fifty years and today." *Internat. J. Psychiat.* 1: 318-19.
111. Slater, E. Obituary notice, F.J. Kallmann. *Brit. Med. J.* 1: 1440.
112.* Slater, E. and Glithero, E. A follow-up of patients diagnosed as suffering from "Hysteria." *J. Psychosom. Res.* 9: 9-13. [20]
113. Coppen, A.J., Cowie, V.A., and Slater, E. Familial aspects of "neuroticism" and "extraversion." *Brit. J. Psychiat.* 111: 70-83.

1966

114.* Slater, E. Expectation of abnormality on paternal and maternal sides: a computational model. *J. Med. Genet.* 3: 159-61. [24]
115. Slater, E. Pain and the psychiatrist. Letter in *Brit. J. Psychiat.* 112: 329.
116. Crome, L., Cowie, V.A., and Slater, E. A statistical note on cerebellar and brain-stem weight in mongolism. *J. Ment. Defic. Res.* 10: 69-72
117.* Shields, J., and Slater, E. La similarité du diagnostic chez les jumeaux et le problème de la spécificité biologique dans les névroses et les troubles de la personnalité [Diagnostic similarity in twins and the problem of biological specificity in the neuroses and personality disorders]. *Evolut. Psychiat.* 31: 441-51. [21]
118. Slater, E. (unsigned). The genetics of schizophrenia. In *Medical Research Council Annual Report, April 1965–March 1966*, pp. 54-61. London: Her Majesty's Stationery Office.

1967

119.* Slater, E. Distinguishing the effects of heredity and environment. Discussion of "The psychogenesis of schizophrenia: a review of the literature" by Hans Kind. *Internat. J. Psychiat.* 3: 416-17. [14]
120.* Slater, E. Review of *On Aggression* by Konrad Lorenz. *Brit. J. Psychiat.* 113: 803-6. [3]
121. Shields, J., and Slater, E. Genetic aspects of schizophrenia. *Hosp. Med. (Lond.)* 1: 579-84.
122. Slater, E. Genetics of criminals. *World Med.* 2(12): 44-45.
123.* Slater, E. Vote of thanks to Dr. A.H. Halsey on the occasion of the Galton lecture 1967. *Eugen. Rev.* 59: 149. [28]
124. Slater, E. Genetic factors and schizophrenia. Transcript of the Symposium on Biological Research in Schizophrenia (Moscow, November 28– December 2, 1967), ed. D. Lozovskii, pp. 109-13 (Russian) and 244-48 (English). Moscow: Akademia Meditsinskikh Nauk SSSR. Also in *Vestn. Acad. Med. Nauk SSSR (1969)* 4: 75-9 (in Russian).
125. Shields, J., Gottesman, I.I., and Slater, E. Kallmann's 1946 schizophrenic twin study in the light of new information. *Acta Psychiat. Scand.* 43: 385-96.

1968

126. Slater, E. Review of *ESP: A Scientific Evaluation* by C.E.M. Hansel. *Brit. J. Psychiat.* 114: 653-58.
127. Slater, E., and Tsuang, M-t. Abnormality on paternal and maternal sides: observations in schizophrenia and manic-depression. *J. Med. Genet.* 5: 197-99.
128. Slater, E. Mental disorders: genetic aspects. In *International Encyclopedia of the Social Sciences*, pp. 127-33. New York: MacMillan and Free Press.

129. Cowie, V.A., and Slater, E. The fertility of mothers of mongols. *J. Ment. Defic. Res.* 12: 196-208.
130. Cowie, J., Cowie, V.A., and Slater, E. *Delinquency in Girls.* London: Heinemann.
131. Slater, E. A review of earlier evidence on genetic factors in schizophrenia. In *The Transmission of Schizophrenia,* eds. D. Rosenthal and S.S. Kety, pp. 15-26. Oxford: Pergamon. (Also issued as *J. Psychiat. Res.* 6: Suppl. 1, 15-26.)
132. Slater, E. La Herencia en las Psicosis Endogenas [Heredity in the endogenous psychoses], translated by César Pérez de Francisco. *Neurología-Neurocirugía Psiquiatria* 9: 137-49; and *Revistá Gharma* 34: 9-20 (1969).
133. Slater, E. *The Ebbless Sea, Poems 1922-1962.* London: Outposts Publications.
134. Slater, E. A note on terms of art in "Hamlet." *Shakespearean Authorship Review* 20: 1-4.

1969

135. Slater, E., and Shields, J. Genetical aspects of anxiety. In *Studies of Anxiety,* ed. M.H. Lader, pp. 62-71. *Brit. J. Psychiat.,* Special Publn. No. 3. Ashford (Kent): Headley.
136. Slater, E., and Moran, P.A.P. The schizophrenia-like psychoses of epilepsy: relation between ages of onset. *Brit. J. Psychiat.* 115: 599-600.
137. Slater, E., and Roth, M. *Mayer-Gross, Slater and Roth Clinical Psychiatry,* 3rd. ed. London: Baillière, Tindall and Cassell.
138. Slater, E. Choosing the time to die. In *Proceedings, 5th International Conference on Suicide Prevention,* London 1969, ed. R. Fox, pp. 269-72. Vienna: International Association for Suicide Prevention.

In press or current

139. Slater, E. The problems of pathography. *Studies Dedicated to Erik Essen-Möller. Acta Psychiat. Scand.* Suppl. 219:209-15 (1970).
140. Slater, E. The case for a major partially dominant gene. In *Genetic Factors in Schizophrenia,* ed. A.R. Kaplan. Springfield, Ill.: Charles C. Thomas.
141. Slater, E. A psychiatric view of Shakespeare's sonnets. *An. Port. Psiquiat.,* volume in honour of Prof. Barahona Fernandes.
142. Slater, E., and Cowie, V. *The Genetics of Mental Disorders.* London: Oxford University Press.
143. Slater, E. "Autobiographical Sketch" and "Retrospect." This volume.
144. Slater, E. Schizophrenia-like illnesses of epilepsy. In *Current Problems in Neuropsychiatry,* ed. R.N. Herrington, pp. 77-81. *Brit. J. Psychiat.,* Special Publication No. 4. Ashford (Kent): Headley (1969).
145. Kahn, J., Carter, W.I., Dernley, N., and Slater, E. Chromosome studies in remand home and prison populations. In *Criminological Implications of Chromosome Abnormalities,* ed. D.J. West, pp. 44-48. Cambridge: Institute of Criminology (1970).
146. Slater, E., Maxwell, J., and Price, J.S. Distribution of ancestral secondary cases in bipolar affective disorders. *Brit. J. Psychiat.* 118: 215-18 (1971).
147. Slater, E. The social value of an elite. Paper read at the symposium *Human Differences and Social Issues* (London, Aug. 1970). In press.
148. Slater, E. Psychiatry, science and non-science: the second Mapother lecture, 1970.

REFERENCES[1]

Abe, K., and Moran, P. A. P. 1969. Parental age of homosexuals. *Brit. J. Psychiat*. 115: 313–17.

Abel-Smith, B., and Stevens, R. 1968. *In search of justice*. London: Allen Lane, The Penguin Press.

Abraham, G. 1954. In *Grove's Dictionary of Music*, ed. E. Blom, 5th ed., vol. 7. London: Macmillan.

Alanen, Y. O. 1966. The family in the pathogenesis of schizophrenia and neurotic disorders. *Acta Psychiat. Scand*. Suppl. 189.

Allen, G. 1960. The M quadruplets. II. The interpretation of quantitative differences. *Acta Genet. Med. (Roma)* 9: 452–65.

Alley, M., and Alley, J. 1956. *A passionate friendship: Clara Schumann and Brahms*, tr. by M. Savill. London: Staples.

Baeyer, W. von. 1935. *Zur Genealogie psychopathischer Schwindler und Lügner*. Leipzig: Thieme.

Banse, J. 1929. Zum Problem der Erbprognosebestimmung (Die Erkrankungsaussichten der Vettern und Basen von Manisch-Depressiven). *Z. Ges. Neurol. Psychiat*. 119: 576–612.

Bartlet, J. E. A. 1957. Chronic psychosis following epilepsy. *Amer. J. Psychiat*. 114: 338–43.

Basch, V. 1931. *A life of suffering*. New York: Tudor.

Beard, A. W., and Slater, E. 1962. The schizophrenic-like psychoses of epilepsy (abridged). *Proc. Roy. Soc. Med*. 55: 311–16.

Bennett, E. 1945. Some tests for the discrimination of neurotic from normal subjects. *Brit. J. Med. Psychol*. 20: 271–77.

Berlit, B. 1931. Erblichkeitsuntersuchungen bei Psychopathen. *Z. Ges. Neurol. Psychiat*. 134: 382–498.

Bernard, J. 1935. Some biological factors in personality and marriage. *Hum. Biol*. 7: 430.

Billings, E. G., Ebaugh, F. G., Morgan, D. W., O'Kelley, L. I., Short, G. B., and Golding, F. C. 1943. Comparison of one hundred Army psychiatric patients and one hundred enlisted men. *War Med*. 4: 283–98.

Blacker, C. P. 1952. *Eugenics: Galton and after*. London: Duckworth.

Bleuler, M. 1941. *Krankheitsverlauf, Persönlichkeit und Verwandtschaft Schizophrener und ihre gegenseitigen Beziehungen*. Leipzig: Thieme.

---

[1]This consolidated list of works cited does not include publications of which Eliot Slater was sole or first author.

Böök, J. A. 1953. Schizophrenia as a gene mutation. *Acta Genet. (Basel)* 4: 133–39.

Bostroem, A. 1935. Wichtige Entscheidungen aus der Rechtsprechung der Erbgesundheitsgerichte und Erbgesundheitsobergerichte. *Fortschr. Neurol. Psychiat.* 7: 271–81.

Braconi, L. 1961. Le psiconevrosi e le psicosi nei gemelli. *Acta Genet. Med. (Roma).* 10: 100–36.

Braun, A. 1940. *Krankheit und Tod im Schicksal bedeutender Menschen.* Stuttgart: Enke.

Brion, M. 1956. *Schumann and the romantic age.* London: Collins.

Brown, F. W. 1942. Heredity in the psychoneuroses. *Proc. Roy. Soc. Med.* 35: 785–90.

Brugger, C. 1935. Untersuchungen an Kindern, Neffen, Nichten und Enkeln von chronischen Trinkern. *Z. Ges. Neurol. Psychiat.* 154: 223–41.

Burch, P. R. J. 1964. Schizophrenia: some new aetiological considerations. *Brit. J. Psychiat.* 110: 818–24.

Burgess, E. W., and Wallin, P. 1943. Homogamy in social characteristics. *Amer. J. Sociol.* 49: 109.

Burt, C. 1946. *Intelligence and fertility.* London: Hamish Hamilton.

Cameron, K. 1940. Occupation therapy for war neuroses. *Lancet* 2: 659–60.

Carter, C. O. 1965. The inheritance of common congenital malformations. *Progr. Med. Genet.* 4: 59–84.

Chissell, J. 1948. *Schumann.* Master Musicians Series. London: Dent.

Connell, P. H. 1958. *Amphetamine psychosis.* Maudsley Monograph 5. London: Chapman and Hall.

Conrad, K. 1935–36. Erbanlage und Epilepsie. 3 parts. *Z. Ges. Neurol. Psychiat.* 153: 271–326; 155: 254–97; and 155: 509–42.

Coppen, A., Cowie, V., and Slater, E. 1965. Familial aspects of "neuroticism" and "extraversion." *Brit. J. Psychiat.* 111: 70–83.

Curran, D. 1937. The problem of assessing psychiatric treatment. *Lancet* 2: 1005–9.

Curran, R. D., and Mallinson, P. 1940. War-time psychiatry and economy in man-power. *Lancet* 2: 738–43.

Dahlberg, G. 1926. *Twin births and twins from a hereditary point of view.* Stockholm: Tidens.

———. 1941. Rare psychological defects from the point of view of the population. *Proc. Seventh Internat. Genet. Congress (1939),* p. 94. *Suppl. J. Genet.* Cambridge.

Dahlberg, G., and Stenberg, S. 1931. Eine Statistische Untersuchung über die Wahrscheinlichkeit der Erkrankung an verschiedenen Psychosen und über die demographische Häufigkeit von Geisteskrankheiten. *Z. Neurol.* 133: 447–82.

Dawson, G. D. 1954. A summation technique for the detection of small evoked potentials. *Electroenceph. Clin. Neurophysiol.* 6: 65–84.

Debenham, G., Hill, D., Sargant, W., and Slater, E. 1941. Treatment of war neurosis. *Lancet* 1: 107–9.

Dencker, S. J., Hauge, M., Kaij, L., and Nielsen, A. 1961. The use of anthropological traits and blood groups in the determination of the zygosity of twins. *Acta Genet. (Basel)* 11: 265–85.

Du Cann, C. G. L. 1960. *Miscarriages of justice.* London: Muller.

Duncan, A. G., Penrose, L. S., and Turnbull, R. C. 1936. A survey of the patients in a large mental hospital. *J. Neurol. Psychopathol.* 16: 225–38.

Edwards, J. H. 1960. The simulation of Mendelism. *Acta Genet. (Basel)* 10: 63–70.

———. 1963. The genetic basis of common disease. *Amer. J. Med.* 34: 627–38.

Egger, H. 1942. Zum Problem der Gattenwahl Schizophrener. *Z. Ges. Neurol. Psychiat.* 174: 353–96.

Elsässer, G. 1952. *Die Nachkommen geisteskranker Elternpaare.* Stuttgart: Thieme.

Erickson, T. C. 1945. Erotomania (nymphomania) as an expression of cortical epileptiform discharge. *Arch. Neurol. (Chicago)* 53: 226–31.

Ervin, F., Epstein, A. W., and King, H. E. 1955. Behavior of epileptic and non-epileptic patients with "temporal spikes." *Arch. Neurol. (Chicago)* 74: 488–97.

Essen-Möller, E. 1941. Psychiatrische Untersuchungen an einer Serie von Zwillingen. *Acta Psychiat. Neurol. Scand.,* Suppl. 23.

Eysenck, H. J. 1943. Neurosis and intelligence. *Lancet* 2: 362–63.

———. 1947. *Dimensions of personality.* London: Kegan Paul.

Faergeman, P. M. 1963. *Psychogenic psychoses: a description and follow-up of psychoses following psychological stress*. London: Butterworth.

Feis, O. 1910. *Studien über die Genealogie und Psychologie der Musiker*. Wiesbaden: Bergmann.

Ferriman, D. 1941. The genetics of true oxycephaly and acrocephalosyndactyly. *Proc. Seventh Internat. Genet. Congr. (1939)*, p. 120. Cambridge.

Feuchtwanger, E., and Mayer-Gross, W. 1938. Hirnverletzung und Epilepsie. *Schweiz. Arch. Neurol. Psychiat.* 41: 17–99.

Früh, L. 1943. Über die Belastung von Ehegatten Schizophrener. *Z. Ges. Neurol. Psychiat.* 176: 695–741.

Galton, F. 1883. *Inquiries into human faculty*. London: Macmillan.

———. 1908. *Memories of my life*. London: Methuen.

Garrison, F. H. 1934. The medical history of Robert Schumann and his family. *Bull. N. Y. Acad. Med.* 10: 523.

Garrison, R. J., Anderson, V. E., and Reed, S. C. 1968. Assortative marriage. *Eugen. Quart.* 15: 113–27.

Gates, R. R. 1946. *Human genetics*. New York: Macmillan.

———. 1947. "Human Genetics" and the reviewers. *Eugenics Review* 39: 124–27.

Gebbing, M. 1932. Die Erbanlage bei Neurotikern. *Deutsch. Z. Nervenheilk.* 125: 45.

Glaus, A. 1931. Über Kombinationen von Schizophrenie und Epilepsie. *Z. Ges. Neur. Psychiat.* 135: 450–500.

Golla, F., Hutton, E. L., and Walter, W. G. 1943. The objective study of mental imagery: Physiological concomitants. *J. Ment. Sci.* 89: 216–23.

Gottesman, I. I. 1962. Differential inheritance of the psychoneuroses. *Eugen. Quart.* 9: 223–27.

Gottesman, I. I., and Shields, J. 1966a. Contributions of twin studies to perspectives on schizophrenia. In *Progress in experimental personality research*, ed. B. A. Maher, vol. 3, pp. 1–84. New York: Academic Press.

———. 1966b. Schizophrenia in twins: 16 years' consecutive admissions to a psychiatric clinic. *Brit. J. Psychiat.* 112: 809–18.

———. 1967. A polygenic theory of schizophrenia. *Proc. Nat. Acad. Sci. USA* 58: 199–205.

Gruhle, H. W. 1936. Über den Wahn bei Epilepsie. *Z. Ges. Neur. Psychiat.* 154: 395–99.

Gruhle, W. 1906. Brief über Robert Schumanns Krankheit an P. B. Möbius. *Zbl. Nervenheilk.* 29: 805.

Gunther, M., and Penrose, L. S. 1935. Genetics of epiloia. *J. Genet.* 31: 413–30.

Hadfield, J. A. 1942. War neurosis. *Brit. Med. J.* 1: 281–85, 320–23.

Haldane, J. B. S. 1939. The spread of harmful autosomal recessive genes in human populations. *Ann. Eugen. (London)* 9: 232-37.

———. 1946. The interaction of nature and nurture. *Ann. Eugen.* 13: 197–205.

Halperin, S. L., and Curtis, G. M. 1942. The genetics of gargoylism. *Amer. J. Ment. Defic.* 46: 298–301.

Halsey, A. H. 1967. Sociology, biology and population control. *Eugen. Rev.* 59: 155–64.

Halstead, H. 1943. An analysis of the matrix (Progressive Matrices) test results on 700 neurotic (military) subjects, and a comparison with the Shipley Vocabulary Test. *J. Ment. Sci.* 89: 202–15.

Hart, B., and Spearman, C. 1912. General ability, its existence and nature. *Brit. J. Psychol.* 5: 51–84.

Heston, L. L. 1966. Psychiatric disorders in foster home reared children of schizophrenic mothers. *Brit. J. Psychiat.* 112: 819–25.

Higgins, J. V., Reed, E. W., and Reed, S. C. 1962. Intelligence and family size: a paradox resolved. *Eugen. Quart.* 9: 84–90.

Hill, D. 1944. Cerebral dysrhythmia: its significance in aggressive behaviour. *Proc. Roy. Soc. Med.* 37: 317–28.

———. 1953. Psychiatric disorders of epilepsy. *Med. Press* 20: 473–75.

———. 1968. Depression: Disease, reaction, or posture? *Amer. J. Psychiat.* 125: 445–57.

Hill, D., Pond, D., Symonds, C. 1962. The schizophrenic-like psychoses of epilepsy (Discussion). *Proc. Roy. Soc. Med.* 55: 314–16.

Hillbom, E. 1960. After-effects of brain injuries. *Acta Psychiat. Neurol. Scand.* Suppl. 142.

Hoenig, J. 1967. The prognosis of schizophrenia. In *Recent developments in schizophrenia*, eds. A. Coppen and A. Walk, *Brit. J. Psychiat.* Spec. Publn. 1, pp. 115–32. Ashford (Kent): Headley.

Hoffmann, H. 1921. *Die Nachkommenschaft bei endogenen Psychosen. Monogr. Neurol. Psychiat.* 26. Berlin: Springer.

Holt, S. B. 1961. The inheritance of dermal ridge patterns. In *Recent advances in human genetics*, ed. L. S. Penrose, pp. 101–19. London: Churchill.

Huber, G. 1961. *Chronische Schizophrenie: Synopsis klinischer und neuroradiologischer Untersuchungen an defektschizophrenen Anstaltspatienten.* Heidelberg.

Hubert, W. H. de B. 1941. Acute nervous illness in active warfare. *Lancet* 1: 306–8.

Ihda, S. 1960. A study of neurosis by twin method. *Psychiat. Neurol. Jap.* 63: 861–892. (Japanese; English summary).

Jackson, D. D. 1960. A critique of the literature on the genetics of schizophrenia. In *The etiology of schizophrenia*, ed. D. D. Jackson, pp. 37–87. New York: Basic Books.

Jasper, H. H., Fitzpatrick, C. P., and Solomon, P. 1939. Analogies and opposites in schizophrenia and epilepsy. *Amer. J. Psychiat.* 95: 835–51.

Jervis, G. A. 1939. The genetics of phenylpyruvic oligophrenia. *J. Ment. Sci.* 85: 719–62.

_____. 1941. Juvenile amaurotic family idiocy. Six cases of its occurrence in siblings. *Amer. J. Dis. Child* 61: 327–38.

Jones, E. 1956. The nature of genius. *Brit. Med. J.* 2: 257–62.

Juda, A. 1939. Neue psychiatrisch-genealogische Untersuchungen an Hilfsschulzwillingen und ihren Familien: I. Die Zwillingsprobanden und ihre Partner. *Z. Ges. Neurol. Psychiat.* 166: 365–452.

_____. 1953. *Höchstbegabung: Ihre Erbverhältnisse sowie ihre Beziehungen zu psychischen Anomalien.* Munich: Urban & Schwarzenberg.

Juel-Nielsen, N. 1965. Individual and environment. *Acta Psychiat. Scand.* Suppl. 183.

Kallmann, F. J. 1938. *The genetics of schizophrenia.* New York: Augustin.

_____. 1941. The operation of genetic factors in the pathogenesis of mental disorders. *New York State Med. J.* 41: 1352–57.

_____. 1946. The genetic theory of schizophrenia. *Amer. J. Psychiat.* 103: 309–22.

_____. 1948. Heredity and constitution in relation to the treatment of mental disorders. In *Failures in psychiatric treatment*, ed. P. H. Hoch, pp. 132–49. New York: Grune and Stratton.

_____. 1953. *Heredity in health and mental disorder.* New York: W. W. Norton.

Kallmann, F. J., and Anastasio, M. M. 1947. Twin studies on the psychopathology of suicide. *J. Nerv. Ment. Dis.* 105: 40–55.

Kallmann, F. J., and Reisner, D. 1943. Twin studies on the significance of genetic factors in tuberculosis. *Amer. Rev. Tuber.* 47: 549–74.

Karagulla, S., and Robertson, E. E. 1955. Psychical phenomena in temporal lobe epilepsy and psychoses. *Brit. Med. J.* 1. 748–52.

Karn, M. N. 1952. Birth weight and length of gestation of twins, together with maternal age, parity and survival rate. *Ann. Eugen.* 16: 365–77.

Kemp, T. 1947. Danish experiences in negative eugenics. *Eugen. Rev.* 38: 181–86.

Kety, S. S., Rosenthal, D., Wender, P. H., and Schulsinger, F. 1968. The types and prevalence of mental illness in the biological and adoptive families of adopted schizophrenics. In *The transmission of schizophrenia*, eds. D. Rosenthal and S. S. Kety, pp. 345–62. Oxford: Pergamon.

Kind, H. 1966. The psychogenesis of schizophrenia, a review of the literature. *Brit. J. Psychiat.* 112: 333–49.

Klein, M. 1935. *Wer ist erbgesund und wer ist erbkrank?* Jena: Verlag G. Fischer.

Kleist, K. 1921. Die autochthonen Degenerationspsychosen. *Z. Ges. Neurol. Psychiat.* 69: 1.

Kolle, K. 1932. Die Nachkommenschaft von Trinkern mit "Eifersuchtswahn." *Mschr. Psychiat. Neurol.* 83: 127.

Koller, S. 1939. Über den Erbgang der Schizophrenie. *Z. Ges. Neurol. Psychiat.* 164: 199–228.

Kranz, H. 1936. *Lebensschicksale krimineller Zwillinge.* Berlin: Springer.

Krapf, E. 1928. Epilepsie und Schizophrenie. *Arch. Psychiat. Nervenkr.* 83: 547–86.

Kraulis, W. 1931. Zur Vererbung der hysterischen Reaktionsweise. *Z. Ges. Neurol. Psychiat.* 136: 174–258.

391

Krauss. 1903. Über die Vererbung von Geisteskrankheiten. *Allg. Z. Psychiat.* 60: 224–231.

Kreitman, N. 1968. Married couples admitted to mental hospitals. *Brit. J. Psychiat.* 114: 699–718.

Kringlen, E. 1966. Schizophrenia in twins: an epidemiological-clinical study. *Psychiatry* 29: 172–84.

——. 1967. *Heredity and environment in the functional psychoses: an epidemiological-clinical twin study.* London: William Heinemann Medical Books.

Labhardt, F. 1963. *Die schizophrenieähnlichen Emotionspsychosen.* Berlin: Springer-Verlag.

Lader, M. H., and Wing, L. 1966. *Physiological measures, sedative drugs and morbid anxiety.* Maudsley Monograph 14. London: Oxford University Press.

Lamy, M., Frézal, J., de Grouchy, J., and Kelley, J. 1957. Le nombre de dermatoglyphes dans un échantillon de jumeaux. *Ann. Hum. Genet.* 21: 374–96.

Landolt, H. 1960. *Die Temporallappenepilepsie und ihre Psychopathologie.* Basel: Karger.

Lange, J. 1929. *Verbrechen als Schicksal; Studien an kriminellen Zwillingen.* Leipzig: Thieme.

Lange-Eichbaum, W. 1956. *Genie, Irrsinn und Ruhm.* 4th ed. Munich: Reinhardt.

Leistenschneider, P. 1938. Beitrag zur Frage des Heiratskreises der Schizophrenen. *Z. Ges. Neurol. Psychiat.* 162: 289–326.

Lennox, W. G., Gibbs, E. L., and Gibbs, F. A. 1939. Inheritance of epilepsy as revealed by electro-encephalograph. *J. Amer. Med. Assoc.* 113: 1002–3.

——. 1940. Inheritance of cerebral dysrhythmia and epilepsy. *Arch. Neurol. Psychiat.* 44: 1155–83.

——. 1942. Twins, brain waves and epilepsy. *Arch. Neurol. Psychiat.* 47: 702–6.

Lenz, J. 1937. Mendeln die Geisteskrankheiten? *Z. Indukt. Abstamm.* 73: 559–64.

Leonhard, K. 1934. Atypische endogene Psychosen im Lichte der Familienforschung. *Z. Ges. Neurol. Psychiat.* 149: 520–62.

Lewis, A. J. 1936. Problems of obsessional illness. *Proc. Roy. Soc. Med.* 29: 325–36.

——. 1967a. *Inquiries in psychiatry; clinical and social investigations.* London: Routledge and Kegan Paul; and New York: Science House.

——. 1967b. *The state of psychiatry; essays and addresses.* London: Routledge and Kegan Paul; and New York: Science House.

Lewis, A., and Slater, E. 1942. Neurosis in soldiers. *Lancet* 1: 496–98.

Lidz, T. 1952. Some remarks concerning the differentiation of organic from so-called "functional" psychoses. In *The biology of mental health and disease*, p. 322. New York: B. B. Hoeber.

Litzmann, B. 1918. *Clara Schumann: Ein Künstlerleben.* 5th ed. Leipzig: Breitkopf & Härtel.

——. 1927. *Letters of Clara Schumann and Johannes Brahms.* London: Arnold.

Ljungberg, L. 1957. Hysteria: A clinical, prognostic and genetic study. *Acta Psychiat. Neurol. Scand.* Suppl. 112.

Loewenstein, J. 1947. *Treatment of impotence, with special reference to mechanotherapy.* London: Hamish Hamilton.

Lorenz, K. 1966. *On aggression*, trans. M. Latzke. London: Methuen.

Luther. 1914. Erblichkeitsbeziehungen der Psychosen. *Z. Ges. Neurol. Psychiat.* 25: 12.

Luxenburger, H. 1928. Vorläufiger Bericht über psychiatrische Serienuntersuchungen an Zwillingen. *Z. Ges. Neurol. Psychiat.* 116: 297–326.

——. 1930. Psychiatrische-Neurologische Zwillingspathologie. *Zbl. Ges. Neurol. Psychiat.* 56: 145–80.

——. 1932. Erbprognose und praktische Eugenik im cyclothymen Kreise. *Nervenarzt* 5: 505–18.

——. 1933. Berufsgliederung und soziale Schichtung in den Familien erblich Geisteskranker. *Eugenik* 3: 34–40.

——. 1934. Einige für den Psychiater besonders wichtige Bestimmungen des Gesetzes zur Verhütung erbkranken Nachwuchses. *Nervenarzt* 7: 437–56.

——. 1935a. Der Begriff der "Belastung" in der Eheberatungstätigkeit des Arztes. *Erbarzt.*

——. 1935b. Untersuchungen an schizophrenen Zwillingen und ihren Geschwistern zur Prüfung der Realität von Manifestationsschwankungen. *Z. Ges. Neurol. Psychiat.* 154: 351–94.

——. 1937. Bemerkungen zu dem Vortrag von F. Lenz. *Z. Indukt. Abstamm.* 73: 565.

McArthur, N. 1953. *Genetics of twinning.* Canberra.

McKellar, P. 1957. *Imagination and thinking.* London: Cohen and West.

MacMaster, H. 1928. La folie de Robert Schumann. Thesis. Paris.

Mayer-Gross, W. 1925. Grundsätzliches zur psychiatrischen Konstitutions- und Erblichkeits-forschung. Eine Erwiderung auf den gleichnamigen Aufsatz von Hermann Hoffmann (Bd. 97 dieser Zeitschrift, S.541). *Z. Ges. Neurol. Psychiat.* 100: 467–73.

Medawar, P. 1960. *The future of man*. London: Methuen.

Menninger, K. 1966. *The crime of punishment*. New York: The Viking Press.

Möbius, P. J. 1906. *Über Robert Schumanns Krankheit*. Halle: Marhold.

Morton, L. T. 1956. Daniel McNaughton's signature. *Brit. Med. J.* 1: 107–8.

Newman, H. H., Freeman, F. N., and Holzinger, K. J. 1937. *Twins: A study of heredity and environment*. Chicago: University of Chicago Press.

Nixon, W. L. B. 1956. On the diagnosis of twin-pair ovularity and the use of dermatoglyphic data. In *Novant' anni delle Leggi Mendeliane*, ed. L. Gedda, pp. 235–45. Rome: Istituto Gregorio Mendel.

Nixon, W. L. B., and Slater, E. 1957. A second investigation into the children of cousins. *Acta Genet. (Basel)* 7: 513–32.

Nussbaum, F. 1923. *Der Streit über Robert Schumanns Krankheit*. Dissertation. Cologne.

Ødegaard, Ø. 1963. The psychiatric disease entities in the light of a genetic investigation. *Acta Psychiat. Scand.*, Suppl. 169: 94–104.

Panse, F. 1942. *Die Erbchorea*. Leipzig: Thieme.

Pare, C. M. B. 1956. Homosexuality and Chromosomal sex. *J. Psychosomat. Res.* 1: 247–51.

Pascal. 1908. Les maladies mentales de Robert Schumann. *J. Psychol. Norm. Path.* 5: 98.

Patzig, B. 1937. Untersuchungen zur Frage des Erbgangs und der Manifestierung schizophrener Erkrankungen. *Zbl. Ges. Neurol. Psychiat.* 87: 707.

Pearson, K. 1896. Regression, heredity and panmixia. *Philosoph. Trans.* 187A: 253 and 318.

———. 1914–30. *The life, letters and labours of Francis Galton*. 4 vols. London: Cambridge University Press.

Penrose, L. S. 1942. Auxiliary genes for determining sex as contributory causes of mental illness. *J. Ment. Sci.* 88: 308–16.

———. 1944. Mental illness in husband and wife: a contribution to the study of assortative mating in man. *Psychiat. Quart. Suppl.* 18: 161.

———. 1961. Parental age and non-disjunction. In *Human chromosomal abnormalities*, ed. W. M. Davidson and D. R. Smith, pp. 116–22. London: Staples.

Pohlisch, K. 1934. *Die Kinder männlicher und weiblicher Morphinisten*. Leipzig: Thieme.

Pond, D. A. 1957. Psychiatric aspects of epilepsy. *J. Ind. Med. Prof.* 3: 1441–51.

Pond, D. A. 1962. *See* Hill, Pond, and Symonds (1962) *supra*.

Rado, S. 1953. Dynamics and classification of disordered behavior. *Amer. J. Psychiat.* 110: 406–16.

Rees, W. L., and Eysenck, H. J. 1945. A factorial study of some morphological and psychological aspects of human constitution. *J. Ment. Sci.* 91: 8–21.

Reinhard, W. 1956. Die Krankheiten Mozarts und Schumanns. *Med. Mschr.* 10: 320.

Registrar-General. 1948. *Statistical review for England and Wales*. London: H.M.S.O.

Rey, J. H., Pond, D. A., and Evans, C. C. 1949. Clinical and electroencephalographic studies of temporal lobe functions. *Proc. Roy. Soc. Med.* 42: 891–904.

Richardson, H. M. 1939. Studies of mental resemblance between husbands and wives and between friends. *Psychol. Bull.* 36: 104–20.

Richter, D. L., and Geisser, S. 1960. A statistical model for diagnosing zygosis by ridge-count. *Biometrics* 16: 110–14.

Riedel, H. 1937. Zur empirischen Erbprognose der Psychopathie (Untersuchungen an Kindern von Psychopathen). *Z. Ges. Neurol. Psychiat.* 159: 597–667.

Rife, D. C. 1950. An application of gene frequency analysis to the interpretation of data from twins. *Hum. Biol.* 22: 136–45.

Ritter, R. 1937. *Ein Menschenschlag. Erbärztliche und erbgeschichtliche Untersuchungen über die – durch siebzehn Geschlechterfolgen erforschten – Nachkommen von "Vagabunden, Gaunern und Räubern."* Leipzig: Thieme.

Roberts, J. A. F. 1939. Intelligence and family size. *Eugen. Rev.* 30: 237–47.

———. 1940. Studies on a child population. V. The resemblance in intelligence between sibs. *Ann. Eugen.* 10: 293–312.

———. 1941. Inheritance of mental deficiency. *Proc. Seventh Internat. Genet. Congr. (1939)*, p. 249–51. Cambridge.

Rodin, E. A., De Jong, R. N., Waggoner, R. W., and Bagchi, B. K. 1957. Relationship between certain forms of psychomotor epilepsy and "schizophrenia." *Arch. Neur. Psychiat.* 77: 449–63.

Röll, A., and Entres, J. L. 1936. Zum Problem der Verarbeitung der Erbprognosebestimmung. Die Erkrankungsaussichten der Neffen und Nichten von Manisch-Depressiven. *Z. Neurol.* 156: 169–202.

Rosanoff, A. J., Handy, L. M., and Plesset, I. R. 1935. The etiology of manic-depressive syndromes with special reference to their occurrence in twins. *Amer. J. Psychiat.* 91: 725–62.

Rosenthal, D. 1959. Some factors associated with concordance and discordance with respect to schizophrenia in monozygotic twins. *J. Nerv. Ment. Dis.* 129: 1–10.

———. 1962a. Problems of sampling and diagnosis in the major twin studies of schizophrenia. *Psychiat. Res.* 1: 116–34.

———. 1962b. Familial concordance by sex with respect to schizophrenia. *Psychol. Bull.* 59: 401–21.

———. 1963. *The Genain Quadruplets.* New York: Basic Books.

Rosenthal, D., and Kety, S. S. (eds.), 1968. *The Transmission of Schizophrenia.* Oxford: Pergamon.

Rosenthal, D., Wender, P. H., Kety, S. S., Schulsinger, F., Welner, J., and Østergaard, L. 1968. Schizophrenics' offspring reared in adoptive homes. In *The transmission of schizophrenia*, eds. D. Rosenthal and S. S. Kety, pp. 377–91. Oxford: Pergamon.

Rüdin, E. 1916. *Zur Vererbung und Neuentstehung der Dementia Praecox.* Berlin: Springer.

———. 1923. Über Vererbung geistiger Störungen. *Z. Ges. Neurol. Psychiat.* 81: 459–96.

Sargant, W. 1967. *The unquiet mind.* London: Heinemann; and Boston: Little, Brown, & Co.

Sargant, W., and Craske, N. 1941. Modified insulin therapy in war neuroses. *Lancet* 2: 212–14.

Sargant, W., and Slater, E. 1940. Acute war neurosis. *Lancet* 2: 1–2.

———. 1941. Amnesic syndromes in war. *Proc. Roy. Soc. Med.* 34: 757–64.

Schröder, H. 1939. Anlage und Umwelt in ihrer Bedeutung für die Verwahrlosung weiblicher Jugendlicher. *Allg. Z. Psychiat.* 112: 224.

Schulz, B. 1932. Zur Erbpathologie der Schizophrenie. *Z. Ges. Neur. Psychiat.* 143: 175–293.

———. 1937. Übersicht über auslesefreie Untersuchungen in der Verwandtschaft Manisch-Depressiven. *Z. Psych. Hyg.* 10: 39–60.

———. 1940. Kinder schizophrener Elternpaare. *Z. Ges. Neurol. Psychiat.* 16: 332–81.

———. 1942. Zur Altersberücksichtigung bei Berechnung der Gefährdungsziffern. *Z. Ges. Neurol. Psychiat.* 174: 135–38.

Schulz, B., and Leonhard, K. 1940. Erbbiologisch-klinische Untersuchungen an insgesamt 99 im Sinne Leonhards typischen beziehungsweise atypischen Schizophrenien. *Z. Ges. Neurol. Psychiat.* 168: 587–613.

Schumann, A., ed. 1917. *Der junge Schumann: Dichtungen und Briefe.* Leipzig: Insel-Verlag.

Serafetinides, E. A., and Falconer, M. A. 1962. The effects of temporal lobectomy in epileptic patients with psychosis. *J. Ment. Sci.* 108: 584–93.

Shields, J. 1962. *Monozygotic twins brought up apart and brought up together.* London: Oxford University Press.

———. 1968. Psychiatric genetics. In *Studies in Psychiatry*, ed. M. Shepherd and D. L. Davies, pp. 168–91. London: Oxford University Press.

Sjögren, T. 1931. Die juvenile amaurotische Idiotie. Klinische und erblichkeitsmedizinische Untersuchungen. *Hereditas (Lund)* 14: 197–426.

———. 1935. Vererbungsmedizinische Untersuchungen über Huntington's Chorea in einer Schwedischen Bauernpopulation. *Z. Menschl. Vererb. Konstitut. Lehre* 19: 131–65.

Slater, P., 1945a. The psychometric differentiation of neurotic from normal men. *Brit. J. Med. Psychol.* 20: 277–82.

———. 1945b. Scores of different types of neurotics on tests of intelligence. *Brit. J. Psychol.* (General Section) 35 (2): 40–42.

Smith, J. C. 1925. Atypical psychoses and heterologous hereditary taints. *J. Nerv. Ment. Dis.* 62: 1–32.

Smith, M. 1941. Similarities of marriage partners in intelligence. *Amer. Sociol. Rev.* 6: 697–701.

——. 1946. A research note on homogamy of marriage partners in selected physical characteristics. *Amer. Sociol. Rev.* 11: 226–28.

Smith, S. M., and Penrose, L. S. 1955. Monozygotic and dizygotic twin diagnosis. *Ann. Hum. Genet.* 19: 273–89.

Stanford, C. V., and Forsyth, C. 1917. *A history of music.* New York: Macmillan.

Steinberg, D. L., and Wittman, M. P. 1943. Etiologic factors in the adjustment of men in the armed forces. *War Med.* 4: 129–39.

Steinwallner, B. 1935. Zwei Jahre Erbgesundheitsgesetz—1½ Jahre Erbgesundheitsgerichtsbarkeit. *Psychiat. Neurolog. Wochenschrift* 37: 325–28.

Stengel, E. 1959. Classification of mental disorders. *Bull. W.H.O.* 21: 601–63.

Stenstedt, A. 1959. Involutional melancholia. *Acta Psychiat. Neurol. Scand.* Suppl. 127.

Stern, K. 1951. *The Pillar of Fire.* London: Michael Joseph.

Strömgren, E. 1935. Zum Ersatz des Weinbergschen "abgekürzten Verfahrens." Zugleich ein Beitrag zur Frage von der Erblichkeit des Erkrankungsalters bei der Schizophrenie. *Z. Ges. Neurol. Psychiat.* 153: 784–97.

Stumpfl, F. 1936. *Die Ursprünge des Verbrechens, dargestellt am Lebenslauf von Zwillingen.* Leipzig: Thieme.

Symonds, C. P. 1943. The human response to flying stress. I. Neurosis in flying personnel. *Brit. Med. J.* 2: 703–6.

——. 1962. *See* Hill, Pond, and Symonds (1962) *supra.*

Thomson, G. H. 1939. *Factorial analysis of human ability.* London: University of London Press.

Tienari, P. 1963. Psychiatric illnesses in identical twins. *Acta Psychiat. Scand.* Suppl. 171.

Timoféeff-Ressovsky, N. W. 1935. Verknüpfung von Gen und Aussenmerkmal. *Wiss. Woche zu Frankfurt/M. (Erbbiologie)* 1:92.

Trivett, J. V. 1959. The coloured sticks. *New Scientist* 6: (160) 1183.

Tsuang, M-t. 1966. Birth order and maternal age of psychiatric in-patients. *Brit. J. Psychiat.* 112: 1131–41.

——. 1967. A study of pairs of sibs both hospitalized for mental disorder. *Brit. J. Psychiat.* 113: 283–300.

Van Reeth, P. C., Dierkens, J., and Luminet, D. 1958. L'hypersexualité dans l'épilepsie et les tumeurs du lobe temporal. *Acta Neurol. Psychiat. (Belg.)* 58: 194–218.

Wasiclewski, W. J. von. 1906. *Robert Schumann.* 4th cd. Leipzig: Breitkopf & Härtel.

Weinberg, I., and Lobstein, J. 1936. Beitrag zur Vererbung des manisch-depressiven Irreseins. *Psychiat. Neurol. Bl. (Amst.).* Ia: 339–72.

Wendt, G. G. 1955. Der individuelle Musterwert der Fingerleisten und seine Vererbung. *Acta Genet. Med. (Roma)* 4: 330–37.

Wilmanns, K. 1922. Die Schizophrenie. *Z. Ges. Neurol. Psychiat.* 78: 325–72.

Wilson, P. T., and Jones, H. E. 1932. Left-handedness in twins. *Genetics* 17: 560–71.

Wimmer, A. 1916. Psykogene Sindssygdomsformer [Psychogenic varieties of mental diseases]. *St. Hans Hospital 1816–1916 Jubilee Publication*, pp. 85–216. Copenhagen: Gad.

World Health Organization. 1957. *International Classification of Diseases and Causes of Death.* Geneva.

Wörner, K. H. 1949. *Robert Schumann: Ein letzter Zukunftsblick.* Zurich: Atlantis.

Young, P. M. 1957. *Tragic muse: the life and work of Robert Schumann.* London: Hutchinson.

Zazzo, R. 1960. *Les jumeaux, le couple et la personne.* 2 vols. Paris: Presses Universitaires de France.

——. 1963. Les jumeaux et la psychologie. *Proc. Second Internat. Cong. Hum. Genet. (Rome, Sept. 6–12, 1961)* pp. 1692–1700. Rome: Istituto Gregorio Mendel.

Zehnder, M. 1940. Über Krankheitsbild und Krankheitsverlauf bei schizophrenen Geschwistern. *Mschr. Psychiat.* 103: 230–77.

395

NAME INDEX

Abe, K., 259
Abel-Smith, B., 369
Abraham, G., 351, 360
Alanen, Y. O., 377
Allen, G., 266
Alley, J., 349
Alley, M., 349
Anastasio, M. M., 112
Anderson, E., 13–14

Baeyer, W. von, 217
Banse, J., 44–45, 50
Bartlet, J. E. A., 133
Basch, V., 349
Beard, A. W., 70, 131, 136–37, 139, 149,
     161–62
Bell, J., 86
Bennett, E., 225–27
Berlit, B., 217
Bernard, J., 229
Billings, E. G., 229
Blacker, C. P., 306, 310
Bleuler, E., 53, 133
Bleuler, M., 70–71, 107, 175, 279
Böök, J. A., 125, 128
Bostroem, A., 285, 292
Braconi, L., 256
Bramwell, Lord, 334
Braun, A., 349
Brion, M., 349
Brown, M. A., 90, 124, 217, 220
Brugger, C., 217
Burch, P. R. J., 377
Burden, G., 69, 73
Burgess, E. W., 323
Burt, C., 299

Cameron, K., 204
Carmichael, E. A., 130
Carter, C. O., 272
Cassels, Justice, 334, 336
Chissell, J., 361–62
Collier, J., 10
Connell, P. H., 170
Conrad, K., 19, 90
Coppen, A., 256
Cowie, J., 278
Cowie, V., 256, 259, 277–78
Craike, W. H., 69, 73–74
Craske, N., 187, 204
Creak, M., 13
Curran, D., 13, 20, 206, 334
Curran, R. D., 217
Curtis, G. M., 218
Curtius, F., 21

Dahlberg, G., 20, 59, 86, 262, 323
Darwin, C., 302, 310–12
Dawson, G. D., 303–04
Debenham, G., 187, 204
Dencker, S. J., 266
Du Cann, C. G. L., 344–45
Duncan, A. G., 54

East, N., 335
Edwards, J. H., 70, 272
Egger, H., 327
Elkington, J. S., 4
Elsässer, G., 127
Entres, J. L., 44, 63–65, 67
Erickson, T. C., 241
Ervin, F., 133

397

SUBJECT INDEX

THE JOHNS HOPKINS PRESS
Designed by Arlene J. Sheer
Composed in Baskerville text and display
by Jones Composition Company, Inc.

Printed on 60 lb. Perkins and Squier, R
by Universal Lithographers, Inc.
Bound in Columbia Riverside Linen RL 3435
by L. H. Jenkins, Inc.